Healthmaking in Ancient Egypt

Culture and History of the Ancient Near East

VOLUME 138

The titles published in this series are listed at *brill.com/chan*

Healthmaking in Ancient Egypt

The Social Determinants of Health at Deir el-Medina

By

Anne E. Austin

BRILL

LEIDEN | BOSTON

The Library of Congress Cataloging-in-Publication Data is available online at https://catalog.loc.gov
LC record available at https://lccn.loc.gov/2024020392

Typeface for the Latin, Greek, and Cyrillic scripts: "Brill". See and download: brill.com/brill-typeface.

ISSN 1566-2055
ISBN 978-90-04-70086-4 (hardback)
ISBN 978-90-04-70087-1 (e-book)
DOI 10.1163/9789004700871

This book is printed on acid-free paper and produced in a sustainable manner.

Contents

Acknowledgments

Writing a book about health has given me a deep appreciation for the transformative impact of support from my family, friends, colleagues, and institutions.

To my beautiful wife and inquisitive son—thank you for your patience, support, and love. I began writing this book in earnest in 2021. In the years since, we faced some of our hardest challenges as a family: personal health struggles, the loss of a beloved brother, and a global pandemic. Completing a book during this time was only possible because of the grace and selflessness that you each possess. Jen, thank you for loving me when I'm traveling, stressed, tired, and hangry. Thank you for prioritizing me when I asked and even when I didn't. To August—thank you for getting me through the stress of an uncertain academic future during a global pandemic. The two months I got to spend with you during the beginning of the pandemic filled me with so many unexpected laughs, experiments, cuddles, and loving memories.

To my parents and sister—thank you for inspiring me to pursue archaeology. The day I finished my last semester in college, we talked on the phone about my future. Dad—you made a point of telling me that I should pursue graduate school, and that you would support me whatever that looked like. Thank you. Mom, thank you for your unshakable faith in me and for caring for Jen, August, and me even from a distance. Adrienne, you have inspired me to live a healthier life. Your proactive health journey these past few years has helped me see how I can do more too, and you have helped me see ways I can put the lessons I learned from writing this book into practice.

To Emily Cole, thank you for more than just your hours editing and revising. You are one of the most intelligent people I know, and navigating life post-graduate school has been so much easier because you are in it. The quality of this book is far better because of your input.

To Mélie Louys, thank you for your months of data collection at Deir el-Medina since 2019. Your attention to detail, hard work ethic, and ability to rise to any challenge in the field make you a wonderful colleague and friend. Thank you, as well, for the laughter and songs that have gotten us through thousands of data entries.

To the reviewers of this book, thank you for your detailed and supportive suggestions. Reviewing is an unrewarding task, yet I received feedback that showed close attention and a sincere attempt to make this book better.

Finally, I would like to thank the institutions that made the research for this book possible. Thank you to the Egyptian Ministry of Tourism and Antiquities for allowing me to conduct my fieldwork. Thank you to the Institut Français d'Archéologie Orientale for permission to join the mission at Deir el-Medina, and more specifically, to Cédric Gobeil and Cédric Larcher for directing our fieldwork. Thank you to institutions who funded fieldwork at Deir el-Medina over the 2013–2022 seasons, including the University of California Humanities Research Institute, American Research Center in Egypt, Andrew W. Mellon Foundation, and University of Missouri.

Figures

Tables

CHAPTER 1

Introduction

1 A Mythical History of Human Health

How would you describe the history of human health from 3,000 years ago to the present? I asked this question to many friends, students, and colleagues, and as I heard their responses, I noticed a prevalent myth about the history of health that tells us our ability to control our health and fight disease is a modern phenomenon. This myth begins with the idea that any society prior to the Greeks was, at best, fated to lack any control over their health and, at worst, prone to irrational decisions that were directly deleterious to it. And while rational Greek thinkers like Hippocrates founded Western medicine, their practices were lost in time and only revisited during the European Enlightenment. As Gustav Born, a prominent German pharmacologist, described it: "It is surely no accident that natural science germinated only twice in human history: for the first time in Athenian Greece, where it did not survive; and for the second time in post-Reformation Europe, where it did."[1] The myth thus suggests that human health has steadily progressed over time with significant leaps in health outcomes owed to the contributions of Greek and European medicine.

While many scholars offer more pluralistic histories that incorporate Mesopotamian, Chinese, Arab, and other medical traditions, we still see this myth in some earlier scholarship on the history of health and medicine. Seminal volumes on the topic mention medical traditions outside of Europe only in passing, treating Greece as the true ancient origin of European (i.e., Western) science. As Nutton states, in Greek medicine "are to be found the beginnings of Western science and medicine in its gradual emancipation from religious and folk healing; observation and argument replace prayer and panaceas."[2] Similarly, Porter argues that Hippocratic medicine was important because doctors were "no longer pretending to be an intercessor with the gods," and instead, "the true doctor would be the wise and trusty bedside friend of the sick."[3] These connections carry with them the connotation that other past people were respond-

1 Gustav V.R. Born, "The Wide-Ranging Family History of Max Born," *Notes and Records of the Royal Society of London* 56, no. 2 (2002): 238.

2 Vivian Nutton, *Ancient Medicine*, 2nd ed. (London: Routledge, 2012), 12.

3 Roy Porter, *Blood and Guts: A Short History of Medicine* (London: Allen Lane, 2002), 25.

 | DOI:10.1163/9789004700871_002

ing to illnesses with treatments that were neither rational nor effective, making them false and untrustworthy caretakers. When other medical traditions were rooted in religion, by that logic, they would not have made meaningful impacts on the history of human health.

The myth continues by arguing that the advent of biomedicine, particularly in Europe, marked the beginning of reason-based approaches that markedly improved human health. Through understanding health as the presence of disease, key medical advances were suddenly possible. Bacterial infections could now be more easily treated with penicillin, cancerous cells with chemotherapy, and dangerous viruses with more harmless vaccines. As Rathbun and Steckel argue, "In the absence of a reliable theory of disease causation, the rich and the well-educated did not know how to spend their wealth to improve health."[4] According to this myth, prior to germ theory even the wealthy were incapable of controlling their health outcomes because this could only be accomplished through biomedicine.

The myth ends with the idea that we now live in a world where any health problem can be solved through the next big discovery in biomedicine. Porter states that with increasingly effective and scientifically-evidenced medical breakthroughs, the public began to think of medicine as "a fairy godmother who would, it was hoped, grant everybody's wishes."[5] We can see this in the way some authors write about the future of medicine and its relationship to health. In his book on the future of mankind, Harari wrote that, "In the arms race between doctors and germs, doctors run faster … The era when humankind stood helpless before natural epidemics is probably over."[6] Harari's prediction shows that the myth of human health focuses on scientific discoveries in biomedicine as its sole protagonist, making most health problems obstacles that doctors will eventually overcome.

At its core, this myth is based on a false analogy: that health equals the absence of disease and, therefore, biomedical discoveries that treat disease are the only way we can improve health outcomes. Furthermore, since it argues that it is only by treating disease that we can solve health problems, it also suggests that only those trained in biomedicine can improve our population health.

---

4 Ted A. Rathbun and Richard H. Steckel, "The Health of Slaves and Free Blacks in the East," in *The Backbone of History: Health and Nutrition in the Western Hemisphere*, ed. Richard H. Steckel and Jerome C. Rose (Cambridge: Cambridge, 2002), 219.

5 Porter, *Blood and Guts*, 155–156.

6 Yuval Noah Harari, *Homo Deus: A Brief History of Tomorrow* (New York: Harper Collins, 2017), 19.

Many readers may already see how this myth can quickly unravel. The emergence of Covid-19 made it clear that pandemics are still a concern of the present, killing over 3 million people in 2020 alone.[7] Researchers quickly developed effective vaccines, yet many people hesitated or refused to get them resulting in dramatically different vaccination rates that largely correlate with social factors like urban vs. rural areas, political affiliations, and years of formal education.[8] Clearly, biomedicine alone cannot save us from disease.

The Covid-19 pandemic and its economic fallout also revealed many of the small, daily decisions people make to impact their and their loved ones' health outcomes and the disparities of choice many face. Daily, people chose when and whether to wear a mask, how to support a friend who lost a job, what to do when childcare is suddenly unavailable, whether to work from home, and more. For many, the ability to make these choices was limited by jobs, economic circumstances, and social networks. These various non-medical factors are deeply influential in health outcomes yet hard to quantify.

Researchers have also found that the history of human health was far from a linear progression. Disease, culture, and medicine are intertwined, leading Porter to argue that health history is far from a "pageant of progress." Instead, "disease is a social development no less than the medicine that combats it."[9] Major changes in human lifestyle like the advent of agriculture and the Industrial Revolution led to a variety of costly health outcomes including the spread of infectious diseases.[10] And these costs were not evenly distributed across populations, leading to key differences in health outcomes both within and between populations. In writing about the history of health, authors emphasize how the growth of civilizations often led to worse health outcomes. The health of past peoples ebbed and flowed based on agriculture, urbanization, and industry, but comparatively less is known about how past people responded to these changes to better their and their loved ones' health.

---

7 "The True Death Toll of COVID-19: Estimating Global Excess Mortality," accessed May 16, 2023, https://www.who.int/data/stories/the-true-death-toll-of-covid-19-estimating-global-excess-mortality.

8 Yue Sun and Shannon M. Monnat, "Rural-Urban and within-Rural Differences in COVID-19 Vaccination Rates," *The Journal of Rural Health* 38, no. 4 (2022): 916–922, https://doi.org/10.1111/jrh.12625; Xinyuan Ye, "Exploring the Relationship between Political Partisanship and COVID-19 Vaccination Rate," *Journal of Public Health*, October 23, 2021, https://doi.org/10.1093/pubmed/fdab364.

9 Roy Porter, *The Greatest Benefit to Mankind: A Medical History of Humanity* (New York: W.W. Norton & Company, 1998), 15.

10 Mark Nathan Cohen, *Health and the Rise of Civilization* (New Haven: Yale University Press, 1989).

2 Correcting the Myth by Redefining Health and Disease

Given that human health has not progressed linearly over time, nor is it merely a reflection of medical care, it is essential to look across human history to more realistically understand how people responded to disease and consider how past people attempted to control their health outcomes. Such research has the potential to not only correct the myth but also replace it with a more nuanced history of human health that makes past people dynamic actors in their own health stories. To do so, it is important to think about health as more than merely the absence of disease. This means redefining health and disease through a social lens.

During the first half of the 20th century, there was a movement to broaden medical treatment to include a more holistic approach, giving rise to the World Health Organization (WHO)'s definition of health when it was founded as "a state of complete physical, mental and social well-being and not merely the absence of disease or infirmity."[11] The breadth of this definition allows one to look at a person's social context to understand health. This makes it possible to think about diseases like diabetes as treatable not only through medication but also by addressing underlying causes including insufficient housing, limited nutrition, and barriers to accessing health care services.[12]

In the decades following the creation of the WHO, researchers refined the definition by differentiating between the terms disease, illness, and sickness:[13] "While 'disease' refers to the medical or pathological source of a problem, 'illness' generally refers to the individual experience of being ill ... the term 'sickness' can be used to draw attention to the social-structural causes of unwellness."[14] Although these definitions vary in exact wording throughout the disci-

---

11 Daniel Callahan, "The WHO Definition of 'Health,'" *The Hastings Center Studies* 1, no. 3 (January 1, 1973): 77–87, https://doi.org/10.2307/3527467.

12 Jacqueline Hill, Marcia Nielsen, and Michael H. Fox, "Understanding the Social Factors That Contribute to Diabetes: A Means to Informing Health Care and Social Policies for the Chronically Ill," *The Permanente Journal* 17, no. 2 (2013): 67–72, https://doi.org/10.7812/TPP/12-099.

13 For example, Lester S. King, "What Is Disease?," *Philosophy of Science* 21, no. 3 (July 1954): 193–203; Arthur Kleinman, Leon Eisenberg, and Byron Good, "Culture, Illness, and Care: Clinical Lessons from Anthropologic and Cross-Cultural Research," *Annals of Internal Medicine* 88, no. 2 (February 1978): 251–258, https://doi.org/10.7326/0003-4819-88-2-251; Andrew C. Twaddle, "Influence and Illness: Definitions and Definers of Illness Behavior among Older Males in Providence, Rhode Island" (Ph.D Dissertation, Providence, Brown University, 1968).

14 Elisa Janine Sobo and Martha O. Loustaunau, *The Cultural Context of Health, Illness, and Medicine*, 2nd ed. (Santa Barbara: Praeger, 2010), xv.

plines, many scholars maintain the distinction of disease as biological, illness as phenomenological, and sickness as more broadly cultural.[15] By differentiating these three terms, researchers could also disentangle health's biological, psychological, and social origins.

This separation of disease and illness is also important when studying health in past populations where our data limit our interpretations of health. While skeletal lesions may give us indications of disease, they offer far more ambiguous evidence of experiences such as pain. Conversely, historical texts may include an individual's experience of an illness, but we should be wary of projecting modern definitions of diseases onto a past narrative given differences in how cultures describe and understand disease processes.[16] Delineating between these terms is particularly important when we attempt to understand health in the past because they allow us to consider illnesses and diseases simultaneously, while also recognizing the differences between them both in terms of our evidence and their implications for health.

3 How to Understand Health in the Past

Using these definitions, we can now turn to correcting the myth of the history of human health through studies of health, illness, and disease in the past. One of the primary ways researchers have studied the history of health is through biological studies of human remains. Such studies inform us about physical experiences in the past, but without a broader social context, they can only limitedly explain how a culture responded to illness. As a result, we often lack interpretations of the relationship between physiological health and social health outcomes. To resolve this problem, researchers have used interdisciplinary models for studying past health that incorporate both biological and social factors to analyze not only how individuals died, but also what helped them to survive in the past.

---

15 For example, Kenneth M. Boyd, "Disease, Illness, Sickness, Health, Healing and Wholeness: Exploring Some Elusive Concepts," *Medical Humanities* 26 (June 2000): 9–17, https://doi.org/10.1136/mh.26.1.9; Ann McElroy and Patricia K. Townsend, *Medical Anthropology in Ecological Perspective*, 3rd ed. (Boulder: Westview Press, 1996); Allan Young, "The Anthropologies of Illness and Sickness," *Annual Review of Anthropology* 11 (1982): 257–285.

16 Piers D. Mitchell, "Retrospective Diagnosis and the Use of Historical Texts for Investigating Disease in the Past," *International Journal of Paleopathology* 1, no. 2 (October 2011): 81–88, https://doi.org/10.1016/j.ijpp.2011.04.002.

In most contexts, however, this is no easy task. Artifacts documenting how past people responded to illnesses are often scarce or ambiguous, and even when they can be identified, they may not offer sufficient information to explain health patterns. Pathological case studies, for example, can suggest the integration of the disabled into society, but these unique cases cannot explain how a culture accommodated short-term illness or temporary impairment. Research documenting different health patterns in an entire population may signal that individuals were experiencing more biological and social stress than their peers, but these do not show how and when communities responded to these stressors in order to improve overall health.

Egyptologists are particularly well-positioned to study past relationships between health and society owing to myriad scholars who have examined the paleopathology of human remains in Egypt and medicine in the Egyptian textual record. Yet even in Egyptology, much of the paleopathological literature is focused on royal human remains, leaving a noticeable gap in the study of illness and care among the vast majority of ancient Egyptians.[17] Recent bioarchaeological research on broader Nile Valley populations at sites like Amarna and Tombos have diversified the bioarchaeological record,[18] yet paradoxically, individuals in these studies are not as well represented in the textual record, making the forms of care they received less accessible.

---

17 Jane E. Buikstra, B.J. Baker, and D.C. Cook, "What Diseases Plagued Ancient Egyptians? A Century of Controversy Considered," in *Biological Anthropology and the Study of Ancient Egypt*, ed. W. Vivan Davies and Roxie Walker (London: British Museum Press, 1993), 24–53.

18 For example, Michele R. Buzon, "Health of the Non-Elites at Tombos: Nutritional and Disease Stress in New Kingdom Nubia," *American Journal of Physical Anthropology* 130, no. 1 (2006): 26–37, https://doi.org/10.1002/ajpa.20303; Michele R. Buzon, "Tombos during the Napatan Period (~750–660 BC): Exploring the Consequences of Sociopolitical Transitions in Ancient Nubia," *International Journal of Paleopathology* 7 (December 2014): 1–7, https://doi.org/10.1016/j.ijpp.2014.05.002; Gretchen R. Dabbs, "Bioarchaeology of the Non-Elite North Tombs Cemetery at Amarna: A Preliminary Assessment of the Non-Elite Individuals of the North Tombs Cemetery at Tell El-Amarna, Egypt," *Bioarchaeology International* 3, no. 3 (2019): 174–186, https://doi.org/10.5744/bi.2019.1012; Gretchen R. Dabbs and Melissa Zabecki, "Abandoned Memories. A Cemetery of Forgotten Souls," in *Remembering the Dead in the Ancient Near East*, ed. Benjamin W. Porter and Alexis T. Boutin (Boulder: University Press of Colorado, 2014), 217–250; Barry Kemp et al., "Life, Death and beyond in Akhenaten's Egypt: Excavating the South Tombs Cemetery at Amarna," *Antiquity* 87, no. 335 (March 2013): 64–78, https://doi.org/10.1017/S0003598X00048626; Katie Marie Whitmore, Michele R. Buzon, and Stuart Tyson Smith, "Living on the Border: Health and Identity during Egypt's Colonization of Nubia in the New Kingdom Period," in *Bioarchaeology of Frontiers and Borderlands*, ed. Cristina I. Tica and Debra L. Martin (Gainesville: University of Florida Press, 2019), 135–159.

4 A Case Study on the History of Health at Deir el-Medina

This book bridges the gap between research on royal and non-royal ancient Egyptians through a case study that integrates bioarchaeological research at the New Kingdom village of Deir el-Medina with the site's unusually robust historical records. At its core, this book is based on a decade of bioarchaeological research I have conducted at Deir el-Medina since 2012. This work was conducted as part of the mission of the *Institut Français d'Archéologie Orientale* and with the permission of the Egyptian Ministry of Tourism and Antiquities. It represents the most comprehensive synthesis of the study of human remains from the site to date. This book is also based on hundreds of ancient Egyptian papyri and ostraca from the site. These include absence from work records, personal letters referencing health and care, as well as other categories of texts from the site that specifically address health and illness, such as rations for medical professionals, legal investigations into treatment of the sick, and medical prescriptions.

By combining a traditional bioarchaeological approach with a textual analysis of letters, medical texts, and state documents, this book evaluates health experiences at Deir el-Medina and how people responded to illnesses and stressors. While osteological analyses document the physiological health histories of the Deir el-Medina population, textual sources inform the social mechanisms that structured how people could combat illness in the village.

This book relies on some of the same evidence as my dissertation, which similarly explored health and disease at Deir el-Medina, but is fundamentally different because it incorporates broader evidence, a more integrated structure, and a more applicable theoretical orientation. First, the dataset of human remains from the site is far more comprehensive, offering a fuller picture of health during the New Kingdom by allowing the comparison of contemporaneous family tombs. The book also includes some of the only complete human remains so far found at Deir el-Medina. These individuals represent the relatively under-documented 18th Dynasty occupation of the site, allowing for a more comprehensive comparison of health across Deir el-Medina both by family and period.

Second, this book better integrates evidence from human remains and texts throughout its chapters rather than separating the two into independent sections. I prioritized placing these two datasets side-by-side in many of the following chapters. While some scholars may be inclined to focus only on sections related to their field, I invite readers to consider the book in its entirety in the hopes that doing so may bridge some of the divides in scholarship and citation across disciplines. An interdisciplinary approach is essential for a study on human health. Therefore, I wrote this book with myriad readers in mind, attempting to make Egyptological and bioarchaeological scholarship legible and accessible to non-specialists.

Finally, this book uses a more robust theoretical approach that expands on how we can explain health discrepancies in the past. This approach forefronts the *Social Determinants of Health*—a variety of social factors used to explain health patterns in modern populations—to differentiate the emic ways that Egyptians reacted to illness and improved health. Rather than a veneer of change, using the *Social Determinants of Health* fundamentally reoriented my inquiry, allowing me to incorporate more Egyptian texts by asking how factors beyond healthcare could have impacted health. This forced me to reconsider issues untouched in my dissertation like the impacts of the late Ramesside collapsing economy on health outcomes at the site.

Before delving into *how* we can study health history at Deir el-Medina, it is important to understand *why* this site is such an optimal case study. Deir el-Medina, a UNESCO world heritage site, was the home of the workmen who cut and decorated the royal tombs during the New Kingdom (1550–1080 B.C.E.). This archaeological site, excavated primarily in the 20th century by Bernard Bruyère and the *Institut Français d'Archéologie Orientale*,[19] is unusual in Egypt as it consists of both the village and its surrounding cemeteries, giving us access to information from the human remains and from the settlement itself. During his excavations, Bruyère unearthed a giant pit filled with thousands of ostraca—limestone flakes or pottery fragments used for writing. These copious texts make Deir el-Medina "the community of the ancient world about which we know the most."[20] While a review of all of the research on daily life at Deir el-Medina is beyond the scope of this introduction,[21] the following summary outlines how Deir el-Medina's unique physical, socioeconomic, and political place within broader Thebes makes it exceptionally suitable for correcting the myth on the history of human health.

---

19 Cédric Gobeil, "The IFAO Excavations at Deir El-Medina," *Oxford University Press*, Oxford Handbooks Online, 2015, https://doi.org/10.1093/oxfordhb/9780199935413.013.32.

20 Steven Snape, "Sennedjem: Building and Buying at Deir El-Medina," in *Ancient Egyptian Tombs: The Culture of Life and Death* (Chichester: Wiley-Blackwell, 2011), 233.

21 Several key overviews of Deir el-Medina include Guillemette Andreu, *Les Artistes de Pharaon: Deir El-Médineh et La Vallée Des Rois* (Paris: Brepols Publishers, 2002); Morris L. Bierbrier, *The Tomb-Builders of the Pharaohs* (London: British Museum Publications, 1982); Jaroslav Černý, *A Community of Workmen at Thebes in the Ramesside Period*, Bibliothèque d'étude 50 (Cairo: Institut français d'archéologie orientale, 1973); Dominique Valbelle, *Les ouvriers de la Tombe*, Bibliothèque d'Étude 96 (Cairo: Institut français d'archéologie orientale du Caire, 1985).

The location of Deir el-Medina—situated in the western Theban hills among the mortuary temples and tombs of Egyptian royalty and elite—gives us unusual access to the daily landscape negotiated by the villagers and their families. Ancient Thebes, modern-day Luxor, was naturally divided into two sides by the Nile, with the vast majority of its denizens living on the East bank. The opposing West bank, and more specifically its limestone cliffs and valleys, was an unpopulated landscape of rock-cut tombs. Deir el-Medina's location, in this relatively barren landscape, allows us to use the remnants of the villagers' movements to reconstruct the exact areas where they would have traveled daily.

While we are unsure why the ancient Egyptian government chose the exact location for Deir el-Medina, we can say that it was placed far enough from the royal tombs to warrant the construction of a smaller set of stone-built "huts" for temporary living during the work week.[22] Numerous graffiti and artifacts distributed between the village and the huts have elucidated the path trekked by the residents of Deir el-Medina, and small shrines around the Theban hills have demarcated the areas the villagers once traveled. Topographical terminology also delimits the areas they visited, including references to local mortuary complexes and the marketplace at the Nile riverbank.[23] Modeling health at Deir el-Medina can consequently include the impact of movement to and from these locations, as well as the limitations these spaces would have placed on people with disabilities.

The unique socioeconomic position of Deir el-Medina also gives us unusual access to healthcare. The actual labor required to cut and decorate a tomb took its toll on the villagers.[24] Simultaneously, the villagers had access to many atypical amenities from the Egyptian government. The state provided the workmen and their families with homes, food, water, service personnel, and enslaved labor. Consequently, though they were workers, they likely had unprecedented access to the spectrum of healthcare and medicine only reserved for the wealthy elite.

22 For more information about the workmen's huts, see Andreas Dorn, *Arbeiterhütten im Tal der Könige: ein Beitrag zur altägyptischen Sozialgeschichte aufgrund von neuem Quellenmaterial aus der Mitte der 20. Dynastie (ca. 1150 v. Chr.)*, 3 vols., Aegyptiaca Helvetica 23 (Basel: Schwabe Verlag, 2011).

23 Černý, *A Community of Workmen at Thebes in the Ramesside Period*, 94–95.

24 Anne E. Austin, "The Cost of a Commute: A Multidisciplinary Approach to Osteoarthritis in New Kingdom Egypt," *International Journal of Osteoarchaeology* 27, no. 4 (July 2017): 537–550, https://doi.org/10.1002/oa.2575.

While the elevated status of the workmen created a bevy of opportunities for complex responses to illnesses, the social differentiation within the workforce also allows us to consider how socioeconomic status would have impacted access to care and medicine. Previous studies on the Deir el-Medina community have already established a social hierarchy within the town through analysis of the titles and occupations of its residents.[25] The workmen were divided into two sides, each being led by a foreman and his deputy, and the entire crew was accounted for by one to two scribes. Extensive support staff also provided the workmen with the various resources necessary to live relatively far from the Nile and to enable their work on the royal tomb to continue uninterrupted.[26] These various positions were not only paid different wages, but the scribes and foremen were also given more important social roles in village politics. These highest officials in the workforce were likely part of the top two percent of the Egyptian population.[27] Comparison of these different subdivisions within the workforce at Deir el-Medina can thus elucidate socioeconomic differences in healthcare access.

Finally, the incredibly detailed textual record reflects how Deir el-Medina's position within Egyptian bureaucracy can give us unusually specific access to health histories and healthcare. As an extension of the office of the vizier, the administrators of Deir el-Medina were required to record a variety of administrative documents such as monthly ration distributions, absences from work, and the use of state supplies. These bureaucratic texts can tell us incredibly detailed information about health usually unavailable, such as when a specific workman was sick, how much medical professionals were paid, and the amount of provisions given to specific members of the workforce.

---

25 For example, see Černý, *A Community of Workmen at Thebes in the Ramesside Period*; Benedict Davies, *Who's Who at Deir El-Medina. A Prosopographic Study of the Royal Workmen's Community*, Egyptologische Uitgaven 13 (Leiden: Nederlands Instituut voor het Nabije Oosten, 1999); Jac J. Janssen, *Village Varia: Ten Studies on the History and Administration of Deir El-Medina*, Egyptologische Uitgaven 11 (Leiden: Nederlands Instituut voor het Nabije Oosten, 1997).

26 Kathrin Gabler, *Who's who around Deir el-Medina. Untersuchungen zur Organisation, Prosopographie und Entwicklung des Versorgungspersonals für die Arbeitersiedlung und das Tal der Könige*, Egyptologische Uitgaven 31 (Leiden: Peeters Publishers, 2018).

27 Andrea G. McDowell, *Village Life in Ancient Egypt: Laundry Lists and Love Songs* (New York: Oxford University Press, 1999), 7.

5 The Path toward Understanding Illness and Care at Deir el-Medina

To understand how the people of Deir el-Medina responded to illnesses, it is first necessary to learn the theoretical models underpinning how we can study health patterns in past populations. Chapter 2 provides theoretical and methodological approaches to defining and identifying health using the WHO's broader definition of health. It focuses on the issues identified in the *Osteological Paradox*, a landmark article describing limitations in studying health patterns in the past. In particular, *hidden heterogeneity in frailty* is a key limitation to studies of health in past peoples that has yet to be fully addressed. The chapter partly resolves this by bridging traditional bioarchaeological studies of physical stress responses with the *Social Determinants of Health*.

Chapter 3 then focuses on the people and place of Deir el-Medina to further explain why this particular village offers an exemplary case study in the study of health patterns in the past. This chapter outlines in more depth the nature of the village and its community, demonstrating that texts and human remains from the site are important evidence for health patterns and health experiences in the village. The chapter concludes with a description of the specific tombs studied for this book and the potential dates of use and demography of each tomb. These people represent the broader occupation of the village and are a more representative population than texts traditionally allow owing to the more abundant presence of women, children, and the elderly.

Chapter 4 presents six skeletal stress indicators from Deir el-Medina to evaluate how health experiences varied both within the village and across ancient Egyptian sites where other scholars have collected similar data. These six indicators of stress—enamel hypoplasias, cranial porosities, stature, trauma, degenerative joint disease, and periosteal reactions—are organized by their representation of health experiences throughout the life course, helping to evaluate how health changed from childhood to adolescence to adulthood. This chapter challenges one aspect of the myth of human health: the notion that prior to germ theory, people did not know how to use their wealth to protect their health. By comparing evidence from sites ranging in burial wealth, occupation, time, and location, the chapter identifies when during the life course the ancient Egyptians were able to use their wealth to make health.

Following this, the next three chapters focus on specific *Social Determinants of Health* to evaluate if they are present in the village and how they could have impacted health outcomes at the site. Each chapter evaluates textual evidence for a different *Social Determinant of Health* and assesses how it operated in the community. By including research on how these impact health today and examples of how they could have impacted health at Deir el-Medina, the chapters identify the ways the *Social Determinants of Health* explain health patterns in past populations and how past people could control their health outcomes. While Chapter 5 accomplishes this by looking at social support and interpersonal care, Chapter 6 does so by evaluating the ways people could access healthcare at the site and the degree of medical literacy present within the village. Finally, Chapter 7 evaluates the role of economic stability in ensuring positive health outcomes for the villagers and the agency the villagers had in maintaining their economic stability amid crumbling state infrastructure.

The conclusion, Chapter 8, returns to a bird's eye view of the book's central question: how did the people of Deir el-Medina control their health outcomes? By coalescing evidence across the previous chapters, the conclusion focuses on the ways the *Social Determinants of Health* structure how we can answer that question. However, Deir el-Medina did not exist in a vacuum, and this research should not either. The conclusion, therefore, draws on insights from Deir el-Medina to inform how and why other studies should integrate the *Social Determinants of Health* into explanations for past health patterns.

As these chapters demonstrate, in ancient Egypt, just as today, wealth made health. However, the kinds of wealth available to the people of Deir el-Medina and the variety of ways they creatively used their wealth to improve their health reveal the complex ways wealth and health are intertwined in the past just as much as in the present.

6 A Note on Translations and Names

Because this book crosses disciplines and invites readers who are specialists within the fields of bioarchaeology, Egyptology, and Health Studies, ancient Egyptian texts will frequently include both translations and, where necessary, transliterations. Whenever I provide translations without additional citation, they are my own and based on cited hieroglyphic transcriptions and transliterations. When important, I also reference database entries in the extensive Thesaurus Linguae Aegyptiae (TLA) to clarify definitions of key terms.[28]

Additionally, the names of members of the community of Deir el-Medina are transliterated rather than anglicized.[29] While this is more difficult for those unfamiliar with ancient Egyptian language to read, it offers more consistent

28 Tonio Sebastian Richter et al., "Thesaurus Linguae Aegyptiae, Corpus Issue 17, Web App Version 2.1.0," October 13, 2023, https://thesaurus-linguae-aegyptiae.de/.

29 Name transliterations follow conventions used in the Deir el-Medina Database.

spelling of names than anglicized phonetic renderings, making it more useful for Egyptologists. Anglicized, phonetic renderings are plagued with issues like ambiguous short vowels, double consonants, and multiple ways of rendering Egyptian phonemes that result in multiple spellings for the same Egyptian name (e.g., Qenhirkhopshef, Qenherkhopshef, Qenherkhopeshef, Qeniherkhepeshef, Kenherkhopshef). For Deir el-Medina specialists, this problem is compounded by the need to represent names consistently while also aligning them with their phonetic rendering in Davies' *Who's Who at Deir el-Medina*.[30] Consequently, the index of this book includes both the transliteration and anglicized rendering of names based on Davies' spellings with individuals of the same name differentiated when possible.

30 *Who's Who at Deir El-Medina.*

CHAPTER 2

A New Theoretical Approach to Ancient Health

Even in modern populations, modeling health and explaining differences in health patterns across communities is a debated and difficult task. While the WHO definition of health allows for a broader range of factors to explain health patterns, it also makes these patterns harder to measure and explain. This is even more difficult when looking at past populations where evidence is both limited and inconsistent. How do we explain *past* health patterns if we are beginning with such a broad and all-encompassing definition of health and not simply looking for the absence of disease?

This chapter presents the broader ways researchers have attempted to define and explain health inequalities both in the present and past to answer this question. Scholars focused on modern health disparities have used the biopsychosocial model—a theoretical approach that layers biology, psychology, and social context—to explain the impacts of health experiences more holistically. Their work also led to a broader acceptance that social context can have an outsized influence on health outcomes. To explore how specific aspects of social context impact health outcomes, researchers focused on the *Social Determinants of Health*, a set of social factors demonstrated to influence health inequalities in meaningful ways connected to health patterns seen today.

Researchers specializing in health in past populations have followed a similar trajectory by studying evidence of stress in skeletal remains as a proxy for a broader definition of health. Bioarchaeologists have, however, had to contend with the *Osteological Paradox*—a set of key issues that complicate whether and how health is reflected in skeletal lesions—making it difficult to compare and explain health inequalities within and across populations. To resolve the issues brought up in the *Osteological Paradox*, bioarchaeological research needs to include a greater focus on communities with homogenous contexts as well as a clearer understanding of the variety of factors influencing health outcomes.

As a new way forward, this book applies the *Social Determinants of Health* to respond to the *Osteological Paradox* at Deir el-Medina. These social determinants are often used to describe health patterns in modern populations but have yet to be used to evaluate whether and how these same social determinants may have impacted past health patterns. By applying the *Social Determinants of Health*, this book offers concrete causal explanations for how the people at Deir el-Medina could control some of their health outcomes. These social determinants also help to explain past health patterns by identifying

 | DOI:10.1163/9789004700871_003

how various factors (e.g., social networks, socioeconomic status, and healthcare access) would have influenced health outcomes in ancient Egypt.

1 The Biopsychosocial Model as a Scalar Approach to Health

In 1977, George Engel published a landmark article on his "biopsychosocial model,"[1] which combined the biological, psychological, and social impacts on health into separate yet overlying layers.[2] Engel's approach argued that even though fully quantifying these variables is complex, such measurements are theoretically possible by considering multiple systemic layers affecting health. Engel's biopsychosocial model is a systems theory approach to medicine that was influenced by the broader development of systems theory in the second half of the 20th century.[3] Importantly, it offers a means to connect the different aspects of biology, psychology, and social context into a unified system that works together to explain health outcomes.

This model evolved over the following decades and was incorporated by the WHO into its theoretical framework for the International Classification of Impairment, Disability, and Handicap.[4] In their version of the biopsychosocial model, five mutually exclusive layers of interactions create a complete understanding of the relationship between an individual and their body, culture, and environment:[5]

1. *Physiological abnormality or losses*: Physiological manifestations of disease or trauma
2. *Impairment*: Functional limitations caused by the physiological abnormality or losses
3. *Activity limitation*: Activities an individual can no longer complete due to their impairment

---

1 "The Need for a New Medical Model: A Challenge for Biomedicine," *Science* 196, no. 4286 (April 8, 1977): 129–136, https://doi.org/10.1126/science.847460.

2 For further discussion on the role of Engel in developing and disseminating the biopsychosocial model, see White *Biopsychosocial Medicine: An Integrated Approach to Understanding Illness* (Oxford: Oxford University Press, 2005), 3–6.

3 Ludwig von Bertalanffy, *General System Theory: Foundations, Development, Applications* (New York: George Braziller, 1969).

4 "International Classification of Functioning, Disability and Health (ICF)," 2012, http://www.who.int/classifications/icf/en/.

5 These layers are most frequently discussed in detail in disability studies. For example, see Albrecht, Seelman, and Bury, eds., *Handbook of Disability Studies*, 1st ed. (Thousand Oaks: Sage Publications, Inc, 2001).

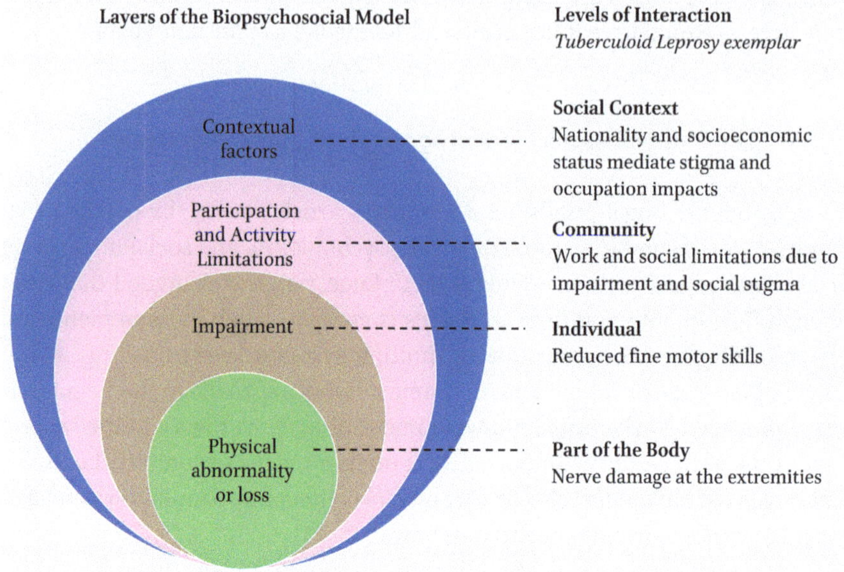

FIGURE 1 Layers of the Biopsychosocial Model

4. *Participation limitation*: Societal expectations that inhibit an individual with specific physiological abnormality or losses from participating
5. *Contextual factors*: The surrounding context of an individual which forms their social identity and cultural perceptions

Together, these five components identify and explain how biology, environment, and society intersect to affect an individual's health status. Using tuberculoid leprosy as an example, we can think of these layers as interacting on four levels (Figure 1). First, at its smallest level, one or more pathological lesions form, primarily as nerve lesions at the extremities.[6] These cause nerve damage and create a physical impairment with a loss or reduction of fine motor skills. When that individual then tries to interact with their community and space, they are limited both by cultural activities that require fine motor skills and by social stigma surrounding leprosy. Finally, when we place this individual within their socioeconomic context, their social status and identity dictate the opportunities and treatment they can receive as someone with leprosy. An individual's nationality and socioeconomic status, for instance, could impact how they are viewed and their access to medical care.[7] In this example, the

6 Arthur C. Aufderheide, Conrado Rodríguez-Martín, and Odin Langsjoen, *The Cambridge Encyclopedia of Human Paleopathology* (Cambridge: Cambridge University Press, 1998), 146.

7 For an example of this contextual approach for leprosy, see Jane Buckingham, "Indian and

health outcomes of leprosy are not simply their biological impacts (i.e., nerve damage leading to reduced fine motor skills). The same physical impairment could have myriad health outcomes because they are regulated by social context (i.e., social stigma and socioeconomic status reducing opportunities for work and healthcare).

The biopsychosocial model also accommodates the different definitions of disease, illness, and sickness discussed in the last chapter. While disease is represented most directly by observations of physiological abnormalities or losses, illness can be parallel to impairments and activity limitations because they focus on the experience of an individual. Sickness, then, embodies both the participation limitations and contextual factors that affect and are affected by broader socio-cultural processes. Thus, the biopsychosocial model allows us to define both health and the myriad ways it can be negatively impacted.

The biopsychosocial model is advantageous because it treats its constituent layers as separate yet overlying elements, allowing a study of health in the past through integrating multiple avenues of evidence independently. This is particularly important since evidence around illness experiences and diseases may come from different sources in archaeological and historical datasets. For example, if we wanted to understand the health impacts of walking disabilities in ancient Egypt, we could approach this through several distinct datasets, including (1) bioarchaeological examples of traumatic injuries, amputations, and pathological impairments in the legs; (2) artistic depictions of leg injuries and deformities; (3) archaeological evidence of walking aids; (4) textual descriptions of individuals with walking disabilities; and/or (5) geospatial analyses of walked terrain. Independently, each example evidences that walking impairments existed in the past. However, when we combine them, it becomes clear how those impairments changed an individual's career trajectory, inclusion/exclusion within a community, and the spaces they could physically access. This makes the biopsychosocial model particularly powerful because by considering each layer independently and looking at how they influence each other, it is possible to assess these distinct datasets, either combined or separately. This approach, therefore, takes advantage of the interdisciplinary opportunities to study health at a site like Deir el-Medina where we have access to information about village life from texts, archaeological excavations, depictions in tombs, and human remains.

British Concepts of Leprosy and of the Leprosy Sufferer," in *Leprosy in Colonial South India: Medicine and Confinement* (London: Palgrave Macmillan, 2002), 7–35, https://doi.org/10.1057/9781403932730_2.

2 Quantifying Health in Bioarchaeology through Stress Models

Although the biopsychosocial model allows archaeologists and historians to evaluate health impacts on individuals, it does not resolve a central issue around studying health: how can we quantify and compare health between individuals in a way that also recognizes the variety of ways in which health can be impacted biologically, socially, and psychologically? Researchers on health more broadly, including bioarchaeologists, have addressed this issue by measuring stress.

Concurrent with the development of new definitions of health in the early 20th century, there was also a growth in stress models. While the word stress is commonplace today, it originally only referred to a physical property between a force and its resistance until Selye redefined it in *The Stress of Life*.[8] In this work, Selye defines stress as, "the sum of all the non-specific effects of factors (normal activity, disease-producers, drugs, etc.), which can act upon the body. These agents themselves are called stressors, when we refer to their ability to produce stress."[9] Selye notes that his interest in stress grew out of a need to understand the consistent pattern in which the body responds to a multitude of diseases. Inflammation, for example, is part of a patterned response to disease but on its own is a non-specific indicator—it can occur as a result of a variety of different diseases.

This stress model is advantageous as it explains how the body physiologically responds to stress, but it does not completely explain how social factors can act as stressors. A variety of scholars addressed social factors through more holistic theoretical stress models[10] and quantitative studies on the importance of cultural stressors.[11] For example, Moss demonstrates how social communication networks can introduce psychological and social stressors that can cause measurable negative physiological impacts; simultaneously, these communication networks can also supply therapies to increase physiological immunity and relief.[12] Essentially, Moss clarifies how Selye's stress model not only offers a means to explain the mechanisms in the body responding to these differ-

---

8 *The Stress of Life* (New York: McGraw-Hill, 1956).

9 Selye, 42.

10 For example, Harold G. Wolff, *Stress and Disease*, American Lecture Series 166 (Springfield: Thomas, 1953).

11 For example, James P. Spradley and Mark Phillips, "Culture and Stress: A Quantitative Analysis," *American Anthropologist* 74, no. 3 (June 1972): 518–529, https://doi.org/10.1525/aa.1972.74.3.02a00190.

12 *Illness, Immunity, and Social Interaction: The Dynamics of Biosocial Resonation.* (New York: Wiley, 1973).

ent stressors, but also suggests that quantifying stress allows us to evaluate and compare the multiple layers of biological, social, and psychological health between individuals.

While the WHO definition of health is unmeasurable, physiological responses to stressors act as a proxy for health because they are responsive to the many layers of the biopsychosocial model. For example, if an individual experiences an illness that prevents them from working, they may also have reduced access to food because of minimal social support and increased psychological stress when looking for employment. In this example, biological, psychological, and social factors can all act as stressors, resulting in a cumulative physiological impact. Measuring stress then measures not just the impact of the illness but also the anxiety around searching for work and the lack of social support.

Developments in bioarchaeology during the 20th century allowed the discipline to adapt stress models for the analysis of health patterns within and across ancient populations. While population-based studies of health status in the past began with Hooton who assessed epidemiological patterns in the burials at Pecos Pueblo,[13] the broader application of such research arguably did not begin in archaeology until the 1960s.[14] At this time, multiple publications in *Science* on paleopathology made the study of disease in antiquity accessible to a public, scientific audience.[15] Focusing on the Nile Valley, Armelagos' research on diachronic Nubian health patterns exemplifies how population-based studies make it possible to compare relative health across different cultural groups.[16]

Methodologically, studies of ancient health also developed in the 1960s and 1970s, with a growth in research on ways non-specific stress manifests in human remains.[17] These methods provided the foundations for a broader analysis of

13 *The Indians of Pecos Pueblo: A Study of Their Skeletal Remains* (New Haven: Yale University Press, 1930).

14 Della Collins Cook and Mary Lucas Powell, "The Evolution of American Paleopathology," in *Bioarchaeology: The Contextual Analysis of Human Remains*, ed. Jane E. Buikstra and Lane A. Beck (Amsterdam: Academic Press, 2006), 313.

15 J. Lawrence Angel, "Porotic Hyperostosis, Anemias, Malarias, and Marshes in the Prehistoric Eastern Mediterranean," *Science* 153, no. 3737 (1966): 760–763; George J. Armelagos, "Disease in Ancient Nubia," *Science* 163, no. 3864 (1969): 255–259; Saul Jarcho, "Paleopathology," *Science* 147, no. 3662 (1965): 1160–1163; Ellis R. Kerley and William M. Bass, "Paleopathology: Meeting Ground for Many Disciplines," *Science* 157, no. 3789 (1967): 638–644.

16 Armelagos, "Disease in Ancient Nubia."

17 For example, Angel, "Porotic Hyperostosis, Anemias, Malarias, and Marshes in the Prehistoric Eastern Mediterranean"; George J. Armelagos et al., "Bone Growth and Development in Prehistoric Populations from Sudanese Nubia," *Journal of Human Evolution* 1, no. 1

generalized stress in bioarchaeology, which was crystalized at a much grander scale in the conference volume *Paleopathology at the Origins of Agriculture*.[18] In this volume, the "systemic stress model" was formalized by Goodman and colleagues.[19] Since then, this model has been adapted and most prominently utilized at an international scale in the *Global History of Health Project*, a comprehensive diachronic study on health that began in the Western Hemisphere and has since expanded into Europe and Asia.[20] These studies use multiple non-specific stress markers evidenced in the skeleton (e.g., stature, degenerative joint disease, enamel hypoplasias, and cribrotic lesions) to identify and quantify stress in human remains. In theory, these markers offer physiological evidence of stress as defined by the project as "a measurable physiological disruption or perturbation that has consequence for individuals and populations."[21]

Chapter 4 of this book outlines these specific stress markers and their etiology. Here, it is important to understand how skeletal stress markers provide a means of measuring past health that aligns with its broader definition. Stress is assumed to be inversely correlated to health, where better health is affiliated with lower amounts of stress. By modeling skeletal lesions resulting from stress, it is possible to assess the overall stress an individual experienced rather than looking for the specific etiologies of individual diseases. This is advantageous as it (1) does not require correct identification of specific diseases in order to assess health status; (2) considers the multiple and compounding effects of more than one stressor on an individual; and (3) allows consideration of the many stressors which do not result in diagnostic skeletal lesions. In essence, the systemic stress model is an ideal metric for the WHO definition of health

(1972): 89–119; Edward A. Sweeney et al., "Factors Associated with Linear Hypoplasia of Human Deciduous Incisors," *Journal of Dental Research* 48, no. 6 (1969): 1275–1279.

18 Mark Nathan Cohen and George J. Armelagos, eds., *Paleopathology at the Origins of Agriculture*, Proceedings of the Conference on Paleopathology and Socioeconomic Change at the Origins of Agriculture (New York: Academic Press, 1984).

19 "Indicators of Stress from Bones and Teeth," in *Paleopathology at the Origins of Agriculture*, ed. George J. Armelagos and Mark Nathan Cohen (New York: Academic Press, 1984), 13–49.

20 Richard H. Steckel and Jerome C. Rose, eds., *The Backbone of History: Health and Nutrition in the Western Hemisphere* (New York: Cambridge University Press, 2002); Richard H. Steckel et al., eds., *The Backbone of Europe: Health, Diet, Work and Violence over Two Millennia*, Cambridge Studies in Biological and Evolutionary Anthropology 80 (Cambridge: Cambridge University Press, 2018).

21 Alan Goodman and Debra Martin, "Reconstructing Health Profiles from Skeletal Remains," in *The Backbone of History: Health and Nutrition in the Western Hemisphere*, ed. Richard H. Steckel and Jerome C. Rose (Cambridge: Cambridge University Press, 2002), 12.

and the biopsychosocial model because it measures overall health through cumulative biological, psychological, and social stress experienced in a lifetime.

We should consider some caveats, however, when evaluating the utility of stress models as proxies for health. First, researchers should be cautious about using stress markers as proxies of health at an individual level. Research on living populations has demonstrated that stress in one individual can impact subsequent generations through the epigenome. This is particularly apparent in research on the effects of maternal stress on newborn health outcomes.[22] Therefore, measurements of stress may reveal transgenerational periods of stress and not simply the experiences of one individual. Additionally, self-perceived health does not always directly align with stress markers; research has found that in some cases, those with markers present (i.e., anemic individuals) report very good health, while in others, those without markers report poor health.[23] Consequently, while stress markers can correlate with overall poorer health in a population, they should not be used to indicate an individual's perceived health.

Second, though these markers offer a means to compare populations, we should also use caution when attempting to categorize and compare populations as "healthy" vs. "non-healthy."[24] Indeed, such terminology implies a binary distribution of health when research has instead shown that health exists as a spectrum. Stress markers also measure specific disruptions in health rather than an accumulation of all health experiences.[25] Consequently, they should not be used to indicate overall comparable health statuses (i.e., as a health index).[26] To resolve this, bioarchaeologists must consider the etiology, timing, and implications of individual stress markers when comparing populations.

22 Nicole C. Rodney and Connie J. Mulligan, "A Biocultural Study of the Effects of Maternal Stress on Mother and Newborn Health in the Democratic Republic of Congo," *American Journal of Physical Anthropology* 155, no. 2 (2014): 200–209.

23 Barbara A. Piperata, Mark Hubbe, and Kammi K. Schmeer, "Intra-Population Variation in Anemia Status and Its Relationship to Economic Status and Self-Perceived Health in the Mexican Family Life Survey: Implications for Bioarchaeology," *American Journal of Physical Anthropology* 155, no. 2 (2014): 210–220.

24 Daniel H. Temple and Alan H. Goodman, "Bioarcheology Has a 'Health' Problem: Conceptualizing 'Stress' and 'Health' in Bioarcheological Research," *American Journal of Physical Anthropology* 155, no. 2 (October 2014): 186–191, https://doi.org/10.1002/ajpa.22602.

25 Laurie J. Reitsema and Britney Kyle McIlvaine, "Reconciling 'Stress' and 'Health' in Physical Anthropology: What Can Bioarchaeologists Learn from the Other Subdisciplines?," *American Journal of Physical Anthropology* 155, no. 2 (2014): 181–185, https://doi.org/10.1002/ajpa.22596.

26 Temple and Goodman, "Bioarcheology Has a 'Health' Problem."

Additionally, inferences about stress markers must be based on a contextual approach to each population.

Finally, the etiologies of skeletal stress markers are still under debate, partly due to their non-specific nature. Recent research has demonstrated that some skeletal stress markers are more sensitive to early childhood stressors,[27] can be inherited through genetics and/or environment,[28] and are more indicative of environmentally-specific factors.[29] Scholars even suggest avoiding using the term "stress" because of its broad use and ambiguity when assessing so-called "stress markers."[30] While fruitful research has been able to explore how these markers interact and correlate,[31] it is also important to consider each marker individually as the absence of one marker may not indicate the absence of stress, but rather that it was not expressed under specific conditions. Additionally, scholars advocate for studying skeletal stress markers through multidisciplinary lenses in order to explain their etiologies better.[32]

---

27 Samantha L. Yaussy and Sharon N. DeWitte, "Patterns of Frailty in Non-Adults from Medieval London," *International Journal of Paleopathology* 22 (September 2018): 1–7, https://doi.org/10.1016/j.ijpp.2018.03.008.

28 Julie Lawrence et al., "Heterogeneous Frailty and the Expression of Linear Enamel Hypoplasia in a Genealogical Population," *American Journal of Physical Anthropology* 176, no. 4 (2021): 638–651.

29 Such as the correlation between malaria and cribra orbitalia as noted by Angel, "Porotic Hyperostosis, Anemias, Malarias, and Marshes in the Prehistoric Eastern Mediterranean"; Rebecca L. Gowland and A. Gaynor Western, "Morbidity in the Marshes: Using Spatial Epidemiology to Investigate Skeletal Evidence for Malaria in Anglo-Saxon England (AD 410–1050)," *American Journal of Physical Anthropology* 147, no. 2 (February 2012): 301–311, https://doi.org/10.1002/ajpa.21648; Nicole E. Smith-Guzmán, "Cribra Orbitalia in the Ancient Nile Valley and Its Connection to Malaria," *International Journal of Paleopathology* 10 (September 2015): 1–12, https://doi.org/10.1016/j.ijpp.2015.03.001.

30 Marija Edinborough and Carolyn Rando, "Stressed Out: Reconsidering Stress in the Study of Archaeological Human Remains," *Journal of Archaeological Science* 121 (September 2020): 105197, https://doi.org/10.1016/j.jas.2020.105197.

31 For example, Amy B. Scott and Robert D. Hoppa, "The Subtleties of Stress: A Comparative Analysis of Skeletal Lesions between the Medieval and Post-Medieval Black Friars Cemetery Population (13th to 17th Centuries)," *International Journal of Osteoarchaeology* 28, no. 6 (2018): 695–702; Samantha L. Yaussy, Sharon N. DeWitte, and Rebecca C. Redfern, "Frailty and Famine: Patterns of Mortality and Physiological Stress among Victims of Famine in Medieval London," *American Journal of Physical Anthropology* 160, no. 2 (2016): 272–283; Yaussy and DeWitte, "Patterns of Frailty in Non-Adults from Medieval London"; Samantha L. Yaussy, "The Intersections of Industrialization: Variation in Skeletal Indicators of Frailty by Age, Sex, and Socioeconomic Status in 18th- and 19th-Century England," *American Journal of Physical Anthropology* 170, no. 1 (2019): 116–130, https://doi.org/10.1002/ajpa.23881.

32 Temple and Goodman, "Bioarcheology Has a 'Health' Problem."

3 The *Osteological Paradox* and its Impact on Interpreting Health Patterns in the Past

Previous research measuring non-specific stress in human remains has demonstrated its power to compare systemic stress markers at a global scale and over thousands of years, as is most clearly visible in *The Backbone of History*[33] and its follow-up volume *The Backbone of Europe*.[34] Yet, measuring stress only documents differences in the rates of these markers; it does not explain *why* these differences exist and *how* they relate to health. A landmark article by Wood and colleagues put this issue into sharp relief by pointing out that when bioarchaeologists study health patterns in the past, they may actually be making incorrect and even paradoxical inferences comparing health across populations.[35] This *Osteological Paradox* makes it difficult to discern when and how skeletal lesions reflect meaningful differences in the health experiences of two or more populations.

Wood and colleagues argue that there are two specific issues for comparative health studies in bioarchaeology.[36] The first is *selective mortality*. Since our data come from a dead and not living population, our datasets are biased. When trying to infer health experiences, we cannot assume that those who died in one age group are representative of a living population. Instead, they are much more likely to die from hazards pertinent to that age group. The second issue is *hidden heterogeneity in frailty*, which refers to the unknown factors causing variation in underlying risk within a population. Wood and colleagues combine these factors to make the broader point that when trying to infer and compare health within and across populations, we can paradoxically mistake healthier populations for less healthy ones because individuals with skeletal lesions had to survive long enough for those lesions to form.

This paradox is best exemplified by three hypothetical groups: (1) a robust group exposed to an elevated risk (e.g., tuberculosis) that exhibits skeletal lesions, (2) a frail group exposed to the same risk that died before manifesting skeletal lesions, and (3) another group (either frail or robust) that was never exposed to that risk and therefore would not have any lesions. Suppose we used skeletal lesions to compare these groups. In that case, we might easily combine

---

33 Steckel and Rose, *The Backbone of History*.

34 Steckel et al., *The Backbone of Europe*.

35 "The Osteological Paradox: Problems of Inferring Prehistoric Health from Skeletal Samples [and Comments and Reply]," *Current Anthropology*, 1992, 343–370.

36 The *Osteological Paradox* also focuses on demographic non-stationarity, but this issue is more relevant when studies focus on demographic differences between populations.

those who were exposed but frail with those who were never exposed because neither would show evidence of skeletal lesions. Consequently, we can only positively identify whether a group was exposed to an elevated risk; we cannot know when groups were not exposed. *Selective mortality* predisposes those individuals who are frailer to die from the risk soon after exposure and prior to the development of skeletal lesions. Consequently, if we used skeletal lesions to identify which populations were healthiest, we could paradoxically identify the robust group exposed to an elevated risk as the least healthy population because that group carries the most skeletal lesions.

Wood and colleagues suggest bioarchaeologists can only address these issues if we first look outside the discipline to modern studies of health. These can inform us about the sources of *hidden heterogeneity in frailty*, their impact on mortality, and their relationship to the pathological processes that form skeletal lesions. The authors continue that bioarchaeologists can take on the *Osteological Paradox* by conducting studies in cases with more homogenous populations (e.g., temporally, genetically, and socially) to control for variation and better reveal *hidden heterogeneity in frailty*.[37]

Since the publication appeared in 1992, several review articles have documented how scholars have progressed in addressing the main points made by Wood and colleagues.[38] Several researchers incorporated improved diagnostic techniques to better understand the etiology of skeletal lesions and their relationship to, for instance, the oral microbiome,[39] parasites,[40] maternal stress,[41] and the presence of viral aDNA.[42] Steckel and Rose focused on addressing selective mortality and the concept that better health makes for worse skele-

37 Wood et al., "The Osteological Paradox," 357–358.

38 Mark Nathan Cohen, "The Osteological Paradox Reconsidered," *Current Anthropology* 35, no. 5 (December 1994): 629–637; Sharon N. DeWitte and Christopher M. Stojanowski, "The Osteological Paradox 20 Years Later: Past Perspectives, Future Directions," *Journal of Archaeological Research* 23 (2015): 397–450, https://doi.org/10.1007/s10814-015-9084-1; Lori E. Wright and Cassady J. Yoder, "Recent Progress in Bioarchaeology: Approaches to the Osteological Paradox," *Journal of Archaeological Research* 11, no. 1 (2003): 43–70, https://doi.org/10.1023/A:1021200925063.

39 Christina Warinner et al., "Pathogens and Host Immunity in the Ancient Human Oral Cavity," *Nature Genetics* 46, no. 4 (April 2014): 336–344, https://doi.org/10.1038/ng.2906.

40 Piers D. Mitchell, ed., *Sanitation, Latrines and Intestinal Parasites in Past Populations* (London: Routledge, 2016), https://doi.org/10.4324/9781315607603.

41 Julia Gamble and Gillian Bentley, Developmental origins of health and disease (DOHaD): perspectives from bioarchaeology (2022).

42 Kirsten I. Bos et al., "A Draft Genome of Yersinia Pestis from Victims of the Black Death," *Nature* 478, no. 7370 (2011): 506–510, https://doi.org/10.1038/nature10549.

tons.[43] They conducted a regression analysis comparing rates of skeletal lesions with life expectancies to see if they exhibited, as predicted by the *Osteological Paradox*, an inverse correlation, where longer-lived, healthier individuals survived and accumulated skeletal indicators of stress. They found that, overall, "it is incorrect to think that substantial deception from the paradox is commonplace, literally hiding under every rock."[44] They emphasize that contextual analysis clarifies when the paradox may be present, and they argue that it is most likely to occur in cases where population health changes dramatically, such as their own study of a poorhouse in Rochester, New York. They consequently suggest that the *Osteological Paradox* is a non-issue, stating: "Whenever time and resources were adequate to bury the dead with some ceremony, unassisted from the outside (unlike the poorhouse), then the possibility of substantial deception is unlikely when good contextual information is available."[45]

Despite the variety of studies addressing the *Osteological Paradox, hidden heterogeneity in frailty* still remains a critical problem that bioarchaeologists rarely address directly.[46] DeWitte and Stojanowski make clear that "understanding the nature of human frailty and how it relates to social inequality and social complexity is a highly relevant topic that crosscuts disciplinary boundaries ... yet bioarchaeologists have largely, though not entirely, avoided explorations of the topic."[47]

4 Explaining Health Patterns at Scale: The Goldilocks Problem

When studies have attempted to explain *hidden heterogeneity in frailty*, they have often been either too small (i.e., at the scale of the individual) or too big (i.e., across populations), making it difficult to reveal *hidden heterogeneity in frailty*. The confines of individual-level analyses hide the heterogeneous risk of frailty. Bioarchaeologists, for instance, have used osteobiographies to

43 Steckel and Rose, *The Backbone of History*.

44 Richard H. Steckel and Jerome C. Rose, "Conclusions," in *Backbone of History: Health and Nutrition in the Western Hemisphere*, ed. Richard H. Steckel and Jerome C. Rose (Cambridge: Cambridge University Press, 2002), 586.

45 Steckel and Rose, 586.

46 As discussed by DeWitte and Stojanowski, "The Osteological Paradox 20 Years Later"; for a more recent example of a focus on heterogeneous frailty, see Yaussy, "The Intersections of Industrialization."

47 "The Osteological Paradox 20 Years Later," 428.

conduct individual-level analyses of health in order to infer social impacts on health through modeling care,[48] such as in the "bioarchaeology of care."[49] Tilley's "index of care"[50] acts as a framework for determining whether or not care was required and available for an individual in the past. This approach is particularly suited to identifying how care helped individuals with physical limitations in past populations, demonstrating that "archaeology can show disabled people that their experiences are not uniquely contemporary."[51] These individual-level analyses offer unique examples of often extreme pathologies and disabilities, but cannot inform about heterogeneous frailty because they are difficult to extrapolate to broader groups of people.

At the other end of the scale, researchers used several key demographic and ecological variables to identify and possibly explain correlations in shifting health patterns over the broad chronology and geography in the *Backbone of History*.[52] The researchers chose ecological variables that could be compared between sites (e.g., elevation, settlement pattern, climate, topography, subsistence strategy). Looking at these traits over time, however, they found that especially as sites became more socially complex, these ecological constraints were poorly correlated to their health index, suggesting that ecological factors alone cannot reveal *hidden heterogeneity in frailty*.[53] The book's epilogue suggests that as social complexity evolved, so too did large disparities in health and wealth. Armelagos and Brown describe social stratification as a kind of "macroparasitism" in which the wealthy exploit and deprive the poor, leading to a lack of access to food, clean water, medical care, and shelter.[54] Their arguments suggest possible connections between health and wealth, but because

48 For an overview, see, Lauren Hosek and John Robb, "Osteobiography: A Platform for Bioarchaeological Research," *Bioarchaeology International* 3, no. 1 (2019): 1–15, https://doi.org/10.5744/bi.2019.1005.

49 Lorna Tilley, *Theory and Practice in the Bioarchaeology of Care*, Bioarchaeology and Social Theory (New York: Springer, 2015).

50 Lorna Tilley and Tony Cameron, "Introducing the Index of Care: A Web-Based Application Supporting Archaeological Research into Health-Related Care," *International Journal of Paleopathology* 6 (September 2014): 5–9, https://doi.org/10.1016/j.ijpp.2014.01.003.

51 Morag Cross, "Accessing the Inaccessible: Disability and Archaeology," in *Disability and Archaeology*, ed. Nyree Finlay (New York: Routledge, 1999), 8.

52 Steckel and Rose, *The Backbone of History*.

53 Richard H. Steckel and Jerome C. Rose, "Patterns of Health in the Western Hemisphere," in *The Backbone of History: Health and Nutrition in the Western Hemisphere*, ed. Richard H. Steckel and Jerome C. Rose (Cambridge: Cambridge University Press, 2002), 574.

54 George J. Armelagos and Peter J. Brown, "The Body as Evidence; the Body of Evidence," in *The Backbone of History* (Cambridge: Cambridge University Press, 2002), 600.

these comparisons are between sites that are so disparate in period, location, and social structure, these hypotheses are difficult to evaluate. Essentially, the populations are too big to reveal *hidden heterogeneity in frailty* because there are far too many variables across sites.

Given this assumed connection between social and health inequality, evaluating how social inequality contributed to heterogeneous frailty would seem promising. However, the variety of cultures, technologies, and social organizations in the sites covered by the *Backbone of History* project makes any social contributions to *hidden heterogeneity in frailty* challenging to extricate. Some of the authors of the *Backbone of History* further dismiss the connections between health and wealth because "in the absence of a reliable theory of disease causation, the rich and the well-educated did not know how to spend their wealth to improve health."[55] By dismissing socioeconomic status, the authors suggest that people in the past were too ignorant to use their wealth to control their health without biomedicine. This logic falls into some of the traps of the myth of the history of health described in the introduction, and such an overarching assumption dismisses other ways people could use their wealth to improve health beyond biomedicine. *Hidden heterogeneity in frailty* remains hidden because scholars have prematurely dismissed social factors impacting health despite acknowledging that the ecological factors used in the study cannot fully explain the variety of health outcomes seen as sites become increasingly socially diverse.

In considering the potential for bioarchaeologists to reveal *hidden heterogeneity in frailty*, DeWitte and Stojanowski write that "it is the ability of bioarchaeology to move between analytical scales—from the individual to the family to the community—that is so powerful. But ... these kinds of analyses require a more contextualized, particularistic consideration of health at the site and community level."[56] Moving from the individual to the community in a scalar approach allows us to identify health patterns in the past, but also allows researchers to explain those health patterns by layering on social context. This means studying communities that fit the Goldilocks' rule—individuals are too small, populations are too large, but communities with rich and knowable context are just right. In proceeding with this approach, however, we must consider carefully the variety of ways an individual's social and communal context can impact their health.

55 Steckel and Rose, *The Backbone of History*, 219.
56 DeWitte and Stojanowski, "The Osteological Paradox 20 Years Later," 428.

5 Revealing *Hidden Heterogeneity in Frailty* with the *Social Determinants of Health*

As Wood and colleagues suggested, one way bioarchaeologists can think more critically about *hidden heterogeneity in frailty* is by looking at modern health studies, and in public health, psychology, and medicine, we have seen a growing area of research focusing on how social factors impact frailty. These *Social Determinants of Health* include a variety of non-medical factors impacting health and have become a critical way that public health organizations study, explain, and address health disparities worldwide.[57]

The *Social Determinants of Health* emerged in response to the shifting view of health as a product of biological, psychological, and social processes. This last point—the social nature of health—was already documented during the Industrial Revolution, when it became increasingly apparent that an individual's social context (e.g., occupation and neighborhood) exposed them to different health risks.[58] As stress theory gained ground, public health researchers better understood the biological pathways of social and psychological behaviors and risk factors. Over the past thirty years, researchers have focused on understanding how to characterize, separate, and create policies for specific *Social Determinants of Health*.[59] In the United States, public health policies have aimed to address inequalities in *Social Determinants of Health* through a framework that identifies five key *Social Determinants of Health* (Figure 2): (1) education access and quality, (2) healthcare access and quality, (3) neighborhood and built environment, (4) social and community context, and (5) economic stability.

---

57 For key early volumes, see Robert G. Evans, Morris L. Barer, and Theodore R. Marmor, eds., *Evans, Robert G., Barer, Morris L. and Marmor, Theodore R.. Why Are Some People Healthy and Others Not?: The Determinants of Health of Populations*, Social Institutions and Social Change (Boston: De Gruyer, 1994), https://doi.org/10.4324/9781315135755; and Michael Marmot and Richard G. Wilkinson, *Social Determinants of Health*, 2nd ed. (Oxford: Oxford University Press, 2006); For its adaptation to major research and policy changes, see Commission on Social Determinants of Health, *Closing the Gap in a Generation: Health Equity through Action on the Social Determinants of Health: Commission on Social Determinants of Health Final Report* (Geneva: World Health Organization, 2008).

58 John W. Frank and J. Fraser Mustard, "The Determinants of Health from a Historical Perspective," *Daedalus* 123, no. 4 (1994): 1–19.

59 While contributions preceded it, Marmot and Wilkinson, *Social Determinants of Health* offered a landmark comprehensive contribution to the field.

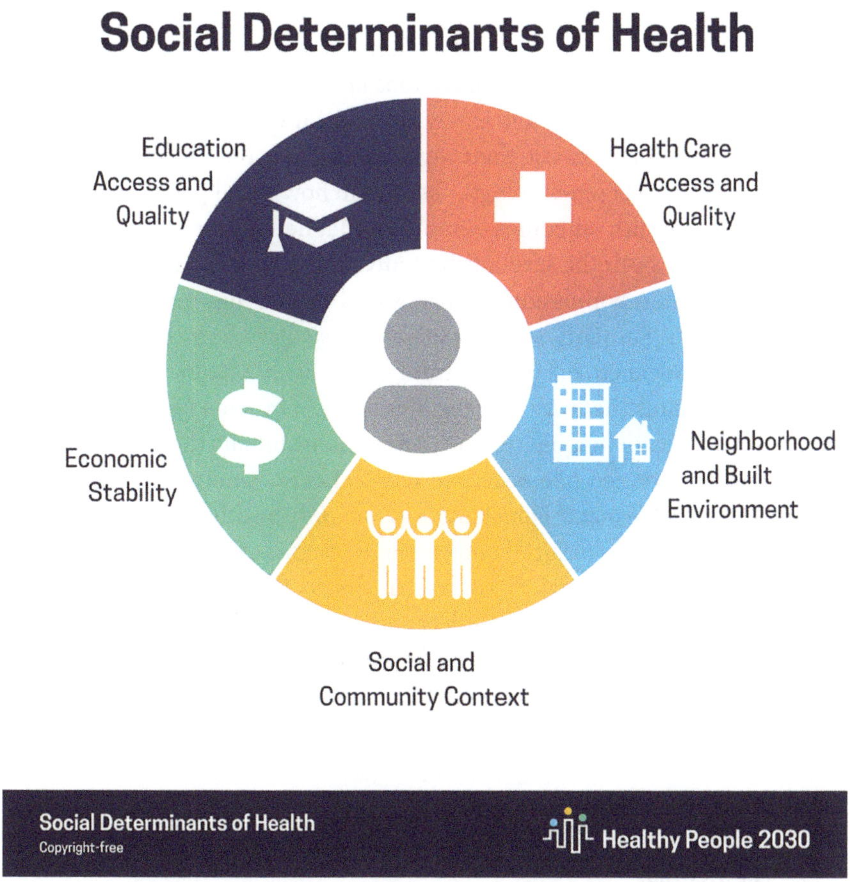

FIGURE 2 The Framework for the Social Determinants of Health used for the Healthy People 2030, U.S. Department of Health and Human Services, Office of Disease Prevention and Health Promotion
RETRIEVED APRIL 11, 2023, FROM HTTPS://HEALTH.GOV/HEALTHYPEOPLE/OBJECTIVES-AND-DATA/SOCIAL-DETERMINANTS-HEALTH

However, the relationship between health and wealth is far more complex than simply using one's means to acquire more goods or access medicine. If health inequalities were solely the product of deprivation—an inability to get adequate access to food, water, shelter, and medicine—we would expect to find a bimodal distribution in health where only those in poverty experienced significantly worse health outcomes than the rest of society. Researchers have, instead, repeatedly found that health disparities exist as a gradient across the socioeconomic spectrum and not merely as a result of deprivation.[60] This

60 Richard G. Wilkinson, *Unhealthy Societies: The Afflictions of Inequality* (Routledge, 2002).

gradient is not only caused by unequal access to material goods but likely includes other social features like education and social status.[61] Consequently, when considering the possible connections between wealth and health in the past, we should recognize that access to medical care is only one of many actions people can take to use their wealth to improve their health.

Research in social epidemiology—studies in how social position and social context impact health outcomes—indicates that heterogeneous frailty should be considered at both the level of the individual and at the scale of broader subgroups within a population because social context has major impacts on health outcomes. Similarly, social epidemiologists have framed differences in health as "heterogeneities," demonstrating that health status correlates with social determinants that vary over the life course.[62] In some cases, these social factors impact health inequalities much more substantially than areas we have traditionally prioritized like access to medical care, genetic predispositions, and individual behaviors.[63] For example, U.S. county health rankings give twice as much weight (40%) to social and economic factors as they do to access and quality of health care (20%).[64] Given that the *Social Determinants of Health* can be used to explain a large portion of the health inequalities visible in modern populations, bioarchaeologists and historians cannot dismiss the impacts of these social determinants if we want to understand health patterns in past populations.

6 Studying Health and Care in Past Populations: A Case Study at Deir el-Medina

So far, this chapter has focused on the broader ways researchers have attempted to define and explain health inequalities both in the present and past. In

61 There is still debate about which social features cause this gradient. For an overview, see Alan Davidson, *Social Determinants of Health: A Comparative Approach* (Oxford: Oxford University Press, 2019).

62 C. Hertzman, J. Frank, and Robert G. Evans, "Heterogeneities in Health Status and the Determinants of Population Health," in *Why Are Some People Healthy and Others Not?*, ed. Robert G. Evans, Morris L. Barer, and Theodore R. Marmor (Boston: De Gruyter, 1994), 67–92.

63 Benjamin C. Amick III et al., eds., *Society and Health* (Oxford: Oxford University Press, 1995); J. Michael McGinnis, Pamela Williams-Russo, and James R. Knickman, "The Case for More Active Policy Attention to Health Promotion," *Health Affairs* 21, no. 2 (2002): 78–93.

64 University of Wisconsin Population Health Institute, "2022 Measures," County Health Rankings & Roadmaps, accessed July 14, 2022, https://www.countyhealthrankings.org/2022-measures.

modern populations, researchers rejected the oversimplified definitions of health for a broader and more comprehensive one that includes biological, psychological, and social factors as outlined in biopsychosocial theory. As a result, they also sought better ways to characterize and measure health beyond identifying disease. Scholars have defined the *Social Determinants of Health* to identify how social context impacts health outcomes and found that these have an even bigger influence over health inequalities than traditional areas of focus such as genetics and medicine.

Researchers specializing in health in past populations have followed a similar trajectory by studying evidence of stress in skeletal remains as a proxy for a broader definition of health. However, bioarchaeologists have had to contend with the *Osteological Paradox*, including *selective mortality* and *hidden heterogeneity in frailty*, making it difficult to compare and explain health inequalities within and across populations. *Hidden heterogeneity in frailty* remains a particular problem that requires a greater focus on communities with homogenous contexts as well as a clearer understanding of the variety of factors influencing health outcomes. Given the importance of the *Social Determinants of Health* in explaining health patterns in modern populations, it is time we consider whether and how these may have also impacted health patterns via skeletal stress markers in past populations (Figure 3).

This book focuses on the *Social Determinants of Health* at Deir el-Medina as a response to the need to reveal *hidden heterogeneity in frailty* in the past through a deeper contextual approach at a community scale. Deir el-Medina offers an ideal place to consider social impacts on health in past populations given the relative homogeneity of the village, its smaller communal size, and its rich context, which provides us with a wealth of evidence on social determinants normally unavailable in the ancient world. Pay receipts, work attendance records, legal texts, and personal letters can all offer important data on key *Social Determinants of Health* from Figure 2 like economic stability, social support, and healthcare access. Furthermore, the clear and defined community membership, along with the relatively uniform socioeconomic status of its members, make it a more homogenous sample when comparing health patterns. Its unique location—separated from most other communities in Thebes—further allows us to consider Deir el-Medina's relatively isolated social and physical environment.

It is essential, however, to recognize the limitations of the evidence available at the site. The human remains at Deir el-Medina have been looted since antiquity, and the heavy commingling at the site makes it impossible to analyze complete skeletons. This limits the opportunities for understanding the health of individuals over the life course and how we can interpret isolated

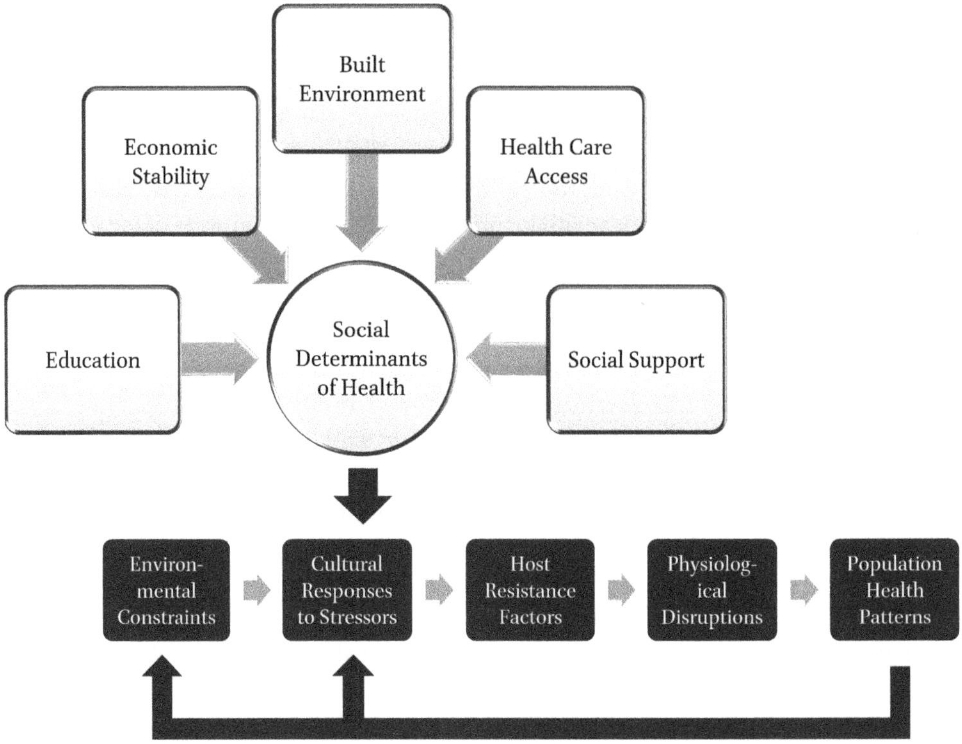

FIGURE 3 A model of the way Social Determinants of Health could impact hidden heterogeneity in frailty for skeletal stress lesions in past populations
MODIFIED FROM ALAN H. GOODMAN AND GEORGE J. ARMELAGOS, "INFANT AND CHILDHOOD MORBIDITY AND MORTALITY RISKS IN ARCHAEOLOGICAL POPULATIONS," WORLD ARCHAEOLOGY 21, NO. 2 (1989)

skeletal lesions. This commingling also makes it impossible to date individual elements beyond the broader dates of use of the tombs. These limitations are not insignificant—if it were possible to compare human remains from the site's early, middle, and late occupations, then it would also be possible to trace how health patterns change and respond to periods of growth, decline, and even state economic collapse.

So, how do we deal with these limitations given the incredibly valuable information offered by Deir el-Medina's rich textual record? The following chapter provides more context on the human remains and tombs from which this research is drawn, as well as the methods used to ensure these commingled remains offer as much robust information as possible on health patterns in Deir el-Medina.

CHAPTER 3

The Place, The Community, and The Evidence

Deir el-Medina offers unusual access to health experiences in the past, allowing this book to tackle aspects of *hidden heterogeneity in frailty*, as it presents a wealth of contextual evidence available at a community scale. Its location gives it a unique place both physically and socially. The community living at Deir el-Medina had relatively high degrees of literacy, limited size, and sociocultural homogeneity, making them ideal for a study of health. The preservation of extensive textual records provides individual accounts of illness and care, making it possible to reconstruct how social determinants would have operated within the village. Human remains from the site give context to these illnesses by providing skeletal evidence of stress experienced during the village's occupation. This allows us to consider how stress changed over the life course and differences in stress among the villagers.

This chapter elucidates these unusual features at Deir el-Medina, focusing in particular on how studying health patterns at Deir el-Medina requires an interdisciplinary combination of texts addressing illness and physiological markers of stress in human remains. For such an interdisciplinary study to work, it is critical to assess how representative the texts and human remains from the site are of the broader community in the village. What are the biases, limitations, and opportunities for each dataset? To answer this question, this chapter outlines the nature of these two datasets, demonstrating their temporal and demographic breadth as representations of the people at Deir el-Medina. This requires even more attention when discussing the human remains from the village, as these have only been partially published. The chapter, therefore, ends with a detailed description of each tomb included in this study and the overall demography of the human remains discussed in this book.

1 The Place

Ancient Thebes, modern-day Luxor, was naturally divided in two by the Nile, with the majority of its denizens living on the East bank of the river. The opposing West bank, specifically its limestone cliffs and valleys, was a landscape of rock-cut tombs. Placed in the middle of this mortuary setting was the village of Deir el-Medina. The Egyptian state founded the village in the early New Kingdom as a permanent residence for the workmen who cut and decorated the

DOI:10.1163/9789004700871_004

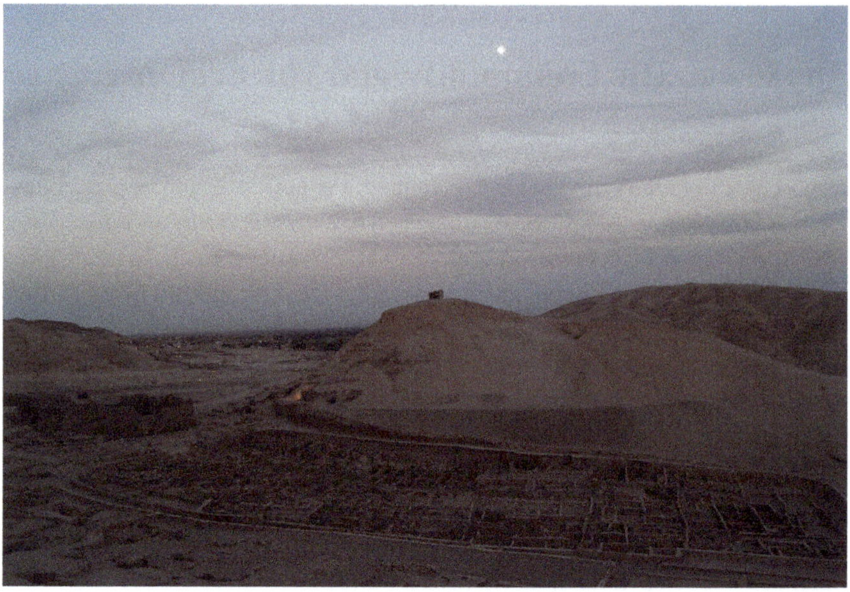

FIGURE 4 A photo of the archaeological site of Deir el-Medina. The village in the foreground of this image is overlooked by the Eastern Cemetery beyond it.

royal tombs in the Valley of the Kings and the Valley of the Queens. In order to have a location for the workmen and their families to live that was near their main worksites, the village was situated at the base of the Theban cliffs in a mostly enclosed desert valley. This location, relatively isolated from the villages and settlements near the Nile, offered an ideal place for a village of its size while also offering easier access to the Valley of the Queens and the Valley of the Kings.

This location also defined the Deir el-Medina community both physically and socially. The desert valley, which the village occupied, was nestled between Eastern and Western hills that became the community's cemeteries and the Theban cliffs bracketed the site to its north (Figure 4). Its physical environment separated the villagers at Deir el-Medina from other Theban populations and limited how much the village could expand. As the size of the crew living at Deir el-Medina grew and shrank based on each ruler's needs, a limited number of new homes were built or remodeled; some houses extended beyond the confines of the village's enclosure wall, though in these circumstances, they butted up against the surrounding cemeteries.[1] At its peak, the village contained sixty-

1 The homes outside the enclosure may also have housed those closely affiliated, but not offi-

eight houses and its population numbered in the hundreds, making Deir el-Medina's community membership physically unambiguous. The ability to live within the enclosure walls was afforded to those families with a member in the workforce. When workmen were removed from the crew, so too was their family's membership as part of the Deir el-Medina community.[2]

The close proximity of homes also lent itself to a community that would be intimately aware of each other's activities; essentially, all community members were neighbors. The tight boundaries of the village, clearly demarcated by both the settlement's enclosure wall and its natural surroundings, meant that homes were placed one next to the other with shared walls and roof spaces. Even today, sounds reverberate easily off the surrounding rock from the cemeteries and cliffs that surround the village.

The people of Deir el-Medina regularly visited other accessible spaces. The site's location in a relatively barren landscape allows us to see the remnants of the villagers' movements (e.g., graffiti, built structures, and discarded texts). We can consequently reconstruct some of the exact areas where they traveled. We know, for example, that the crew often stayed at temporary huts that they built to shorten the distance to their workplace during their work week. These spaces offered each workman a temporary living space in a location that also provided a means to overlook people's movements near and around the royal tombs. While these are archaeologically most visible at the *col station*,[3] a cluster of stone huts placed along the path between the village and the Valley of the Kings, the texts also describe huts closer to the Valley of the Queens. The workforce likely had various temporary huts built as needed as they worked on the royal tombs, including purpose-built spaces outside the tombs and rest areas.[4]

---

cially part of the community at Deir el-Medina, such as the enslaved women who completed household service for the families, retired members of the crew, or divorcees/widows. For a summary, see Benedict G. Davies, *Life Within the Five Walls: A Handbook to Deir El-Medina*, Robb de Peyster Tytus Memorial Series 5 (Wallasey: Abercromby Press, 2018), 108.

2 One clear example of this is when the workforce was cut in half during the reign of Ramesses v. O. Berlin P 12654 indicates that the fired crew was instead placed as part of the support staff (*smd.t*).

3 Dorn, *Arbeiterhütten im Tal der Könige*; Jaana Toivari-Viitala et al., "Preliminary Report of the Work Performed During the Fifth Season in 2012–2013," Workmen's Huts in the Theban Mountains Project (Academy of Finland and University of Helsinki, 2013), https://www.egyptologinenseura.fi/wp-content/uploads/sites/9/2019/09/Report-2012-2013_ACADEMY-OF-FINLAND-AND-UNIVERSITY-OF-HELSINKI_5th-season.pdf.

4 Robert J. Demarée, "A House Is Not a Home—What Exactly Is a Hut?," in *Living and Writing in Deir El-Medine*, ed. Andreas Dorn and Tobias Hofmann, Aegyptiaca Helvetica 19 (Basel: Schwabe Verlag, 2006), 57–66.

In addition to their specific places of work in the Valley of the Kings and Valley of the Queens, the workmen also explored the surrounding Theban necropolis encompassing Deir el-Bahari, intervening wadis, and remote cliffs. The abundant graffiti, which were often written by members of the Deir el-Medina workforce, are the most direct evidence of their explorations. Community members who were not part of the workforce are unattested in graffiti, suggesting they were not allowed or unable to explore these spaces.[5]

Members of the village also regularly visited spaces on the Theban West bank, journeying away from the cliffs and closer to the flood plain, which held fields for livestock and the socially active Nile riverbank (*mr.yt*).[6] The shifting geological landscape of the region makes it difficult to determine with certainty where the Nile riverbank was located during the New Kingdom, but there may have been a river canal which skirted the desert near the mortuary temples east of Deir el-Medina.[7] Texts mentioning the Nile riverbank present it as either a place to buy and sell goods or to receive legal punishment, making it one space where residents of Deir el-Medina could interact with the broader social nexus of Thebes.[8] Depictions of the riverbank in Theban Tomb (TT) 217 as well as textual accounts also demonstrate that it was a space that both women and men could occupy. These texts describe workmen maintaining private huts at the riverbank and women selling goods such as cloth.[9]

2 The Community

These different spaces illustrate how the social and physical spaces available to the people of Deir el-Medina varied based on features like gender and employment. A workman's experience at Deir el-Medina was significantly different than his wife's because of major differences over time in the physical spaces

5 Sławomir Rzepka, *Who, Where and Why: The Rock Graffiti of Members of the Deir El-Medina Community* (Warsaw: Pro-Egipt, 2014).

6 Černý, *A Community of Workmen at Thebes in the Ramesside Period*, 94–97.

7 Willem H.J. Toonen et al., "Holocene Fluvial History of the Nile's West Bank at Ancient Thebes, Luxor, Egypt, and Its Relation with Cultural Dynamics and Basin-Wide Hydroclimatic Variability," *Geoarchaeology* 33, no. 3 (2018): 273–290, https://doi.org/10.1002/gea.21631.

8 Andrea G. McDowell, *Jurisdiction in the Workmen's Community of Deir El-Medîna*, Egyptologische Uitgaven 5 (Leiden: Nederlands Instituut voor het Nabije Oosten, 1990), 219–223; Valbelle, *Les ouvriers de la Tombe*, 249–250.

9 Christopher J. Eyre, "The Market Women of Pharaonic Egypt," in *Le Commerce En Égypte Ancienne*, ed. Nicolás Grimal and Bernadette Menu, Bibliothèque d'étude 121 (Cairo: Institut Français d'Archéologie Orientale, 1998), 173–191.

they occupied. Over a lifetime, an individual may also have experienced these spaces differently after gaining or losing status as a member of the crew. Therefore, it is important to understand Deir el-Medina as a community that, on the one hand, is composed of families with similar socioeconomic standing and occupations, and on the other hand, has key differences to help us explore how identities like gender and age may have impacted their health outcomes.

Membership in the community was an important social feature of Deir el-Medina because of the numerous benefits that the state afforded and on which the continued existence of the community was entirely dependent. Because the village was established for the production of the royal tombs, the state provided the infrastructure necessary for the village to exist in its desert location. Both the houses inside the village and the workmen's huts were state property only awarded to workmen and their families so long as they were actively part of the crew. The state also took care of many chores necessary for daily life in the village by staffing the *smd.t*—a workforce dedicated to supporting Deir el-Medina that included water carriers, woodcutters, fishermen, gardeners, launderers, potters, and more.[10] While members of the *smd.t* were not housed within the village, they were a constant presence due to the variety of tasks they needed to complete for the residents of Deir el-Medina. In some cases, people belonging to the *smd.t* were related to members of the Deir el-Medina community or had previously been workmen in the crew. The state also supplied forced labor for the community, allotting each house a designated number of days of service each month.[11] The state supplied each of these groups—the workmen, *smd.t*, and forced laborers—with monthly rations. These various benefits formed a social system in which the villagers were reliant on the state for food, services, and shelter, which allows us to consider the role of broader political and social structures in impacting health outcomes at the site.

Though all members of the workforce at Deir el-Medina received these benefits, there was also a clear social hierarchy within the crew.[12] The workmen were divided into two sides, each led by a foreman, and a scribe kept track of the entire crew.[13] These various positions were not only paid different wages,

10 Gabler, *Who's Who around Deir el-Medina*.

11 Davies, *Life Within the Five Walls*, 313–315; Erika Endesfelder, "Sklaven (Hmw) in Der Nekropole von Deir El Medine," *Altorientalische Forschungen* 5, no. JG (1978): 17–24, https://doi.org/10.1524/aofo.1978.5.jg.17.

12 Černý, *A Community of Workmen at Thebes in the Ramesside Period*; Davies, *Who's Who at Deir El-Medina*; Janssen, *Village Varia*, 1997.

13 This position was expanded in the 20th Dynasty, so that there were two scribes overseeing the workforce. See Jac J. Janssen, *Commodity Prices from the Ramessid Period: An Economic Study of the Village of Necropolis Workmen at Thebes* (Leiden: Brill, 1975), 461–462.

but the scribes and foremen were also given more important social roles in village politics. Within their ranks, the workmen used titles (e.g., draftsman) to differentiate among themselves even when such titles may not have designated different pay grades. These differences also point to different skills and required degrees of literacy depending on a workman's role on the workforce. A comparison of these subdivisions within the workforce at Deir el-Medina adds granularity to how factors like socioeconomic status and social rank would have impacted health differences within the village.

3 Texts as Evidence for Health Patterns and Health Experiences at Deir el-Medina

Given that the function of the Deir el-Medina workforce was to cut and decorate the royal tombs, the community also had an unusually high degree of literacy in combination with an abundance of bureaucratic records. As an extension of the office of the vizier, the scribes of Deir el-Medina were required to record monthly ration distributions, absences from work, and the use of state supplies. These bureaucratic texts provide incredibly detailed data usually unavailable in ancient Egyptian populations such as when a specific workman was sick. Fortunately, archaeologists recovered many of these records in the *grand puits*—a 30-meter wide and 50-meter deep pit dug in antiquity just outside the village. On their own, the dossier of materials from the *grand puits* is astonishing, but combined with the texts recovered within the village, near the workmen's huts, and stored in the tombs, we have an exceptionally vivid record of daily life at Deir el-Medina.

This abundance of texts allows us to identify specific health experiences at the site and reconstruct how the community responded to illnesses as well as the various ways the *Social Determinants of Health* operated in this community.[14] Medical texts at the site inform us about the illness experiences that the people of Deir el-Medina attempted to control and their ideas about the causes and cures of illnesses. Bureaucratic records, like ration distributions and

14 Modern tools and archival projects have made these materials broadly accessible. The majority of ostraca and papyri in this book were compiled in the invaluable Deir el-Medina Database (see Joris F. Borghouts et al., "The Deir El-Medina Database," The Deir el-Medina Database, 2023, https://dmd.wepwawet.nl/.), and many were transcribed in the detailed Deir el-Medine Online (see "Deir El Medine Online," 2009, https://dem-online.gwi.uni-muenchen.de/.). These databases provide detailed descriptions and bibliographies of over 4,000 texts. Readers should turn to these resources to find extensive bibliographies of published texts.

absence-from-work records, evidence the frequency of missed workdays, rates of illness, and relative pay of the workforce. Personal letters present individual illness experiences and how individuals responded to stressors in their daily lives. Legal texts from the village offer insights into the legal structures that villagers could use to control their health outcomes and enforce community norms. And literary texts from Deir el-Medina also speak to the social values of the villagers and the potential roles those values could play in combatting sickness.

While these texts offer many advantages to accessing health and health patterns, it is important to understand their biases and limitations. Texts are not facsimiles of the past. Rather, they are cultural actors intended for specific audiences and purposes. They, therefore, carry with them biases in authorship, use, and preservation that can limit our understanding of health experiences at Deir el-Medina. A clear example is in the disproportionate number of textual records of working-age men, which is the result of scribes focusing largely on documenting workforce-related activities. The identities of women, on the other hand, are relatively harder to trace and their illness experiences are far less frequently documented, although they do appear in, author, and were the intended audience for some texts in the village. Children and the elderly are far more frequently found at the margins than at the center of texts from the site. Those with more disabling conditions would also have left little or no record in the bureaucratic texts at Deir el-Medina because those individuals would have disappeared from workforce records as soon as their disability prevented them from working on the royal tombs. Being conscious of this tilt towards a working-age male population is helpful but cannot overcome the gaps in the record.

The same can be said for our knowledge of diachronic change given the uneven distribution of texts from the centuries the village was in use. Relatively few texts from the 18th Dynasty have been identified with increasing numbers in the 19th Dynasty and the highest representation in the 20th Dynasty.[15] Not only are there more texts overall as time progresses, but many of the formal letters and legal texts from the village date to the 20th Dynasty, suggesting that

15 Haring indicates that of the original set of texts in the Deir el-Medina Database, their dating is distributed as follows: 17% from the 19th Dynasty, 31% from the 20th Dynasty, 10% from either the 19th or 20th Dynasty, and only 1% from the 18th and 21st Dynasties. Those dating from the 19th Dynasty primarily come from its second half and those dating from the 20th Dynasty primarily come from its first half. Ben J.J. Haring, "From Oral Practice to Written Record in Ramesside Deir El-Medina," *Journal of the Economic and Social History of the Orient* 46, no. 3 (2003): 254.

certain genres of texts increased in popularity as the villagers became more literate over time.[16] This distribution likely also reflects changing rates of literacy and expectations for record-keeping in the village with oral practices (e.g., legal oaths) increasingly being recorded in writing.[17] It is therefore difficult to disentangle whether differences in the prevalence of legal matters and personal letters reflect changing practices around health or simply increased literacy at the site.

Other genres of text such as bureaucratic records also shift over time due to the changing bureaucratic methods of the scribes and their individual recording practices. For example, the "daybook"—a type of bureaucratic text recording daily deliveries and workmen's rosters—was first used in the late 19th Dynasty and continued in use until the mid-20th Dynasty,[18] leaving comparatively less information about daily activities of the workforce for the 18th to early 19th Dynasties. Similarly, the late 20th Dynasty is relatively underrepresented, potentially because scribes transitioned to using papyrus more frequently than ostraca for recording, and preservation bias prevents archaeologists from finding these records with similar frequencies.[19] This period is also when state control diminished and the workforce relocated to Medinet Habu, changing where documents were both created and stored. These dynamic changes in writing practices in the village are a reminder that diachronic analyses of texts at Deir el-Medina must be undertaken critically given the dynamic changes in writing practices over time.

The general issues associated with working on an incomplete record are compounded by more specific biases related to the documentation of health. Egyptian texts rarely discuss the nature of death and dying. Death was often referred to indirectly through euphemisms such as departing on a journey, being at rest, or going to sleep.[20] This makes texts referencing the circumstances of death rare at Deir el-Medina.

When illnesses are mentioned in medical texts from Deir el-Medina, they rarely tell us the efficacy of different treatments. The medical papyri and ostraca from Deir el-Medina were compiled from previous treatments. Most of these texts acted as pharmacological compendia that focus more on ingredi-

16 Haring, "From Oral Practice to Written Record in Ramesside Deir El-Medina."
17 Haring.
18 Christopher J. Eyre, *The Use of Documents in Pharaonic Egypt.*, Oxford Studies in Ancient Documents (Oxford: Oxford University Press, 2013), 240.
19 Haring, "From Oral Practice to Written Record in Ramesside Deir El-Medina."
20 John H. Taylor, *Death and the Afterlife in Ancient Egypt*, 1st ed. (University Of Chicago Press, 2001), 38.

ents than on a patient's symptoms or eventual outcomes. Medical papyri and ostraca outside Deir el-Medina offer more extensive evidence of treatments—including descriptions of specific symptoms and their outcomes—but we do not know if these same treatments were used at Deir el-Medina. Rarely, an Egyptian scribe may marginalize a favored treatment indicating their opinion on which treatments are more effective,[21] but otherwise treatments are often listed side-by-side in medical compendia making it difficult to know how frequently specific treatments were used. Additionally, illnesses and symptoms that do not require complex combinations of ingredients may have been left unrecorded. This means that some important and ubiquitous medical care, like assisting in childbirth, is missing from the textual record. More common treatments that do not require a written memory aid would be less likely to appear in such texts. Finally, among the amuletic texts from Deir el-Medina, we can see that many of the written words were meant to be spoken.[22] Amulets that consisted only of magical drawings, over which words were presumably spoken, would provide little information about what they were intended to treat. Consequently, both medical compendia and amulets often lack a direct connection between an illness experience and its treatment.

Consequently, the textual record offers a limited means for accessing information about morbidity and mortality patterns at Deir el-Medina. Texts were far less likely to address severe illness experiences or the most common ones. They also do not equally represent the experiences of people who were not on the workforce including women, children, the disabled, and the elderly.

4 Human Remains at Deir el-Medina

One way to address these limitations in the textual record at Deir el-Medina is through an interdisciplinary analysis of health experiences and health patterns with human remains at the site. Because the tombs at Deir el-Medina consist of family burials, men and women are more likely to be equally represented in human remains. Children and their health experiences are also visible in both

---

21 This can be done by noting a text as the "right method" (*šs mꜣꜥ*), but also through glosses like "better" (*nfr nfr*). For additional discussion, see Tanja Pommerening, "Heilkundliche Texte aus dem Alten Ägypten: Vorschläge zur Kommentierung und Übersetzung," in *Translating Writings of Early Scholars in the Ancient Near East, Egypt, Greece and Rome: Methodological Aspects with Examples*, ed. Annette Imhausen and Tanja Pommerening, Beiträge zur Altertumskunde 344 (De Gruyter, 2016), 271.

22 For example, P. DEM 40. See Yvan Koenig, "Les Effrois de Keniherkhepeshef (Papyrus Deir El-Médineh 40)," *Revue d'Egyptologie Paris* 33 (1981): 29–37.

the human remains of those who died young and lesions that are still visible in adult skeletons, representing childhood health problems in those who survived (e.g., enamel hypoplasias). Similarly, the human remains at the site can provide new information about elderly and disabled people as well as both the common and extreme health conditions experienced by the villagers. Fatal injuries and conditions that impact the skeleton such as traumatic fractures are highly visible, informing us about some circumstances of death that may otherwise not be recorded in writing. A study of health through these human remains at the site complements the textual record by providing a much more holistic record of health and illness.

Given these advantages, it is clear why we need to include a study of the human remains at Deir el-Medina. However, while many scholars have focused on the texts at Deir el-Medina, comparatively little work has been conducted on the human remains. During the excavations of the cemeteries, Bruyère commented on the state of mummification and occasionally the age and state of human remains in the tombs, but the field of bioarchaeology had not yet developed, and looting in the tombs since antiquity had left the human remains heavily commingled. Consequently, prior to the research leading to this book, the New Kingdom human remains on the site were unstudied with many unanswered questions, such as how many individuals are currently buried in the tombs, which tombs still contain human remains, and what is the overall demography of the population.

This book addresses this gap in our knowledge for the first time, drawing information on health patterns from human remains studied over six seasons of bioarchaeological research with the *Institut Français d'Archéologie Orientale* (IFAO) mission at Deir el-Medina.[23] These data were primarily collected by myself, with the help of Mélie Louys in the 2019–2022 field seasons. Together, these data are derived from at least 134 people and over 1,725 elements. These individuals vary greatly demographically with evidence from neonates to the elderly, men and women, as well as those who died in the earliest history of settlement at the site to those who died soon after it was abandoned. Given this wide range of individuals, the remainder of this chapter gives an overview of who the people included in this book were and how representative they are of the broader health experiences of Deir el-Medina's denizens.

23 This research was conducted under the permission of the Egyptian Ministry of Tourism and Antiquities during the 2013–2015, 2019–2020, and 2022 field seasons. This research was funded through grants from the American Research Center in Egypt, Mellon Foundation, University of California Humanities Research Institute, Antiquities Endowment Fund, and the University of Missouri Strategic Investment Program.

This book focuses on the human remains from three Theban Tombs (TT): TT 217, 290, and 298.[24] These three tombs were chosen as they still contained human remains after their initial discovery and study during Bruyère's excavations. They also offer a nearly complete overview of the occupation of the village of Deir el-Medina and appear to date to the New Kingdom use of the site rather than later Ptolemaic and Coptic reuse. To demonstrate this, it is important to understand how I assessed the date of the human remains found in each tomb. Artifacts found among the human remains are common, but Bruyère and his team removed many larger artifacts such as coffin fragments, decorated stelae, and burial furniture. Looting since antiquity also means that human remains were potentially moved between tombs, and individuals were fragmented and left commingled inside tombs. These disturbances mean that dating the use and possible reuse of a tomb from the site requires combining evidence from the tomb's construction, prior excavation records, burial objects, and mummification styles present in the funerary assemblage, all of which help us reconstruct the lives of the tombs well after their initial excavation and decoration through periods of abandonment, reuse, and looting.

The extensive commingling also requires that we determine a minimum number of individuals (MNI) based on the most frequently repeated element in the assemblage,[25] with consideration of any age and sex information that could be recorded for the human remains found in each tomb.

These three tombs represent all of the individuals currently at Deir el-Medina that I have securely dated to the New Kingdom occupation of the site. More human remains are still unstudied at Deir el-Medina, with many commingled and assembled together in magazine 12 (P. 1022). Additionally, looters assembled numerous individuals in the caves connected to TT 6 before Bruyère's excavations. While some of these individuals likely date to the New Kingdom, their commingling with later Greco-Roman and Coptic human re-

24 In addition to the descriptions below, readers should also review the photographs and information available through IFAO on the tombs of Deir el-Medina. This database includes valuable information including tomb plans, recent photographs, bibliographies, and citation links to the Griffith Institute's Digital Topographical Bibliography. Institut français d'archéologie orientale au Caire, "Tombes de Deir el Medina," October 19, 2015, https://www.ifao.egnet.net/bases/archives/ttdem/.

25 For fragments, I also record features and shaft completeness as discussed in previous studies on commingled remains. See Sherry C. Fox and Kathryn Marklein, "Primary and Secondary Burials with Commingled Remains from Archaeological Contexts in Cyprus, Greece, and Turkey," in *Commingled and Disarticulated Human Remains*, ed. Anna J. Osterholtz, Kathryn M. Baustian, and Debra L. Martin (Springer New York, 2014), 193–211, http://link.springer.com/chapter/10.1007/978-1-4614-7560-6_11.

mains makes it impossible to date them securely. I have had the opportunity to survey numerous tombs at Deir el-Medina, but many more have not been opened in the past ten years. Future studies could identify more human remains of the New Kingdom in these tombs. Finally, some human remains from the site were sent to museum collections. I have not included these individuals in this book, but hopefully, future research can yield comparable data to integrate them into the bioarchaeological research conducted at the site.[26]

4.1 *Theban Tomb 217 and the Burials of the 18th Dynasty*

TT 217 belonged to the sculptor *ʾIpwy* (i) and is one of the most well-known tombs from Deir el-Medina owing to the detailed daily life scenes decorating the tomb's chapel.[27] New Kingdom human remains in TT 217 were found in the main corridor of the tomb as well as along the western side of the tomb's final chamber. However, none of the human remains in TT 217 belong to the tomb owner or his family. Rather, they were stored there by Bruyère's team during their excavations. For the majority of these individuals, Bruyère included identification cards with information about their original context. Given that we have a relatively good understanding of where these human remains were buried, only those with provenance from the New Kingdom are included in this book.

These individuals in TT 217 were originally buried in tombs of the 18th Dynasty, with the majority from the Eastern necropolis.[28] While earlier research suggested the Eastern necropolis did not belong to the villagers of Deir el-Medina,[29] more recent studies suggest these were, in fact, burials of the ear-

26 Raffaella Bianucci et al., "Shedding New Light on the 18th Dynasty Mummies of the Royal Architect Kha and His Spouse Merit," *PLoS ONE* 10, no. 7 (July 22, 2015): e0131916, https://doi.org/10.1371/journal.pone.0131916; Lisa Sabbahy, "The People of Deir El-Medineh: A Preliminary Paleopathology Study," *Anthropologie* 48, no. 2 (2010): 117–120; Julie Tomsová and Zuzana Schierová, "Skeletal Material from Deir El-Medina in the Egyptological Collection of the Hrdlička Museum of Man in Prague," *Annals of the Náprstek Museum* 37, no. 1 (2016): 41–69.

27 For an extensive publication of the tomb, see Norman de Garis Davies, *Two Ramesside Tombs at Thebes* (New York: The Metropolitan Museum of Art, 1927); for additional bibliography, see Bertha Porter and Rosalind L.B. Moss, *Topographical Bibliography of Ancient Egyptian Hieroglyphic Texts, Statues, Reliefs and Painting Volume I: The Theban Necropolis, Part 1—Private Tombs* (Oxford: Griffith Institute, 1960), 315–317.

28 More specifically, they come from pits: 1352, 1371, 1372, 1380, 1382, 1386, and 1390, and unnumbered pits from the children's cemetery.

29 Geneviève Pierrat-Bonnefois, "Cimetière Est Du Village Ou Cimetière à l'est de Deir El-Médineh?," in *Deir El-Médineh et La Vallée Des Rois. Actes Du Colloque Organisé Par Le*

liest residents of the village.[30] The extremely skeletonized remains suggest that the 18th Dynasty burials at Deir el-Medina were simply wrapped without additional mummification treatments.[31] Of particular note are neonatal human remains collected from the area of the cemetery dedicated to children and infants.

Unlike the other tombs in this study, the individuals in TT 217 were curated by Bruyère and generally represent complete individuals rather than commingled remains. There are at least 18 individuals present among the studied human remains from this tomb.[32] Consequently, while these constitute the only 18th Dynasty human remains so far identified on site, they also allow for more complete osteobiographies of their health experiences. Given the relative paucity of textual records from the 18th Dynasty, these individuals also offer important information about the lived experiences of some of Deir el-Medina's earliest residents.

4.2 *Theban Tomb 290 and Families of the Ramesside Period*

In contrast to TT 217, the individuals from TT 290 were fully commingled by the time Bruyère first worked in the tomb in 1922. His original description of the remains from TT 290, the tomb of *ỉr.y-nfr* (i)—depicting them as heavily commingled and pillaged, with looting activity focused on the crania and thoraxes—matches their current state.[33] Bruyère and Kuentz indicate that this looting was not random, but rather from looters who systematically sorted through human remains in a narrow passageway joining TT 290 with TT 291.[34]

Musée Du Louvre Les 3 et 4 Mai 2002, ed. Guillemette Andreu (Paris: Musée du Louvre, 2003), 49–65.

30 Daniel M. Soliman, "Workmen's Marks in Pre-Amarna Tombs at Deir El-Medina," in *Non-Textual Marking Systems in Ancient Egypt (and Elsewhere)*, ed. Julia Budka, Frank Kammerzell, and Slawomir Rzepka, Lingua Aegyptia Studia Monographica 16 (Hamburg: Widmaier, 2015), 109–132.

31 As also noted by Dodson in comparing the skeletal preservation of previously studied individuals in museum collections including Teti, Kha, Merit, Sennefer, and Neferiyt. Aidan Dodson, "The Late Eighteenth Dynasty Necropolis at Deir El-Medina and the Earliest 'Yellow' Coffin of the New Kingdom," in *Deir El-Medina in the Third Millenium AD: A Tribute to Jac. J. Janssen*, ed. Robert J. Demarée and Arno Egberts, Egyptologische Uitgaven 14 (Leiden: Nederlands Instituut voor het Nabije Oosten, 2000), 98–99.

32 The minimum number of individuals (MNI) for this tomb is based on counting both complete skeletons (primarily of adults that had been moved to there during excavations) and the petrous portion of the temporal bone amongst the infant remains which was differentiated based on size and development.

33 Bernard Bruyère, *Rapport sur les fouilles de Deir el Médineh (1923–1924)*, Fouilles de l'Institut français d'archéologie orientale 2 (Cairo: Institut français d'archéologie orientale, 1925), 25.

34 Bernard Bruyère and Charles Kuentz, *Tombes thébaines: la nécropole de Deir el-Médineh; la*

They go on to argue that during the looting, a fire erupted, perhaps set intentionally, which blocked the passageway into TT 290, leaving both its decorated burial chamber and the commingled human remains intact. The individuals, therefore, likely include family members from both of these tombs. Unlike the curated collection of human remains stored in TT 217, those in TT 290 were found and left there by Bruyère and his colleagues. During or after 2004, the human remains in TT 290 were then assembled and stored in a passageway between TT 290 and 291, perhaps to prepare the tomb for public visitors.[35]

Enough artifacts remain to demonstrate that TT 290 dates later in the occupation of the village; it was first used in the 19th Dynasty and the latest datable material is from the early 21st Dynasty.[36] The decoration of the tomb walls of *ʾIr.y-nfr* (i) date to the 19th Dynasty and among the contents of the tomb was the burial equipment of *ʾIr.y-nfr* (i)'s relative, *Wn-nḫw*, who was a workman during the first half of Ramesses II's reign.[37] Artifacts and mummification styles suggest the tomb was continuously used until the 21st Dynasty, a period consistent with the eventual abandonment of the site by the beginning of the Third Intermediate Period. These include fragments of cosmetic boxes and canopic chests parallel in design and construction to those found in the 19th Dynasty tomb of Sennedjem,[38] a hieratic jar label from the assemblage dating to regnal year 32 and therefore belonging most likely to the reign of Ramesses II or Ramesses III,[39] and an Osiris shroud painted with red ink belonging to *ʾImn-{m}-wiꜣ* which is more characteristic of 21st Dynasty funerary equipment.[40]

---

tombe de Nakht-Min et la tombe d'Ari-Nefer, Mémoires publiés par les membres de l'Institut français d'archéologie du Caire 54 (Cairo: L'Institut français d'archéologie orientale, 1926), 68.

35 This date is based on a newspaper found in one of the boxes that held human remains when I first studied them in 2013. This newspaper was dated February 28, 2004, indicating the remains were assembled there during or after that time.

36 Anne E. Austin, "Living and Dying at Deir El-Medina: An Osteological Analysis of the TT 290 Assemblage," in *Outside the Box: Selected Papers from the Conference "Deir El-Medina and the Theban Necropolis in Contact,"* ed. Andreas Dorn and Stéphane Polis (Liège: Presses Universitaires de Liège, 2018), 27–47.

37 Davies, *Who's Who at Deir El-Medina*, 218.

38 "Cosmetic Box from the Tomb of Sennedjem | New Kingdom, Ramesside," The Metropolitan Museum of Art, accessed February 28, 2023, https://www.metmuseum.org/art/collection/search/544701.

39 Ramesses III's death early in year 32 of his reign was recorded in the Turin Legal Papyrus. Other than Ramesses II and III, no other ruler reached a reign of 32 years in the New Kingdom.

40 Aly Abdalla, "A Group of Osiris-Cloths of the Twenty-First Dynasty in the Cairo Museum," *The Journal of Egyptian Archaeology* 74, no. 1 (1988): 157–164; Herbert Eustis Winlock,

The evolution of mummification styles on display in this tomb is also consistent with a long period of use. Most mummified human remains demonstrate stereotypical mummification of the New Kingdom, including painted eyebrows and desiccation of the body with no subcutaneous packing.[41] Some, however, display characteristics specific to the early Third Intermediate Period, including the presence of a vertical visceral cut and extreme packing of the chest with a mélange of materials. The combined data from the artifacts and mummification style support a terminal use date by the end of the 20th Dynasty or beginning of the 21st Dynasty when the village was being abandoned.

Intrusive Graeco-Roman burials—common features of tombs in the Theban region—do not appear in TT 290 based on the mummification styles, associated linen, and artifacts. During the Greco-Roman period, mummification had shifted towards a preference for painted wrappings, geometrically-patterned bandaging, gilding, and more abundant use of resins and bitumen.[42] Other tombs at Deir el-Medina have Ptolemaic remains with these features, bearing witness to this tendency at Deir el-Medina as well.[43]

"The Museum's Excavations at Thebes," *The Metropolitan Museum of Art Bulletin* 21, no. 3 (March 1926): 5–32, https://doi.org/10.2307/3254817.

41 While there is no one set of criteria universally used to date mummification styles, a variety of sources have offered insights into period-specific practices evidenced in the New Kingdom and Third Intermediate Period including Arthur C. Aufderheide, *The Scientific Study of Mummies* (Cambridge: Cambridge University Press, 2003); Aidan Cockburn, Eve Cockburn, and Theodore A. Reyman, eds., *Mummies, Disease and Ancient Cultures*, 2nd ed. (Cambridge: Cambridge University Press, 1998); Warren Royal Dawson and Peter Hugh Ker Gray, *Catalogue of Egyptian Antiquities in the British Museum: I Mummies and Human Remains*, vol. 1 (London: British Museum Press, 1968); Dodson, "The Late Eighteenth Dynasty Necropolis at Deir El-Medina and the Earliest 'Yellow' Coffin of the New Kingdom"; Françoise Dunand and Roger Lichtenberg, *Mummies And Death in Egypt* (Ithaca: Cornell University Press, 2006); Salima Ikram and Aidan Dodson, *The Mummy in Ancient Egypt: Equipping the Dead for Eternity* (London: Thames & Hudson, 1998); William Peck, "Mummies of Ancient Egypt," in *Mummies, Disease and Ancient Cultures*, ed. Thomas Aidan Cockburn, Eve Cockburn, and Theodore A. Reyman, 2nd ed. (Cambridge: Cambridge University Press, 1998), 15–37; Eugen Strouhal and Luboš Vyhnánek, *Egyptian Mummies in Czechoslovak Collections*, Sbórnik Národního Muzea v Praze 35-B 1–4 (Praha: Národní Muzeum, 1979); John H. Taylor, *Unwrapping a Mummy: The Life, Death and Embalming of Horemkenesi* (Austin: University of Texas Press, 1996); Michael R. Zimmerman, "Mummification Styles as a Guide to the Dating of Egyptian Mummies," in *Dating and Age Determination of Biological Materials*, ed. Michael R. Zimmerman and J. Lawrence Angel (London: Croom Helm, 1986), 166–169; Sarah U. Wisseman, *The Virtual Mummy* (Urbana: University of Illinois Press, 2003).

42 Dunand and Lichtenberg, *Mummies And Death in Egypt*; Ikram and Dodson, *The Mummy in Ancient Egypt*; Peck, "Mummies of Ancient Egypt"; Wisseman, *The Virtual Mummy*.

43 Dominic Montserrat and Lynn Meskell, "Mortuary Archaeology and Religious Landscape

This tomb contains a minimum number of 65 individuals,[44] and its burials range from children under 5 to men and women over 50. As this assemblage contains no evidence of use after the early Third Intermediate Period, it is assumed that all individuals originally died in the New Kingdom or Third Intermediate Period. Their quantity may reflect the fact that human remains come from both TT 290 and neighboring TT 291. In comparison, the intact tomb of Sennedjem (TT 1), which would have been used for relatively less time and presumably only by one family, contained at least 20 individuals the majority of whom were found without coffins.[45] The individuals left in TT 290 are, therefore, most likely the product of continuous family burials of the Ramesside period and representative of the community at Deir el-Medina of that time.

4.3 *Theban Tomb 298 and the Beginning of the 19th Dynasty*

TT 298 was originally the tomb of *Bꜣkỉ*, the foreman at Deir el-Medina under Seti I, and his father *Wn-nfr* (i). The earliest burials in this tomb would, therefore, mark the transition into the 19th Dynasty and bridge the remains of the 18th Dynasty currently in TT 217 with the slightly later Ramesside burials in TT 290.

TT 298 was first excavated by IFAO during the 1917–1918 field season when they found the Book of the Dead of *Bꜣkỉ*, foreign vases from Crete, and several ushabtis.[46] These early reports do not discuss the human remains in the tomb nor does Bernard Bruyère during his study in 1927.[47] During the 2019–2021 field seasons of the IFAO mission at Deir el-Medina, however, our team identified human remains in the ante-chamber and additional rooms of the tomb, though almost no human remains were in the burial chamber. It is likely that during the earlier excavations, some of the human remains were moved out of the burial chamber to make it easier to document the room's monochromatic decoration. Given the deep shaft of the tomb and the fact that all of the

at Graeco-Roman Deir El-Medina," *The Journal of Egyptian Archaeology* 83 (1997): 179–197, https://doi.org/10.2307/3822465.

44 The minimum number of individuals (MNI) is based on the left femoral head, the most abundant landmark identified in the human remains. This total includes all observable skeletonized and mummified elements.

45 Rogério Sousa, *Gilded Flesh: Coffins and Afterlife in Ancient Egypt* (Oxford: Oxbow Books, 2019), https://doi.org/10.2307/j.ctv138wsfh.

46 H. Gauthier, Rapport sur les fouilles de l'Institut français d'archéologie orientale dans les nécropoles thébaines en 1917 et 1918, (ASAE 19; Cairo, 1920) http://archive.org/details/annalesduservice04egypuoft.

47 B. Bruyère, Rapport sur les fouilles de Deir el Médineh (1927), (FIFAO 5; Cairo, 1928).

human remains included come from chambers beyond this shaft's entry point, it is most likely that these remains were buried in TT 298 and represent the use and reuse of this tomb rather than looting or archaeological activity that brought human remains into the tomb from other locations.

The mummification styles in this tomb also resemble what we found in TT 290 with many individuals highly desiccated without subcutaneous packing and relatively few examples of individuals with 21st Dynasty mummification techniques. We also did not find evidence of mummification techniques more common during the Greco-Roman period. Textiles from the tomb appear more consistent with New Kingdom and early Third Intermediate Period traditions with s-spun threads unless used for sewing and no examples of wool fibers.[48] In addition to the published artifacts found in TT 298, we identified other grave goods among the human remains including coffin fragments, jewelry, funerary food offerings (e.g., bread and doum palm fruit), and pottery. Based on this combination of grave goods and mummification styles documented in the tomb, the burial goods and human remains found in TT 298 most likely date from the beginning of the 19th Dynasty until the early 21st Dynasty.

This tomb contains a minimum of 51 individuals and similarly, these burials include both men and women.[49] Individuals ranged from those who died in infancy to elderly adults. The smaller quantity of individuals despite a longer duration of use than TT 290 further suggests that individuals from TT 290 potentially represent burials in TT 290 and neighboring TT 291. Both TT 290 and TT 298 likely contain individuals representative of the Ramesside families living in the village.

5 Demography and Representation in the Human Remains from Tombs 217, 290, and 298

Having established that the people in TT 217, 290, and 298 represent the broader occupation of the site, it is also important to consider what these people can tell us about the community that is otherwise difficult to access via texts. Given

48 Whereas I first reviewed the textiles in TT 290 myself, a sample of those in TT 298 were studied by Amandine Mérat in 2022. See Cédric Larcher et al., "Deir el-Médina (2022)," *Bulletin archéologique des Écoles françaises à l'étranger*, June 1, 2023, https://doi.org/10.4000/baefe.8324.

49 The minimum number of individuals (MNI) is based on the right femoral head which was the most abundant landmark identified in the human remains. This total includes all observable skeletonized and mummified elements.

that these three tombs have men, women, neonates, and the elderly, what do they offer demographically that might not be accessible in the texts which tend to focus on the working men from the village? While subsequent chapters answer this question through assessing health experiences at the site, this chapter focuses on the community's demography. Using age and sex estimates derived from the human remains in these three tombs,[50] it is possible to assess the overall demographic trends across the three tombs.

5.1 *Children in the Tombs at Deir el-Medina*

Because of the extensive commingling of remains, especially in TT 290 and 298, elements were assigned to two age categories: first, they were differentiated as juvenile or adult based on epiphyseal fusion.[51] This preliminary sorting provides an overall estimate of how representative children and teenagers are within the assemblage. Overall, 1,402 elements were identified as adults vs. 200 as juveniles with an additional 122 elements too fragmentary to assess epiphyseal fusion. The ratio of fully fused to unfused elements is therefore around 7:1. Since most elements fully fuse between ages 12–20, this means that of those human remains studied, around 14% belonged to individuals who died as infants, children, or teenagers.

Among the juvenile elements, 145 could be assigned a more exact age based on both epiphyseal fusion and diaphyseal length.[52] These are grouped into elements from those who were under 5 years old, 5–11 years old, and 12–20 years old (Figure 5). There are more elements from 12 to 20-year-olds—an age range that generally represents post-pubescent adolescence—at Deir el-Medina than those who died under 12 even when combining the two younger age categories.[53] In the Ramesside period (TT 290 and TT 298), children under 5 are

---

50 A full description of methods used to estimate age and sex are provided in the Appendix.

51 Epiphyseal fusion aging is based on Louise Scheuer and Sue M. Black, *The Juvenile Skeleton* (London: Elsevier Academic Press, 2004). Since the age of epiphyseal fusion varies by element, this first sorting is a broad overview with more detailed age estimates broken down within the juvenile category.

52 Diaphyseal aging is based on Charlotte Primeau et al., "A Method for Estimating Age of Medieval Sub-Adults from Infancy to Adulthood Based on Long Bone Length," *American Journal of Physical Anthropology* 159, no. 1 (2016): 135–145; Douglas H. Ubelaker, "The Estimation of Age at Death from Immature Human Bone," in *Age Markers in the Human Skeleton*, ed. Mehmet Yaşar İşcan (Springfield: Charles C. Thomas, 1989), 55–70. Fetal age estimates are based on István Gyula Fazekas and F. Kósa, *Forensic Fetal Osteology* (Akadémiai Kiadó, 1978). Because these methods are based on populations from both different periods and regions, the calculated ages were separated into broader age categories.

53 Research at Amarna suggests menarche was achieved by age 14 at the earliest, and more often between ages 15–17. See Gretchen R. Dabbs, "Menarche at Amarna: Timing and the

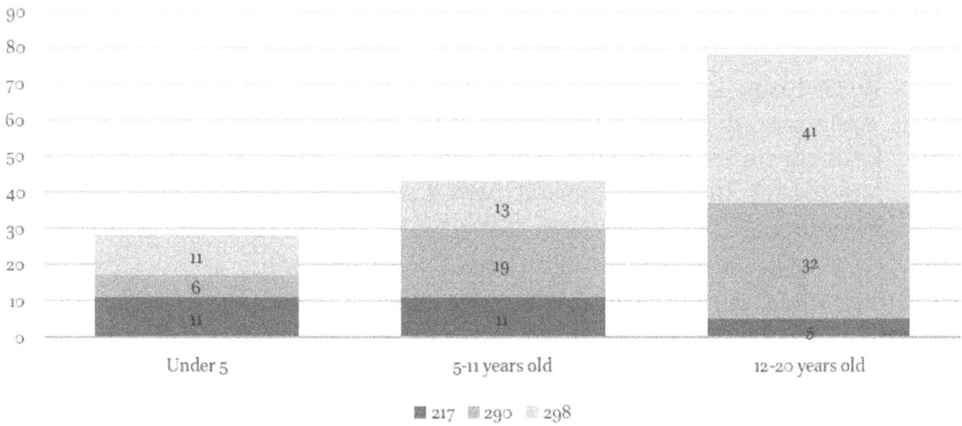

FIGURE 5 Juvenile Age Distribution of Elements by Tomb

the least represented. Conversely, we see relatively more representation of children under 5 in TT 217 since these remains represent those individuals curated by Bruyère from the Eastern cemetery where children's burials were separated from adults. In modern populations, we see the reverse, where children under 5 face a variety of life-threatening risks; once individuals survive this tenuous period, mortality rates drop until adulthood.[54] The relatively higher number of post-pubescent juveniles may point to additional risks at this age such as childbirth. The lack of representation of the youngest people at Deir el-Medina could indicate that fewer individuals died before age 5, but more likely, it suggests that the human remains of infants and toddlers are less likely to be found in the tombs.[55] This could be due to preservation bias, the loss of small bones when looters and archaeologists moved human remains, and different burial treatments. It is noteworthy that in all three tombs, we identified the remains of infants less than a year old wrapped in linen cloth, and thus, intentionally buried in the family tomb.

The relatively few infants and young children found in the tombs can be supplemented by observations made during earlier excavations at the site. When Bruyère first studied the infant burials of the Eastern cemetery, he noted that it

Further Implications," *American Journal of Biological Anthropology* n/a, no. n/a (2023), https://doi.org/10.1002/ajpa.24856.

54 United Nations, *Age and Sex Patterns of Mortality: Model Life-Tables for Under-Developed Countries*, Population Studies 22 (United Nations Department of Social Affairs, Population Branch, 1955).

55 Hervé Guy, Claude Masset, and Charles-Albert Baud, "Infant Taphonomy," *International Journal of Osteoarchaeology* 7, no. 3 (1997): 221–229.

was composed of a series of small pits with no overlying superstructure. Infants were buried within these pits in amphora, baskets, wooden boxes, and coffins.[56] In many cases, they were found in stained cloths, some, according to Bruyère, even containing an amniotic sac as well as a flint knife he proposed could have been used in the surgical operation of delivery or mummification.[57] Even the least ornamented of these burials, which consisted only of a simple form of basketry, would sometimes contain food offerings. In the most elaborate cases, these infants were interred in decorated wooden boxes or coffins, which were then also accompanied by grave goods and burial shrouds.

These 18th Dynasty burials may not represent the same practices of the later Ramesside period, but they demonstrate how the villagers of Deir el-Medina included even very young infants in family burials. Bruyère set aside only a few of these individuals in TT 217, which represent the youngest individuals we have studied so far among the human remains at Deir el-Medina. Several of these individuals would have either been stillbirths or died soon after childbirth. The youngest individual was a male fetus, preserved in the fetal position, who died around 7 months in utero.[58] Found among the infant remains in TT 217 were clay balls and faience-bead bracelets—relatively small burial goods that may have escaped notice during the original excavations, but which demonstrate that even stillbirths and newborns were afforded grave goods in the village.

5.2 *Adults in the Tombs at Deir el-Medina*

While age-at-death for adults is difficult to estimate in commingled remains, it is possible to assign broader age categories to adults (i.e., 20–35 years old, 36–50 years old, over 50 years old) based on aging methods used for the pelvis and skull (Figure 6).[59] Young adults (20–35 years old) are more frequently represented than either middle adults (36–50 years old) or old adults (50+ years old). Like juvenile age ranges which are subject to different rates of preservation, especially when comparing infants and adolescents, previous research has demonstrated that older adults (50+ years old) are less likely to be

56 Bernard Bruyère, *Rapport sur les Fouilles de Deir el Médineh 1934–1935: II*, Fouilles de l'Institut français d'archéologie orientale (Le Caire: L'Institut Français d'Archéologie Orientale, 1937).

57 Bruyère, 12.

58 Age estimation based on partial formation of the tympanic ring, tooth mineralization in both the mandible and maxilla, and diaphyseal lengths. The sex estimation is based on soft tissue still observable in the pelvis.

59 For a more detailed description of aging methods, see the Appendix.

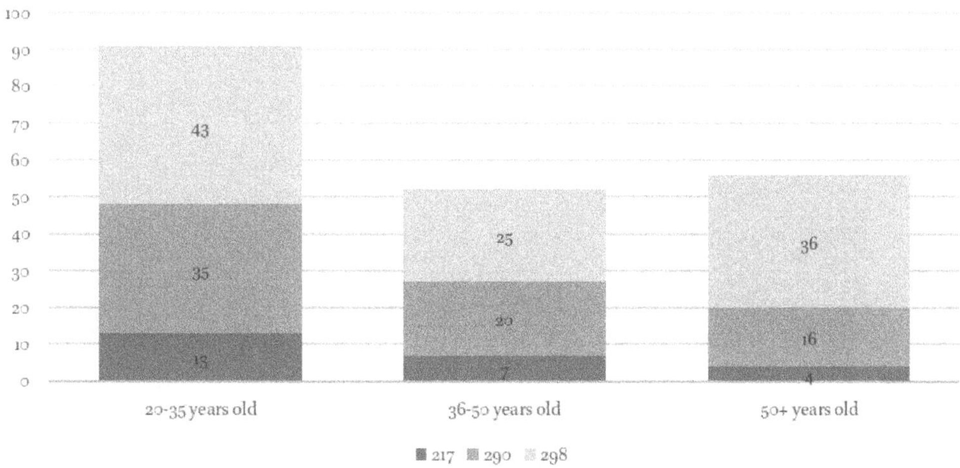

FIGURE 6 Adult Age Distribution of Elements (os coxae and skulls) by Tomb

preserved than young adults (20–35 years old) in other cemetery contexts, though preservation bias is less severe in older adults than it is in infants.[60] It is possible, then, that these represent a real trend in mortality at Deir el-Medina where younger adults are more common than those who make it to either middle or old adulthood. Notably, human remains from TT 217 and TT 290 both show a downward trend where older adults are least represented in their assemblages. TT 298, however, contains comparatively more older adults with 64% (34/53) of skulls and os coxae belonging to individuals who survived past 50.

Adult age distributions can be further compared by estimated sex (Figure 7). Notably, there is no significant difference in representation among young adults when comparing by estimated sex: 40% of males (19/48) and 44% of females (29/66) died in young adulthood.[61] This higher proportion of young adults could be driven by factors like childbirth, as mentioned above, but then we would expect males to be unaffected. Where differences do arise are between middle and old adult categories where fewer males (23%; 11/48) achieve an age over 50 than females (32%; 21/66). These differences cannot be explained by preservation alone. Instead, these data suggest that women at

60 Phillip L. Walker, John R. Johnson, and Patricia M. Lambert, "Age and Sex Biases in the Preservation of Human Skeletal Remains," *American Journal of Physical Anthropology* 76, no. 2 (1988): 183–188, https://doi.org/10.1002/ajpa.1330760206.

61 These values are based on the sum of young adults for both "possible" and "definite" sex estimations.

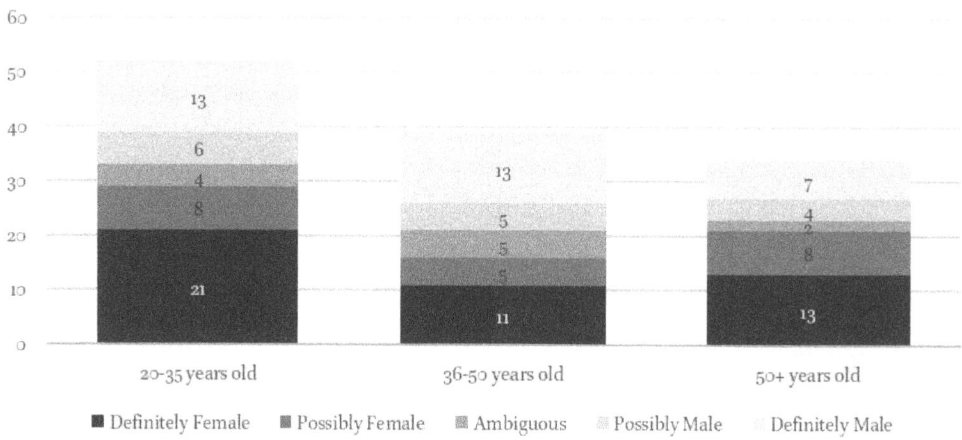

FIGURE 7 Adult age distributions by sex estimation for Os Coxae and Crania from TT 217, 290, 298

Deir el-Medina were more likely to survive to old age than men and that additional factors beyond childbirth are needed to explain mortality among young adults.

While the above graph demonstrates the distribution of os coxae and crania by estimated sex, these values do not include metric sex estimation for long bones. When comparing sex estimations from all elements by tomb (Figure 8), there is an overall even sex ratio in the tombs at Deir e-Medina.[62] The sex ratio is somewhat similar between tombs except in TT 217, where the curated collection of individuals include more females (especially among the adults) than males. This could be in part due to differences in burial during the 18th Dynasty when tombs contained relatively few burials rather than entire families as seen in tombs from the 19th–20th Dynasties.

While texts from the village tend to focus on the experiences of working-age, literate men, the human remains attest to the experiences of a much broader group of inhabitants. The bioarchaeological data gathered from Deir el-Medina and presented in this book correspond to the broader chronology of the site with burials dating from the 18th to the early 21st Dynasty. These individuals also represent the wide variety of community members living at Deir el-Medina, from neonates to the elderly and with a relatively similar representation of men and women.

---

62 One valid critique of metric sex estimation using univariate sectioning points is that the technique tends to lead to a 1:1 sex ratio. An alternative is to compare sex estimates of os coxae. Those estimated to be female (n = 53) outnumber estimates for male (n = 41) by a ratio of 1.3:1. While slightly larger, this ratio still indicates burial assemblages represent both men and women from the village.

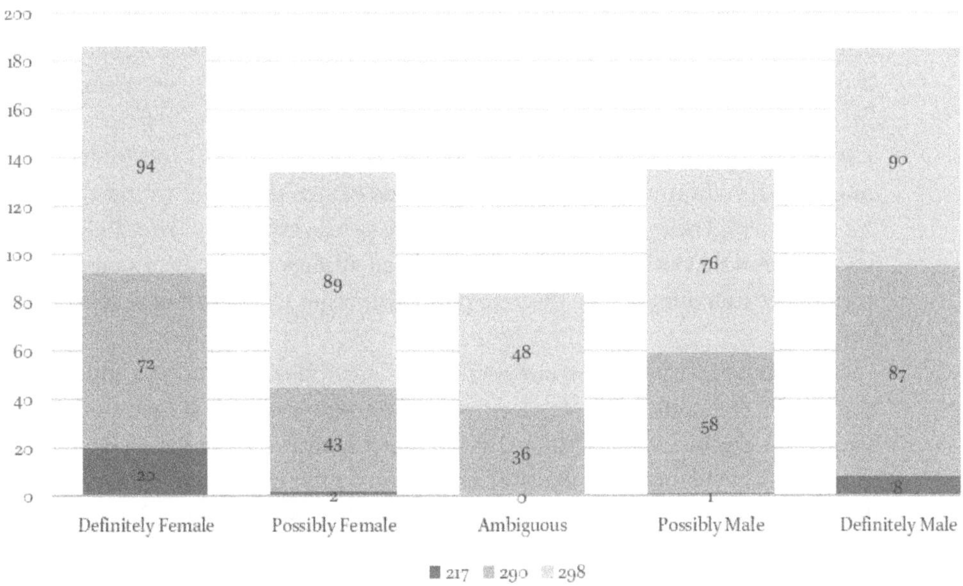

FIGURE 8 Distribution of elements with an estimated sex by tomb

6 Bringing Together the Evidence

At a minimum, this book includes human remains from over 1,700 elements comprising at least 134 people. As you will see in subsequent chapters, individual elements can in some cases tell a complex story about the health experiences at Deir el-Medina. Simultaneously, combining observations across elements and tombs provides a much broader means to understand health and illness at the site by allowing us to trace patterns in health across different ages, sexes, and tombs.

The study of health patterns at Deir el-Medina has limitations, however, as the human remains at the site have been looted since antiquity. The heavy commingling makes complete skeletons rare. This limits the opportunities for understanding the health of individuals over the life course and limits how we can interpret isolated skeletal lesions. Diagnosing diseases usually requires assessing lesions in multiple regions of the skeleton, making it unlikely that specific diseases can be identified in commingled remains. It also makes it impossible to date individual elements beyond the broader dates of village habitation. These limitations are significant; if it were possible to compare human remains from the site's early, middle, and late occupations, then it would be equally possible to trace how health patterns change and respond to periods of growth, decline, and even state economic collapse. Commingling makes it harder to assign estimates for age and sex to most elements as well. Apart from the os coxa and skull, it is impossible to know more about age-at-death than whether an individual reached skeletal maturity. Sex estimates are possible for long bones using metric estimation methods, but these are less reliable than estimating sex from the pelvis. These barriers to accurate age and sex estimation make some key indicators of health harder to trace over the life course. These limitations should cause pause, especially given DeWitte and Stojanowski's call for more contextualized studies that allow researchers to compare individuals from discrete periods in order to assess heterogeneous frailty.

Given these restrictions on our ability to date, estimate age and sex, and analyze whole skeletons, why does Deir el-Medina remain an ideal case study of health patterns in the past? The answer lies in combining the comingled bioarchaeological evidence with the site's texts, which offer important insights into the village as a discrete community with values that likely transcended dynasties. Pay receipts, work attendance records, legal texts, and personal letters offer important data on key *Social Determinants of Health* like economic stability, social support, and healthcare access. Furthermore, the clear and defined community membership and its members' relatively uniform socioeconomic status make it a more homogenous sample when comparing health patterns. Its unique location—separated from most other communities in Thebes—allows us to consider Deir el-Medina's relatively isolated social and physical environment further. These features of the community of Deir el-Medina make it a key case study to consider how the social practices of its inhabitants and context in which they lived impacted their health. But first, it is important to establish a baseline for the health of the village's inhabitants. The following chapter analyzes the human remains from these three tombs by comparing multiple indicators of stress across the life course to document the health experiences of the people at Deir el-Medina.

CHAPTER 4

Finding Health and Stress at Deir el-Medina

Given the demography of the people studied in the three Theban tombs in this book, I now turn to evaluate health within the village. As discussed in Chapter 2, stress provides a useful way to measure and assess health because it can come from a wide variety of sources (e.g., emotional, physical, and environmental) that all leave similar impacts on the body. Consequently, stress markers have become a key means for researchers to assess population health within bioarchaeology.[1] These skeletal indicators not only evidence periods of physical stress but, in some cases, also assess physical stress at different life course stages, making it possible to explore how population health at Deir el-Medina changed from early childhood into old age.

I begin this chapter by presenting comparable sites across the Nile Valley to evaluate how the rates of different stress indicators at Deir el-Medina compare with broader populations. To understand why I chose these sites, their relevance to Deir el-Medina, and their demographies, this chapter opens with an overview of comparable sites in the Nile Valley, including Giza, Amarna, Tombs of the Nobles, and Tombos. In combination, these sites allow us to compare how period, occupation, socioeconomic wealth, and geographic location correlate to health outcomes.

I then present a broader picture of health experiences at Deir el-Medina through six different stress indicators in the skeleton. For each indicator, it is important to explain its etiology, implications for health, and scoring criteria before presenting the data from the human remains at Deir el-Medina. Integrating data from Deir el-Medina with previously published data from other sites in the Nile Valley reveals whether and how each indicator correlates with factors like period, location, socioeconomic status, and occupation.

---

1 Methods of osteological analysis are described in more depth in the Appendix. The identification and scoring of skeletal stress markers in this book are based on guidelines from Richard H. Steckel et al., "Global History of Health Data Collection Codebook," 2006, https://economics.osu.edu/sites/default/files/Codebook-01-24-11-em.pdf; this same codebook was also published in Richard H. Steckel et al., "Data Collection Codebook," in *The Backbone of Europe: Health, Diet, Work and Violence over Two Millennia*, ed. Richard H. Steckel et al., Cambridge Studies in Biological and Evolutionary Anthropology 80 (Cambridge: Cambridge University Press, 2018), 397–427. This allows for broader comparison with the global sites studied as part of the *Global History of Health Project* including those previously published in Steckel and Rose, *The Backbone of History*; and Steckel et al., *The Backbone of Europe*.

 | DOI:10.1163/9789004700871_005

Tracing stress indicators from childhood to adulthood, they tell a story about how stressors impacted the men and women at Deir el-Medina throughout their lives. They suggest that the villagers at Deir el-Medina successfully buffered some of the stress in early childhood and adolescence, especially compared to other sites with working populations. Conversely, as the population aged into the workforce, so too did disparities in their health experiences. Together, osteological data from the Nile Valley more broadly reveal that social context correlates to some but not all health outcomes, with those from working and socioeconomically disadvantaged groups faring worse throughout their lives. The chapter ends with a summary of six trends evidenced in Egyptian bioarchaeology that reveal when wealth could buy health across a variety of places and times in ancient Egypt.

1 Comparing Skeletal Stress Indicators in the Nile Valley and Beyond

There are key advantages and caveats to comparing skeletal stress indicators. The widespread reporting of these values offers biometrics we can compare regardless of cultural affiliation or period. This makes it possible to compare diverse populations, assess differences across groups within a population, and track changes over time. Grouping sites with similar traits helps to evaluate whether differences in health outcomes tend to correlate to factors like period, socioeconomic status, occupation, or geographic region. However, any comparison across periods or regions carries the uncertainty of what these differences represent—an example of *hidden heterogeneity in frailty*. Differences in overall rates of any one lesion could indicate different genetic susceptibilities to specific stress markers, environmental factors, technological changes, or different cultural behaviors across a wide variety of sites. Additionally, reported data come from multiple researchers, leading to interobserver variation and differences in how these data are reported. Contextualizing the results from Deir el-Medina with other sites requires a closer consideration of why differences in reported rates of skeletal stress markers arise.

While this book references various sites with published bioarchaeological data, several sites offer more advantageous comparisons to Deir el-Medina because of similarities in socioeconomic position, period, and/or occupational status. These sites are distributed across the Nile Valley and represent Egyptians who lived in various periods from the Old Kingdom to the Third Intermediate Period.

Amarna, ancient Akhetaten, offers the most relevant direct comparison to Deir el-Medina owing to the overall similarities in its period and population.[2] It was occupied briefly during the 18th Dynasty and included a wide variety of laborers, craftsmen, and elite individuals. Some Amarna residents may have even come from Deir el-Medina when royal craftsmen were moved from Thebes to Amarna as part of a broader political and religious shift under Akhenaten.[3] Research at Amarna has so far revealed three separate cemeteries: the South Tombs Cemetery (STC), North Tombs Cemetery (NTC), and North Cliffs Cemetery (NCC).[4] The STC includes thousands of pit graves with varying degrees of grave goods suggestive of a non-elite population with different levels of socioeconomic access within the cemetery. This cemetery included men, women, and children of varying ages. These individuals may have included skilled laborers, perhaps even some who transferred from Deir el-Medina, as well as a larger proportion of unskilled laborers brought in from elsewhere in Egypt. The NTC—which similarly contains thousands of burials—was almost entirely populated by children and adolescents. Given the high degrees of osteoarthritis and trauma visible in such a young population, these remains likely represent those who worked on the massive building projects required to grow an entire capital within a few short years.[5] The NCC is relatively smaller than either of the other cemeteries at Amarna. It is located near the tombs of elite officials (specifically Panehesy) and may have included individuals related to or serving them. The NCC grave goods show more socioeconomic access than either of the other cemeteries at Amarna. In combination with its location, demography, and grave goods, this suggests that individuals buried there were less likely to be involved in major state-building projects.[6]

Given the labor required to cut and decorate the royal tombs, it is also important to compare Deir el-Medina to other labor-intensive populations beyond Amarna. Cemeteries at Giza contain both the workers from the Giza Southeast Cemetery who built the pyramids and surrounding mortuary complexes as well

---

2 For a general overview of Amarna and its related excavations, see http://amarnaproject.com. Bioarchaeological research at Amarna has been led by Jerry Rose and Gretchen Dabbs. Anna Stevens has led recent excavations of the cemeteries.

3 Miriam Müller, "Deir El-Medina in the Dark—the Amarna Period in the History of the Village," in *Deir El-Medina Studies, Helsinki, June 24–26, 2009. Proceedings*, ed. Jaana Toivari-Viitala, Turo Vartiainen, and Saara Uvanto, The Finnish Egyptological Society Occasional Publications 2 (Helsinki: The Finnish Egyptological Society, 2014), 154–167.

4 Kemp et al., "Life, Death and beyond in Akhenaten's Egypt"; Dabbs, "Bioarchaeology of the Non-Elite North Tombs Cemetery at Amarna"; Anna Stevens et al., "The North Cliffs Cemetery at Amarna," *Egyptian Archaeology*, no. 56 (2020): 4–9. Additionally, the North Desert Cemetery has recently been excavated, but these results are still forthcoming.

5 Dabbs, "Bioarchaeology of the Non-Elite North Tombs Cemetery at Amarna."

6 Stevens et al., "The North Cliffs Cemetery at Amarna."

as high officials from the Giza Western Cemetery.[7] Although these cemeteries date to the Old Kingdom and thus significantly predate Deir el-Medina, they offer a point of comparison between the experiences of a working vs. elite population. Giza, therefore, offers a sounding board for how stress in the skeleton varies by socioeconomic status within one site.

Relatedly, some bioarchaeological data have been published from three Theban tombs (TT 84, TT 85, and TT 95) from the Tombs of the Nobles.[8] These elite tombs of the New Kingdom are located mere kilometers from Deir el-Medina and consequently have the most similar geographic profile to the cemeteries at Deir el-Medina. As a local, elite population with burials dating to the New Kingdom and early Third Intermediate Period, they offer a contemporary counterpoint to Deir el-Medina as local burials of a group of non-working elite families.

Tombos is another site with burials dating to the New Kingdom that is comparable to Deir el-Medina because its inhabitants similarly occupied a middle-ground status socioeconomically. Tombos was a colonial Egyptian fortress near the Third Cataract with a primarily Egyptian population.[9] The Egyptians buried at Tombos were administrators with socioeconomic access and power, but theirs was comparatively less than elite individuals who could afford more elaborate burials. While the administrators at Tombos likely did not have to perform intense manual labor, they also moved from their homeland to the most southern colony of Egypt during the New Kingdom. This required them to form entangled connections with local Nubians as evidenced by their complex mortuary choices and strontium isotopes.[10]

---

7 For additional information about these cemeteries, see Zahi A. Hawass, ed., *The Treasures of the Pyramids* (Vercelli: White Star, 2003); Mark Lehner and Zahi Hawass, *Giza and the Pyramids* (London: Thames Hudson, 2017).

8 Andreas G. Nerlich et al., "Anthropological and Palaeopathological Analysis of the Human Remains from Three 'Tombs of the Nobles' of the Necropolis of Thebes-West, Upper Egypt.," *Anthropologischer Anzeiger* 58, no. 4 (2000): 321–343.

9 Stuart Tyson Smith has led excavations at Tombos, and Michele Buzon has led bioarchaeological research at the site. For an overview of Tombos, see Stuart Tyson Smith, *Wretched Kush: Ethnic Identities and Boundaries in Egypt's Nubian Empire* (London: Routledge, 2003).

10 Michele R. Buzon and Antonio Simonetti, "Strontium Isotope (87Sr/86Sr) Variability in the Nile Valley: Identifying Residential Mobility during Ancient Egyptian and Nubian Sociopolitical Changes in the New Kingdom and Napatan Periods," *American Journal of Physical Anthropology* 151, no. 1 (2013): 1–9, https://doi.org/10.1002/ajpa.22235; Michele R. Buzon, Stuart Tyson Smith, and Antonio Simonetti, "Entanglement and the Formation of the Ancient Nubian Napatan State," *American Anthropologist* 118, no. 2 (2016): 284–300, https://doi.org/10.1111/aman.12524.

Finally, in order to place the broader Nile Valley and Deir el-Medina in context, rates of skeletal stress markers are also compared to the results of the *Global History of Health Project*. The Western Hemisphere module[11] and European module[12] offer unique insights describing what the skeletal markers reflect about population health and how these changed based on location, period, socioeconomic status, or cultural context. Essentially, by including these global values, it is possible to assess when values in the Nile Valley are significantly low or high.[13]

The above Nubian and Egyptian sites provide data from across Pharaonic Egypt that speak to a variety of ways period, region, socioeconomic status, and occupation could reflect health experiences. These factors present four hypothetical outcomes for stress markers. First, if health outcomes were primarily driven by temporal changes (e.g., long-term differences in Nile inundations, technological innovations, or political differences over time), we would expect that stress markers would be largely similar for sites from the New Kingdom (i.e., Tombos, Amarna, Tombs of the Nobles, and Deir el-Medina) in comparison to the Old Kingdom (i.e., Giza). Second, regional differences could reflect different political and environmental hazards along the Nile Valley making data from sites near each other (i.e., Deir el-Medina and the Tombs of the Nobles) similar and distinct from sites in other areas of the Nile Valley. Third, if working conditions instead dictated health outcomes, we would expect data from Deir el-Medina to be more similar to the cemeteries of other state builders at Giza and Amarna and more distinct from their elite counterparts. Fourth, if wealth most impacted health outcomes, we would expect three distinct groupings: working populations with little or no socioeconomic power at Giza and Amarna; sub-elite populations like Deir el-Medina, Tombos, and the NCC at

11 Steckel and Rose, *The Backbone of History*.

12 Steckel et al., *The Backbone of Europe*.

13 Several statistical tests are used in this chapter to compare groups. For continuous observations, such as long bone metrics, averages are compared using a two-sample one-tailed t-test in conjunction with a two-sample F-test to determine equal or unequal variances. Contingency tables showing proportional data (including observations of absence vs. presence of skeletal lesions) are compared using a Chi-Square Goodness-of-Fit test. Fisher's exact tests are used instead when observations are less than 5 in any one cell in a contingency table. An alpha level of .05 is used for all tests. In some cases, chi-squared tests can provide an inaccurate estimate of likelihood when sample sizes are insufficient. To determine the necessary size for a chi-squared test, post-hoc power analyses were also conducted for statistically significant results using the statistical software package G*Power 3.1.9.7. Ideally, power should be higher than 0.8, though given limited sample sizes in archaeological contexts, achieved power may not reach this value.

Amarna with moderate socioeconomic power; and upper elite cemeteries at Tombs of the Nobles and Giza with the highest amounts of socioeconomic power.

Investigating each stress indicator, therefore, affords the opportunity to test which, if any, of these hypothetical scenarios most closely align with the data as well as how those results vary from one indicator of stress to the next. The following sections—organized from childhood to adulthood—also show how these hypothetical scenarios correlate to certain life stages more than others. After reviewing all of the indicators across sites, I return to these hypothetical scenarios to see whether period, location, occupation, and wealth can explain health patterns in ancient Egypt.

2 Indicators of Stress in Childhood

Enamel hypoplasias and cranial porosities occur primarily or exclusively in childhood and, in combination, demonstrate how stress impacts growth during the first eight years of life.[14] They can be particularly important for elucidating what health looked like during infancy and early childhood—a period when illnesses are rarely documented directly. Stress markers developed during childhood are also testaments to survival since, in many cases, they are visible in individuals who survived periods of stress and lived into adulthood. They, therefore, make it possible for us to consider a more nuanced perspective on the *Osteological Paradox* by allowing us to compare the rates of these markers across individuals who survived into adulthood and adolescence. Increasingly, studies demonstrate that early life stress predicts health outcomes later, and consequently childhood health experiences contribute to adult health outcomes.[15] This includes stress experienced in the womb as well as in infancy—

14 A general overview of the age of onset for these conditions can be found in Rebecca Watts, "Childhood Development and Adult Longevity in an Archaeological Population from Barton-upon-Humber, Lincolnshire, England," *International Journal of Paleopathology* 3, no. 2 (2013): 95–104. Additionally, see Lexi O'Donnell et al., "Skeletal Manifestations of Disease Experience: Length of Illness and Porous Cranial Lesion Formation in a Contemporary Juvenile Mortality Sample," *American Journal of Human Biology* 35, no. 8 (2023): e23896, https://doi.org/10.1002/ajhb.2389.

15 More broadly, this has been summarized as the Developmental Origins of Health and Disease (DOHaD) Hypothesis. For additional information about DOHaD and bioarchaeology, see Gamble and Bentley, *Developmental origins of health and disease (DOHaD)*; Rebecca L. Gowland, "Entangled Lives: Implications of the Developmental Origins of Health and Disease Hypothesis for Bioarchaeology and the Life Course," *American Journal of Phys-*

times when health is inextricably linked between a mother and child through gestation and breastfeeding. These earliest indicators of stress, therefore, signal not only the stress experiences of infants and young children but also potentially the stress experiences of their mothers. The intricate implications of early childhood stress on later health outcomes make it clear that a study of stress in infancy and childhood is equally important for understanding health experiences into adulthood.

2.1 *Enamel Hypoplasias*

Enamel hypoplasias develop in early childhood—from soon after birth to around age seven[16]—when the body reduces the production of enamel as a response to a variety of stressors.[17] Frequently, they appear as linear bands on the crown which correspond to the time when stress impacted the development of a tooth's enamel. Multiple hypoplasias on one tooth correspond to multiple discrete periods of stress. While enamel hypoplasias are identified most frequently on the incisors and canines,[18] they can occur in all teeth and be non-linear, with different manifestations potentially indicating differences in etiology.[19] Enamel hypoplasias are associated with a variety of forms of stress

---

ical Anthropology 158, no. 4 (2015): 530–540, https://doi.org/10.1002/ajpa.22820; Haagen D. Klaus, "Frontiers in the Bioarchaeology of Stress and Disease: Cross-Disciplinary Perspectives from Pathophysiology, Human Biology, and Epidemiology," *American Journal of Physical Anthropology* 155, no. 2 (October 2014): 294–308, https://doi.org/10.1002/ajpa.22574; Daniel H. Temple, "Plasticity and Constraint in Response to Early-Life Stressors among Late/Final Jomon Period Foragers from Japan: Evidence for Life History Trade-Offs from Incremental Microstructures of Enamel," *American Journal of Physical Anthropology* 155, no. 4 (December 2014): 537–545, https://doi.org/10.1002/ajpa.22606; Daniel H. Temple, "Bioarchaeological Evidence for Adaptive Plasticity and Constraint: Exploring Life-History Trade-Offs in the Human Past," *Evolutionary Anthropology* 28, no. 1 (January 2019): 34–46, https://doi.org/10.1002/evan.21754.

16 Goodman and Martin, "Reconstructing Health Profiles from Skeletal Remains," 23; D.J. Reid and M.C. Dean, "Variation in Modern Human Enamel Formation Times," *Journal of Human Evolution* 50, no. 3 (March 1, 2006): 329–346, https://doi.org/10.1016/j.jhevol.2005.09.003.

17 Stephen M. Duray, "Dental Indicators of Stress and Reduced Age at Death in Prehistoric Native Americans," *American Journal of Physical Anthropology* 99, no. 2 (1996): 275–286.

18 Alan H. Goodman and Jerome C. Rose, "Assessment of Systemic Physiological Perturbations from Dental Enamel Hypoplasias and Associated Histological Structures," *American Journal of Physical Anthropology* 33, no. S11 (1990): 87, https://doi.org/10.1002/ajpa.1330330506.

19 Ian Towle and Joel D. Irish, "Recording and Interpreting Enamel Hypoplasia in Samples from Archaeological and Palaeoanthropological Contexts," *Journal of Archaeological Science* 114 (February 2020): 105077, https://doi.org/10.1016/j.jas.2020.105077.

including infectious disease, malnutrition, and severe emotional trauma.[20] Recent research suggests that, in some cases, enamel hypoplasias could also be inherited either through environmental factors (e.g., epigenetics, shared household), genetics, or some combination.[21] They may be more sensitive to stressors than cribra orbitalia or porotic hyperostosis as well.[22] This complex etiology suggests that individual life histories should be interpreted carefully since enamel hypoplasias could reflect stressors experienced by an individual's parents and individual genetic susceptibility. Additionally, enamel hypoplasias may be more indicative of acute episodes of stress instead of long, chronic periods of stress.

Enamel hypoplasias were scored as present at Deir el-Medina when a hypoplastic line was visible macroscopically and could be felt with a fingernail.[23] All teeth were observed for the presence of enamel hypoplasias.[24] Of the 113 maxillae and mandibles analyzed from TT 217, 290, and 298, 90 could be observed for enamel hypoplasias (Table 1).[25] Enamel hypoplasias were present on 13% (12/90) of all mandibles and maxillae and 6.6% (38/578) of all observable teeth;[26] however, these values reflect all observable elements and not those with anterior teeth which are most likely to exhibit hypoplasias. When comparing only mandibles and maxillae with one or more anterior teeth present, 29% (10/35) had at least one observable enamel hypoplasia. Enamel hypoplasias were most frequently observed on the canines; 26% (11/42) of observable canines displayed enamel hypoplasias. Canines tend to have enamel hypo-

20 Terrence B. Ritzman, Brenda J. Baker, and Gary T. Schwartz, "A Fine Line: A Comparison of Methods for Estimating Ages of Linear Enamel Hypoplasia Formation," *American Journal of Physical Anthropology* 135, no. 3 (March 1, 2008): 348–361, https://doi.org/10.1002/ajpa.20750; Gary T. Schwartz et al., "A Faithful Record of Stressful Life Events Recorded in the Dental Developmental Record of a Juvenile Gorilla," *International Journal of Primatology* 27, no. 4 (August 2006): 1201–1219, https://doi.org/10.1007/s10764-006-9051-2.

21 Lawrence et al., "Heterogeneous Frailty and the Expression of Linear Enamel Hypoplasia in a Genealogical Population."

22 Yaussy and DeWitte, "Patterns of Frailty in Non-Adults from Medieval London."

23 Steckel et al., *The Backbone of Europe*, 407.

24 Towle and Irish, "Recording and Interpreting Enamel Hypoplasia in Samples from Archaeological and Palaeoanthropological Contexts."

25 Mandibles or maxillae were included so long as they had at least one observable crown that was at least half complete. Cases where mandibles and maxillae were unobservable included edentulous elements, elements with all teeth lost post-mortem, or cases where soft tissue prevents observation of tooth surfaces.

26 These values did not vary significantly between maxillae and mandibles; 7% of maxillary teeth (19/275) and 7% of mandibular teeth (26/275) had enamel hypoplasias present. By element, this was distributed as 17% (7/42) mandibles and 11% (7/63) maxillae.

TABLE 1 Enamel hypoplasias at Deir el-Medina

		Estimated sex			Estimated age				Tomb		
	Total	Male	Female	Unknown	Under 20	20–35	36–50	50+	TT 217	TT 290	TT 298
EH Absent per tooth	540	182	207	79	97	259	61	63	188	160	192
EH Present per tooth	38	7	26	4	1	23	11	0	20	7	11
Total observable teeth	578	189	233	83	98	282	72	63	208	167	203
%EH per tooth	6.6%	3.7%	11.2%	4.8%	1.0%	8.2%	15.3%	0.0%	9.6%	4.2%	5.4%
EH Absent per element	78	25	24	19	10	30	5	13	16	24	38
EH Present per element	12	3	6	2	1	7	3	0	4	3	5
Total observable element	90	28	30	21	11	37	8	13	20	27	43
%EH per element	13.3%	10.7%	20.0%	9.5%	9.1%	18.9%	37.5%	0.0%	20.0%	11.1%	11.6%

plasias more frequently due to their overall morphology.[27] The crowns also take the longest to form, resulting in a record of stress from as early as 6 months to 6 years.[28]

While those estimated to be female had more frequent enamel hypoplasias observed overall, this was primarily driven by the presence of multiple hypoplasias in the same sets of dentition. For example, *Ḥmn*, a woman from the 18th Dynasty originally buried in Pit (P.) 1380,[29] died as a young adult with hypoplasias visible on 12 of her 31 observable teeth (Figure 9). Together with *Nbw- ỉỉ.tỉ* from P. 1382, these two women account for more than half of the teeth displaying hypoplasias from all three tombs studied (53%; 20/38).

It is these same two women who account for all of the enamel hypoplasias observed from the 18th Dynasty, resulting in a higher rate of enamel hypoplasias both per tooth and per element in 18th Dynasty burials (i.e., Eastern cemetery burials moved to TT 217) than those dated to the Ramesside period (TT 290 and 298). This distribution makes it appear that there were higher rates of

27 Alan H. Goodman and George J. Armelagos, "Factors Affecting the Distribution of Enamel Hypoplasias within the Human Permanent Dentition," *American Journal of Physical Anthropology* 68, no. 4 (1985): 479–493, https://doi.org/10.1002/ajpa.1330680404.

28 Reid and Dean, "Variation in Modern Human Enamel Formation Times."

29 Bruyère, *Rapport sur les Fouilles de Deir el Médineh 1934–1935: II*, 175–180.

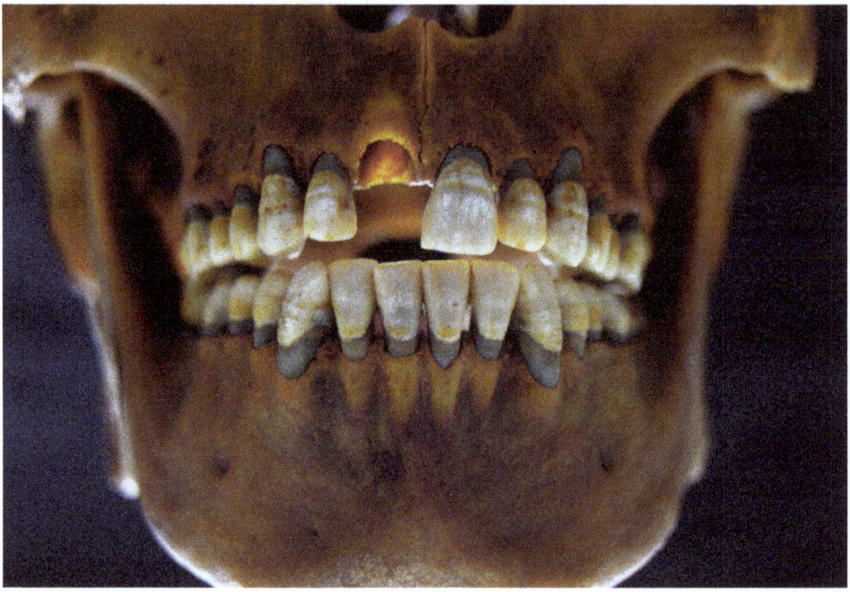

FIGURE 9 Enamel hypoplasias on Ḥmn (DEM 217.19.024), a 20 to 35-year-old woman who was originally buried in P. 1380

enamel hypoplasias in the 18th Dynasty, but this may be due to a smaller sample size. Both tombs from the Ramesside period have similar rates of enamel hypoplasias per tooth and element.

When comparing age groups, enamel hypoplasias appear to be predominantly found in young (20–35) and middle (36–50) adults. Only one enamel hypoplasia was present in juveniles, perhaps due to the smaller sample size of permanent dentition in juvenile skeletal remains (n = 98). No enamel hypoplasias were observed in deciduous dentition (n = 34). Similarly, none were detected in old adults (50+), though due to occlusal wear and antemortem tooth loss, only 63 teeth were observable.

2.1.1 Enamel Hypoplasias in Context

Understanding the relative significance of these rates of enamel hypoplasias requires putting the human remains at Deir el-Medina in a broader context both in reference to comparable sites from the ancient Nile Valley and on a global scale. Several sites from ancient Egypt have data on enamel hypoplasias, and these values are frequently higher than those observed at Deir el-Medina (Table 2).

While several factors may have influenced this distribution of enamel hypoplasias across sites, differences in wealth are noticeably correlated to

TABLE 2 Enamel hypoplasias across the Nile Valley

Per individual with one or more anterior teeth present	Rate	Source
C-Group	19%	Buzon 2006
Tombos	21%	Buzon 2006
Kerma	24%	Buzon 2006
Pharaonic	27%	Buzon 2006
Deir el-Medina	**29%**	**Current Publication**
Memphis	36%	Buzon 2006
Qurneh	39%	Buzon 2006
Amarna North Cliffs	52%	Stevens et al. 2020
Mendes	59%	Lovell and Whyte 1999
Amarna NTC	73%	Stevens et al. 2020
Amarna STC	76%	Stevens et al. 2020

Per Canine	Rate	Source
Deir el-Medina	**26%**	**Current Publication**
Mendes	32%	Lovell and Whyte 1999
Bahriyah	32%	Hussien et al. 2006
Giza High Officials	48%	Hussien et al. 2006
Giza Workers	84%	Hussien et al. 2006

differences in health. This is particularly true in dynastic Egypt. During the transition to agriculture, which likely took a toll on the health outcomes of mothers and young children, rates of enamel hypoplasias fluctuated.[30] As social complexity developed during the Pharaonic period, wealthier groups had noticeably lower rates of enamel hypoplasias both per canine and per individual, even when comparing multiple cemeteries from the same archaeological site (e.g., Giza and Amarna). At Amarna, 73.2% of individuals from the North Tombs Cemetery[31] and 58% of males and 61% of females from the South Tombs Ceme-

30 Anne P. Starling and Jay T. Stock, "Dental Indicators of Health and Stress in Early Egyptian and Nubian Agriculturalists: A Difficult Transition and Gradual Recovery," *American Journal of Physical Anthropology* 134, no. 4 (December 2007): 520–528, https://doi.org/10.1002/ajpa.20700.

31 Dabbs, "Bioarchaeology of the Non-Elite North Tombs Cemetery at Amarna."

tery[32] exhibited enamel hypoplasias—rates that were both notably higher than at the wealthier North Cliffs cemetery. Among Giza workers, they were present in 89% of canines in females and 86% of canines in males, almost double the values seen in the Giza high officials.[33]

While rates of enamel hypoplasias are harder to compare *across* rather than *within* sites, they still show that elite burials tend to have lower rates of enamel hypoplasias than non-elites. Buzon compared rates of enamel hypoplasias per individual across both Nubian and Egyptian sites dating around the New Kingdom.[34] Rates at Tombos are comparable to the wealthy burials at Kerma, Qurneh, and Memphis.[35] Conversely, at Mendes, 59% of non-elite individuals had enamel hypoplasias—a value higher than any of the elite sites documented.[36] These data suggest that wealth had a measurable impact on health in childhood. Contrastingly, the drastically different rates of enamel hypoplasias from neighboring cemeteries in Giza and Amarna, as well as the differences across contemporaneous sites of the New Kingdom, suggest that enamel hypoplasia rates cannot be easily explained by temporal change or regional differences.

Data from Deir el-Medina are much more comparable to—or even lower than—many elite sites. The rate per canine at Deir el-Medina (26%) is the lowest reported, and the rate per individual with one or more anterior teeth (29%) is more comparable to elite cemeteries than working populations. This further suggests that working conditions alone cannot easily explain rates of enamel hypoplasias.

In fact, enamel hypoplasia rates tend to be lower at Deir el-Medina than the majority of sites surveyed in the *Global History of Health Project*;[37] rates

---

32 Dabbs and Zabecki, "Abandoned Memories. A Cemetery of Forgotten Souls."

33 Fawzia H. Hussien, Rokia A. El Banna, and Azza M. Sarry El Din, "Non-Specific Stress Indicators in Ancient Egyptians from Giza and Bahriyah Oasis," *Journal of the Arab Society for Medical Research* 1 (2006): 13–27.

34 Buzon, "Health of the Non-Elites at Tombos."

35 Buzon.

36 Nancy C. Lovell and Ira Whyte, "Patterns of Dental Enamel Defects at Ancient Mendes, Egypt," *American Journal of Physical Anthropology* 110, no. 1 (1999): 69–80.

37 In both the Western Hemisphere module and the European module, only the canines and incisors were scored for enamel hypoplasias. These were reported separately in project data for the Western Hemisphere project based on both tooth type and deciduous vs. permanent dentition. In the European module, data were reported by tooth type and position (i.e., mandibular vs. maxillary). My comparison, therefore, uses only data on permanent dentition and combines evidence from canines and incisors of either maxillae or mandibles to increase the sample size at Deir el-Medina and make data comparable to both Global History of Health databases.

of enamel hypoplasias at Deir el-Medina were lower than 61% (30/49) of sites surveyed in the Western Hemisphere module and 72% (73/102) of sites in the European module. Overall, these demonstrate that Deir el-Medina has lower rates of enamel hypoplasias not just in comparison to relevant sites in Egypt and Nubia, but also more globally including sites that range into more recent historic periods. This suggests that the villagers at Deir el-Medina were particularly effective at protecting its population from childhood and maternal stressors.

To explain this, it is useful to look at trends in data beyond the Nile Valley. To explain the distributions of enamel hypoplasias in Europe, which tend to increase over time, researchers suggested that one driving factor could be rapid population growth.[38] Surprisingly, however, they did not find clear evidence of an "urban penalty" as some urban populations exhibited fewer enamel hypoplasias than their rural counterparts. One suggested reason is that urban populations could buffer the stressors caused by dense living (e.g., higher rates of infectious disease, poor sanitation, and unequal access to food) if urban spaces also had more education, wealth, trade networks, and protection. These factors may help to explain why differences in enamel hypoplasias tend to correlate to differences in wealth in Egypt.

2.2 *Cranial Porosities*

Like enamel hypoplasias, cranial porosities are thought to develop during early childhood when physiological stress causes expansion of the diploë into the outer table resulting in porotic lesions in the orbits (cribra orbitalia) and cranial vault (porotic hyperostosis).[39] El-Najjar and colleagues suggested these expansions were due to iron-deficiency anemia, which requires bone marrow expansion to accommodate for increased red blood cell production and is seen in areas where the overlying outer table is thinnest.[40] Stuart-Macadam found close correlations between clinical examples of anemia and porotic hyperos-

38 Zsolt Bereczki et al., "Growth Disruptions in Children," in *The Backbone of Europe: Health, Diet, Work and Violence over Two Millennia*, ed. Richard H. Steckel et al., Cambridge Studies in Biological and Evolutionary Anthropology 80 (Cambridge: Cambridge University Press, 2018), 175–197.

39 Patty Stuart-Macadam, "Porotic Hyperostosis: Representative of a Childhood Condition," *American Journal of Physical Anthropology* 66, no. 4 (1985), https://doi.org/10.1002/ajpa.1330660407.

40 Mahmoud Y. El-Najjar et al., "The Etiology of Porotic Hyperostosis among the Prehistoric and Historic Anasazi Indians of Southwestern United States," *American Journal of Physical Anthropology* 44, no. 3 (1976): 477–487, https://doi.org/10.1002/ajpa.1330440311.

tosis to support the anemia hypothesis.[41] However, she suggested that the etiology of iron-deficiency anemia in these cases was not due to low levels of iron in the diet, but rather was a defense mechanism due to increased pathological stress.[42] Recent research has also suggested that iron-deficiency anemia is not a viable etiology for expansion of the diploë and that cribra orbitalia and porotic hyperostosis can result from alternative etiologies[43] such as hematogenous infections and excessive blood loss,[44] as well as general inflammation, osteoporosis, and rickets.[45] Malaria as a blood-borne disease is also a possible cause for both conditions because of its impact on red blood cell production.[46] Recent research on living populations has demonstrated a correlation between these lesions and respiratory infections as well as heart conditions.[47] Finally, cribra orbitalia and porotic hyperostosis are often described together because they both relate to the expansion of the diploë, but they may have slightly different underlying etiologies.[48] Within this, orbital porosities without periosteal new bone formation might also be a normal developmental variant,[49] yet most studies do not differentiate between porosities with and without the presence of periosteal new bone formation. Recent work indicates

41 Patty Stuart-Macadam, "Porotic Hyperostosis: New Evidence to Support the Anemia Theory," *American Journal of Physical Anthropology* 74, no. 4 (1987): 521–526, https://doi.org/10.1002/ajpa.1330740410.

42 Patty Stuart-Macadam, "Porotic Hyperostosis: A New Perspective," *American Journal of Physical Anthropology* 87, no. 1 (1992): 39–47, https://doi.org/10.1002/ajpa.1330870105.

43 Phillip L. Walker et al., "The Causes of Porotic Hyperostosis and Cribra Orbitalia: A Reappraisal of the Iron-Deficiency-Anemia Hypothesis," *American Journal of Physical Anthropology* 139, no. 2 (2009): 109–125, https://doi.org/10.1002/ajpa.21031.

44 Megan Brickley and Rachel Ives, *The Bioarchaeology of Metabolic Bone Disease* (Amsterdam: Academic Press, 2008), 3.

45 Ulrike Wapler, Eric Crubézy, and Michael Schultz, "Is Cribra Orbitalia Synonymous with Anemia? Analysis and Interpretation of Cranial Pathology in Sudan," *American Journal of Physical Anthropology* 123, no. 4 (April 1, 2004): 333–339, https://doi.org/10.1002/ajpa.10321.

46 Gowland and Western, "Morbidity in the Marshes"; Smith-Guzmán, "Cribra Orbitalia in the Ancient Nile Valley and Its Connection to Malaria."

47 Lexi O'Donnell et al., "Cribra Orbitalia and Porotic Hyperostosis Are Associated with Respiratory Infections in a Contemporary Mortality Sample from New Mexico," *American Journal of Physical Anthropology* 173, no. 4 (2020): 721–733, https://doi.org/10.1002/ajpa.24131.

48 Frances Rivera and Marta Mirazón Lahr, "New Evidence Suggesting a Dissociated Etiology for Cribra Orbitalia and Porotic Hyperostosis," *American Journal of Physical Anthropology* 164, no. 1 (2017): 76–96, https://doi.org/10.1002/ajpa.23258.

49 Garrard Cole and Tony Waldron, "Cribra Orbitalia: Dissecting an Ill-Defined Phenomenon," *International Journal of Osteoarchaeology* 29, no. 4 (2019): 613–621, https://doi.org/10.1002/oa.2757.

that in cases without new bone formation, the expression of porosities in the orbit might instead be closely connected to anatomical variations in vasculature.[50]

While the etiological debate of these lesions is ongoing, there is a broader consensus that the underlying mechanisms causing expansion of the diploë are likely more complex than just one specific condition and that consequently these lesions can be used as indicators of skeletal stress.[51] They also are most frequently developed during childhood, primarily affecting children from soon after birth to age 8–12,[52] most likely because it is then that marrow tends to transition from red to mixed and eventually yellow marrow in the skull.[53] Afterward, increased red blood cell production only manifests as cribra orbitalia or porotic hyperostosis if there was so much physical demand that the marrow in the skull reconverted into mixed or red marrow.

At Deir el-Medina, observations on cribra orbitalia and porotic hyperostosis were recorded both for their presence and severity following the *Global History of Health Project* Codebook.[54] Because these data are only observed once per individual (unlike enamel hypoplasias), they are more readily compared with other populations despite coming from largely commingled assemblages. Of the 194 crania or cranial fragments studied, 73 had at least one orbit present for observation of cribra orbitalia and 63 had at least one parietal present for observing porotic hyperostosis. Overall, 30% (22/73) of crania observable for cribra orbitalia had the condition, with 41% (9/22) of those exhibiting a more substantial cluster of foramina (more than 1 cm^2). Porotic hyperostosis was less prevalent; only 14% (9/63) of crania showed evidence of the stress indicator, and of these, none have an excessive expansion of the diploë.

---

50 Matthew J. Zdilla et al., "Cribra Orbitalia Is Correlated with the Meningo-Orbital Foramen and Is Vascular and Developmental in Nature," *The Anatomical Record* 305, no. 7 (2022): 1629–1671, https://doi.org/10.1002/ar.24825.

51 Marin A. Pilloud and Al W. Schwitalla, "Re-Evaluating Traditional Markers of Stress in an Archaeological Sample from Central California," *Journal of Archaeological Science* 116 (April 2020): 105102, https://doi.org/10.1016/j.jas.2020.105102.

52 Diane M. Mittler and Dennis P. van Gerven, "Developmental, Diachronic, and Demographic Analysis of Cribra Orbitalia in the Medieval Christian Populations of Kulubnarti," *American Journal of Physical Anthropology* 93, no. 3 (March 1994): 287–297, https://doi.org/10.1002/ajpa.1330930302. O'Donnell et al., "Skeletal Manifestations of Disease Experience."

53 Megan B. Brickley, "Cribra Orbitalia and Porotic Hyperostosis: A Biological Approach to Diagnosis," *American Journal of Physical Anthropology* 167, no. 4 (2018): 896–902, https://doi.org/10.1002/ajpa.23701; Yaussy and DeWitte, "Patterns of Frailty in Non-Adults from Medieval London."

54 Steckel et al., "Global History of Health Data Collection Codebook."

TABLE 3 Cranial porosities at Deir el-Medina

	Estimated sex				Estimated age				Tomb		
	Total	Male	Female	Unknown	Under 20	20–35	36–50	50+	TT 217	TT 290	TT 298
CO Absent	51	13	24	10	6	15	10	9	9	16	26
CO Present	22	4	6	5	7	9	1	1	4	8	10
CO Total	73	17	30	15	13	24	11	10	13	24	36
CO %	30%	24%	20%	33%	54%	38%	9%	10%	31%	33%	28%
PH Absent	54	14	23	10	9	19	9	11	11	16	27
PH Present	9	1	2	4	1	5	0	0	1	4	4
PH Total	63	15	25	14	10	24	9	11	12	20	31
PH %	14%	7%	8%	29%	10%	21%	0%	0%	8%	20%	13%

As evidenced with enamel hypoplasias, the relative frequencies of cribra orbitalia and porotic hyperostosis are similar between crania regardless of estimated sex (Table 3). Cribra orbitalia was present in 20% (6/30) and 24% (4/17) of those estimated to be female and male respectively.[55] Similarly, porotic hyperostosis was identified in similar frequencies between those estimated to be female (8%; 2/25) and male (7%; 1/15). As with enamel hypoplasias, these results suggest that at Deir el-Medina, pre-pubescent girls and boys did not have significant differences in the underlying conditions that lead to stress, such as diet or rates of infectious diseases.

Cribra orbitalia and porotic hyperostosis both vary based on age-at-death. Overall, juveniles are significantly more likely to exhibit cribra orbitalia (54%; 7/13) than adults (23%; 13/56).[56] As with enamel hypoplasias, young adults (38%; 9/24) more frequently had evidence of cribra orbitalia than middle (9%; 1/11) or old adult (10%; 1/10) age categories. While porotic hyperostosis was less commonly found at Deir el-Medina, it was similarly found primarily in young adults (21%; 5/24). These differences may support the idea that those who died as young adults at Deir el-Medina may had more exposure or were more affected by stressors in childhood and early adulthood than those who survived to middle or old adulthood. Alternatively, they may suggest that cranial porosities are most easily detected in juveniles and young adults since the conditions tend to appear when red marrow is still prevalent in the diploë.

55 These values are insignificantly different: $X^2(1, 88) = 0.06$, $p = 0.807$.

56 $X^2(1, 69) = 4.81$, $p = 0.028$. Achieved power is 0.58. Note that the sample size for this excludes individuals with no determinable age.

Finally, neither cribra orbitalia nor porotic hyperostosis varied significantly across the three tombs, implying that the Ramesside families had similar outcomes to the 18th Dynasty individuals in exposure to childhood stressors. Neither *Nbw- ỉỉ.tỉ* nor *Ḥmn*—who accounted for all of the enamel hypoplasias in TT 217—exhibited evidence of porotic hyperostosis and only *Ḥmn* had cribra orbitalia (with fine foramina spanning less than 1 cm^2). The relatively lower rates of both of these stress indicators compared to enamel hypoplasias may be because they are less sensitive indicators of physiological stress and were not as impacted by the stressors children experienced at Deir el-Medina as dental enamel production.[57]

2.2.1 Cranial Porosities in Context

Several scholars compared evidence for cribra orbitalia and porotic hyperostosis[58] at multiple sites ranging periods and locations across the Nile Valley.[59] Table 4 summarizes results for cribra orbitalia from the early dynastic period to the Late Period. While rates of cribra orbitalia and porotic hyperostosis at Deir el-Medina fall in the center of reported rates more broadly from the Nile Valley, we should consider such comparisons carefully. Reported rates vary considerably both within and across periods and geographic locations.[60] When comparing periods, Smith-Guzman found no trend over time or latitude, though she noted that New Kingdom sites with reported rates of cribra orbitalia are generally lower than during most other periods.[61] Latitude may not capture

57 Yaussy and DeWitte, "Patterns of Frailty in Non-Adults from Medieval London."

58 Due to high degrees of interobserver error in reporting severity and healing in these lesions, only the presence or absence of cribra orbitalia and porotic hyperostosis should be evaluated for comparison. Keith P. Jacobi and Marie Elaine Danforth, "Analysis of Interobserver Scoring Patterns in Porotic Hyperostosis and Cribra Orbitalia," *International Journal of Osteoarchaeology* 12, no. 4 (2002): 248–258, https://doi.org/10.1002/oa.619.

59 Corinne Duhig, "'They Are Eating People Here!' Skeletal Indicators of Stress in the Egyptian First Intermediate Period" (Ph.D. Dissertation, Cambridge, University of Cambridge, 2000); S.O.Y. Keita and A.J. Boyce, "Variation in Porotic Hyperostosis in the Royal Cemetery Complex at Abydos, Upper Egypt: A Social Interpretation," *Antiquity* 80, no. 307 (March 2006): 64–73, https://doi.org/10.1017/S0003598X00093261; Ankita Kumar, "Health at Hierakonpolis, a Predynastic Settlement in Upper Egypt" (Ph.D. Dissertation, Fayetteville, University of Arkansas, 2009); Smith-Guzmán, "Cribra Orbitalia in the Ancient Nile Valley and Its Connection to Malaria"; Sarah Musselwhite, "Skeletal Health in Early Egypt," in *Current Research in Egyptology 2012*, ed. Carl Graves et al. (Oxford and Oakville: Oxbow Books, 2013), 128–144.

60 Smith-Guzmán, "Cribra Orbitalia in the Ancient Nile Valley and Its Connection to Malaria."

61 Nicole Elizabeth Smith-Guzmán, "The Paleoepidemiology of Malaria in the Ancient Near East" (Ph.D. Dissertation, Fayetteville, University of Arkansas, 2015).

TABLE 4 Published cribra orbitalia rates from the early dynastic to late period for the Nile Valley

Site	Cemetery/ location	Period(s)	n =	Publication	Rate(s)
Tombos	New Kingdom	New Kingdom	69	Buzon 2014	4%
Kerma	Sacrificial	Classic Kerma	100	Buzon and Judd 2008	11%
Abydos	Northern Cemetery	Middle Kingdom	45	Keita and Boyce 2006	11%
Kerma	Non-Sacrificial	Classic Kerma	189	Buzon and Judd 2008	14%
Tombos	Napatan	Napatan	42	Buzon 2014	19%
Thebes West	TT 85	New Kingdom to Late Period	116	Nerlich et al 2000	20%
Shellal	Cemetery 7	New Kingdom	154	Buzon 2004	20%
Memphis	Duckworth Collection	New Kingdom	306	Buzon 2004	25%
Abusir	Mastaba of Ptahshepses	Old Kingdom	142	Strouhal and Bares 1993	27%
Tell el-Dab'a	SIP	Second Intermediate Period	41	Winkler and Wilfing 1991	27%
Deir el-Medina	**TT 217, TT 290, TT 298**	**New Kingdom to 21st Dynasty**	**73**	**Current Publication**	**30%**
Abydos	Tombs of the Courtiers	Early Dynastic	48	Duhig 2000	33%
Qubbet el-Hawa	FIP	First Intermediate Period	32	Rösing 1990	34%
Abydos	Umm el-Qaab	Early Dynastic	37	Keita and Boyce 2006	35%
Qubbet el-Hawa	LP	Late Period	146	Rösing 1990	36%
Amarna	South Tombs	New Kingdom	103	Smith-Guzman 2015	43%
Dishwasha	OK	Old Kingdom	21	Duhig 2000	43%
Thebes West	TT 95	New Kingdom to Third Intermediate Period	38	Nerlich et al 2000	45%
Qubbet el-Hawa	OK	Old Kingdom	156	Rösing 1990	49%
Qubbet el-Hawa	MK	Middle Kingdom	18	Rösing 1990	50%
Sidmant	MK	Middle Kingdom	15	Duhig 2000	53%
Dendara	FIP	First Intermediate Period	76	Duhig 2000	54%
Tarif	MK	Middle Kingdom	54	Duhig 2000	56%

TABLE 4 Published cribra orbitalia rates from the early dynastic to late period for the Nile Valley (*cont.*)

Site	**Cemetery/ location**	**Period(s)**	n =	**Publication**	**Rate(s)**
Elephantine	Western Cemetery	Old Kingdom	12	Pecotte 1986	58%
Aswan	OK	Old Kingdom	18	Duhig 2000	61%
Qubbet el-Hawa	SIP	Second Intermediate Period	60	Rösing 1990	63%
Qaw el-Kebir	FIP	First Intermediate Period	69	Duhig 2000	64%
Aswan	MK	Middle Kingdom	47	Duhig 2000	64%
Thebes West	TT 84	New Kingdom to Late Period	14	Nerlich et al 2000	64%
Sidmant	FIP	First Intermediate Period	55	Duhig 2000	67%
Qaw el-Kebir	OK	Old Kingdom	27	Duhig 2000	70%
Dakhleh	Ein Tirghi	Late Period	208	Molto 2001	71%
Gebelein	Old Kingdom	Old Kingdom	23	Pecotte 1986	74%
Elephantine	Northern Cemetery	First Intermediate Period	32	Pecotte 1986	75%
Abydos	Middle Cemetery	Old Kingdom	28	Duhig 2000	79%
Gebelein	Trab Nero	First Intermediate Period	47	Pecotte 1986	79%

other geographic factors that could impact cribra orbitalia and porotic hyperostosis such as proximity to the Nile. Because both conditions are more frequently identified in juveniles, the demographics of populations are key considerations for their comparison; for example, at Tombos, while only 4% (3/69) of adults displayed cribra orbitalia, it was present in 43% (6/14) of juveniles.[62] One of the lowest reported rates comes from the sacrificial burials at Kerma (11%), but this sample was entirely composed of adults.[63]

62 Buzon, "Health of the Non-Elites at Tombos."

63 Michele R. Buzon and Margaret A. Judd, "Investigating Health at Kerma: Sacrificial versus Nonsacrificial Individuals," *American Journal of Physical Anthropology* 136, no. 1 (2008): 93–99, https://doi.org/10.1002/ajpa.20781.

Unlike enamel hypoplasias, which tend to correlate with socioeconomic status, cribra orbitalia and porotic hyperostosis seem to vary considerably. For example, 45 % of crania exhibit cribra orbitalia in the elite New Kingdom burials in TT 95 (in the Tombs of the Nobles).[64] In comparison, only 22 % of individuals have cribra orbitalia in the South Tombs Cemetery at Amarna.[65] Meanwhile, in the more middle-class cemetery at Tombos, the rate of cribra orbitalia is 11 % and porotic hyperostosis is almost completely absent.[66] Variation is even visible within sites. Both cribra orbitalia and porotic hyperostosis were significantly higher for individuals buried in the royal tomb at Abydos than the broader funerary enclosure, while enamel hypoplasias are similar between the two areas.[67] In a broader survey of Nile Valley sites, rates of cribra orbitalia were not clearly correlated to either period or latitude.[68]

When comparing rates of cribra orbitalia with broader populations worldwide, both the variation and relatively high values of the Nile Valley are significant.[69] The rate of cribra orbitalia at Deir el-Medina is higher than 67 % (70/104) of sites in the European project with data on one or more individuals. The rate of porotic hyperostosis is higher than 79 % (82/104) of sites. These results are similar when comparing rates at Deir el-Medina with data from the Western Hemisphere where cribra orbitalia and porotic hyperostosis are higher than 77 % (49/63) and 60 % (48/63) of sites respectively. Given that cranial porosities do not vary significantly across socioeconomic groups aside from farmers, researchers have suggested that higher rates of cranial porosities in Europe could be connected to insufficient access to animal proteins as well as environmental stress from malarial parasites.[70]

This may similarly explain the higher rates of cranial porosities in the Nile Valley more broadly along with their irregular distribution (i.e., not correlated to latitude, period, or socioeconomic status) since malaria was endemic

64 Nerlich et al., "Anthropological and Palaeopathological Analysis of the Human Remains from Three 'Tombs of the Nobles' of the Necropolis of Thebes-West, Upper Egypt."

65 Dabbs and Zabecki, "Abandoned Memories. A Cemetery of Forgotten Souls"; This value has alternatively been reported as 43 % Smith-Guzmán, "The Paleoepidemiology of Malaria in the Ancient Near East."

66 Buzon, "Health of the Non-Elites at Tombos."

67 Keita and Boyce, "Variation in Porotic Hyperostosis in the Royal Cemetery Complex at Abydos, Upper Egypt."

68 Smith-Guzmán, "Cribra Orbitalia in the Ancient Nile Valley and Its Connection to Malaria."

69 Smith-Guzmán.

70 Anastasia Papathanasiou et al., "History of Anemia and Related Nutritional Deficiencies," in *The Backbone of Europe: Health, Diet, Work and Violence over Two Millennia*, ed. Richard H. Steckel et al., Cambridge Studies in Biological and Evolutionary Anthropology 80 (Cambridge: Cambridge University Press, 2018), 198–230.

throughout Egypt since before the Predynastic Period.[71] Ancient DNA testing has verified the presence of *P. falciparum*—one of the protozoa responsible for the disease—in mummified remains from the Predynastic Period and beyond.[72] Additionally, Massa and colleagues found that 92% of mummified individuals with malarial antigens also exhibited cribra orbitalia.[73] Smith-Guzmán further suggests that malaria tends "to co-infect with other anemia-causing health factors such as diarrheal diseases."[74] Consequently, even when other factors impact rates of cribra orbitalia, malaria was likely a major factor contributing to morbidity patterns.

If the endemic presence of malaria drove the presence of cranial porosities in the Nile Valley, then one way to explain the varying rates of cribra orbitalia and porotic hyperostosis is by considering malaria the great equalizer. No matter what access an individual had to healthcare, nutrition, or work privileges, there was no way to avoid the fateful bite of a mosquito. The detection of the aDNA of malarial parasites in King Tutankhamun suggests that even royalty were subject to the disease.[75]

3 Adolescent Health at Deir el-Medina

Whereas enamel hypoplasias and cranial vault porosities primarily attest to physiological stress before age 12, adult stature is a more useful way of measuring health disruptions that begin during or continue through adolescence. Even though stature is highly heritable and primarily determined by genetics, an individual's achieved stature is also dependent on their health during child-

71 Smith-Guzmán, "Cribra Orbitalia in the Ancient Nile Valley and Its Connection to Malaria."

72 Raffaella Bianucci et al., "Immunological Evidence of Plasmodium Falciparum Infection in an Egyptian Child Mummy from the Early Dynastic Period," *Journal of Archaeological Science* 35, no. 7 (July 2008): 1880–1885, https://doi.org/10.1016/j.jas.2007.11.019; Zahi Hawass et al., "Ancestry and Pathology in King Tutankhamun's Family," *Journal of the American Medical Association* 303, no. 7 (February 17, 2010): 638–647, https://doi.org/10.1001/jama.2010.121; Andreas G. Nerlich et al., "Plasmodium Falciparum in Ancient Egypt," *Emerging Infectious Diseases* 14, no. 8 (August 2008): 1317–1319, https://doi.org/10.3201/eid1408.080235.

73 E. Rabino Massa, Nicoletta Cerutti, and Martin Savoia, "Malaria in Ancient Egypt: Paleoimmunological Investigation on Predynastic Mummified Remains," *Chungará (Arica)* 32, no. 1 (January 2000), https://doi.org/10.4067/S0717-73562000000100003.

74 Smith-Guzmán, "Cribra Orbitalia in the Ancient Nile Valley and Its Connection to Malaria," 3.

75 Hawass et al., "Ancestry and Pathology in King Tutankhamun's Family."

hood and adolescence. A wide variety of stressors (e.g., nutritional deprivation, infectious disease, parasitic infections) are known to stunt skeletal growth leading to lower achieved stature.[76]

While stature is a sensitive indicator of stressors in the environment, it is also subject to catch-up growth—the ability of an individual to catch up on lost growth after their environment improves.[77] Achieved stature is, therefore, a reflection of chronic and cumulative physiological stress into adolescence when catch-up growth can still impact long bones.[78] If stressors continue throughout this period, however, individuals are more likely to experience irreversible stunted growth once epiphyseal fusion is complete. Consequently, adult stature assesses not only whether growth was interrupted during childhood, but also if that accumulated during adolescence. This period when full stature is achieved can extend from the teenage years into the mid-20s.[79] For the people of Deir el-Medina, this is a critical social age when individuals were likely to get married, experience adolescence, begin a household, join the workforce, and potentially have their first children.[80]

---

76 Lindsay H. Allen, "Nutritional Influences on Linear Growth: A General Review.," *European Journal of Clinical Nutrition* 48 (1994): S75–89; Reynaldo Martorell, "Body Size, Adaptation and Function," *Human Organization* 48, no. 1 (Spring 1989): 15–20; Emily Mosites et al., "Piecing Together the Stunting Puzzle: A Framework for Attributable Factors of Child Stunting," *Paediatrics and International Child Health* 37, no. 3 (2017): 158–165, https://doi.org/10.1080/20469047.2016.1230952; Karoline Schousboe et al., "Twin Study of Genetic and Environmental Influences on Adult Body Size, Shape, and Composition," *International Journal of Obesity* 28, no. 1 (2004): 39–48.

77 R. Martorell, L.K. Khan, and D.G. Schroeder, "Reversibility of Stunting: Epidemiological Findings in Children from Developing Countries," *European Journal of Clinical Nutrition* 48 Suppl 1 (February 1994): S45–57; James L. Sutphen, "Growth As a Measure of Nutritional Status," *Journal of Pediatric Gastroenterology and Nutrition* 4, no. 2 (April 1985): 169–181, https://doi.org/10.1097/00005176-198504000-00004; Caroline C. de Wit et al., "Patterns of Catch-Up Growth," *The Journal of Pediatrics* 162, no. 2 (February 2013): 415–420, https://doi.org/10.1016/j.jpeds.2012.10.014.

78 Andrew M. Prentice et al., "Critical Windows for Nutritional Interventions against Stunting," *The American of Clinical Nutrition* 97, no. 5 (2013): 911–918.

79 Physiological stress can delay the age of final skeletal maturation. Alex F. Roche and Gail H. Davila, "Late Adolescent Growth in Stature," *Pediatrics* 50, no. 6 (December 1, 1972): 874–880, https://doi.org/10.1542/peds.50.6.874.

80 For discussion of the meaning of "marriage" at Deir el-Medina, see Jaana Toivari-Viitala, *Women at Deir El-Medina: A Study of the Status and Roles of the Female Inhabitants in the Workmen's Community during the Ramesside Period*, Egyptologische Uitgaven 15 (Leiden: Nederlands Instituut Voor Het Nabije Oosten, 2001), 49–50. For an estimation of the onset of menarche, see Dabbs, "Menarche at Amarna." For an overview of the transition into adulthood, see Benjamin Samuel Paul Hinson, "Coming of Age or an Age of

Stature is estimated at Deir el-Medina using linear regressions based on Egyptian populations.[81] An advantage to calculating stature from regression equations using long bones is that this method can be used for both commingled assemblages and complete individuals, thus allowing more data to be compared from Deir el-Medina. Maximum lengths were measured to the nearest whole millimeter using an osteometric board for all complete adult femora.[82] While average stature allows us to compare Deir el-Medina to other samples, comparing absolute stature estimates can also reflect other underlying factors such as genetics. It is important to be able to differentiate when differences in achieved stature are due to stress and when they merely reflect different genetic predispositions. Instead of simply comparing average statures, it is also useful to compare variability (i.e., standard deviation) under the assumption that larger disparities in stature reflect lived disparities in physical stress and malnutrition. Individuals who fall well below average stature are more likely to be those who experienced enough stress to stunt their growth, so identifying both differences in standard deviation and those with statures more than two standard deviations below the mean are useful means to assess how stature may have been impacted by stress.[83]

At Deir el-Medina, the average stature was 167 cm (n = 84, S.D. = 5.9) for those estimated to be male and 154 cm (n = 65, S.D. = 2.9) for those estimated

Becoming? The Role of Childhood in Identity Formation at Deir El-Medina, New Kingdom Egypt" (Ph.D. Dissertation, University of Cambridge, 2018), 173–175, https://doi.org/10.17863/CAM.22076. For specific information about joining the workforce, see Kathrin Gabler, "Can I Stay or Must I Go? Relations between the Deir El-Medina Community and Their Service Personnel," in *Outside the Box: Selected Papers from the Conference "Deir El-Medina and the Theban Necropolis in Contact,"* ed. Andreas Dorn and Stéphane Polis (Liège: Presses Universitaires de Liège, 2018), 157–189; Hinson, "Coming of Age or an Age of Becoming?," 98–102.

81 Two methods have been developed to calculate stature for Egyptian populations. Estimates for both are included to make comparisons across populations more viable. Michelle H. Raxter et al., "Stature Estimation in Ancient Egyptians: A New Technique Based on Anatomical Reconstruction of Stature," *American Journal of Physical Anthropology* 136, no. 2 (2008): 147–155, https://doi.org/10.1002/ajpa.20790; Gay Robins and Charles Shute, "Predynastic Egyptian Stature and Physical Proportions," *Human Evolution* 1, no. 4 (August 1986): 313–324, https://doi.org/10.1007/BF02436705.

82 See the Appendix for more information about long bone measurement definitions.

83 Stunted stature is defined as being more than two standard deviations below the mean. This is commonly used in biology to assess health impacts on stature in modern populations, and has recently been applied in bioarchaeology. Giuseppe Vercellotti et al., "Exploring the Multidimensionality of Stature Variation in the Past through Comparisons of Archaeological and Living Populations," *American Journal of Physical Anthropology* 155, no. 2 (2014): 229–242.

to be female. These values were derived from maximum femoral lengths (Figure 10).[84] Although, unsurprisingly, males had higher stature at Deir el-Medina than females, the degree of sexual dimorphism at the site is 9.2%.[85] This value is higher than sexual dimorphism reported in other Egyptian populations which range from 4.9% to 6.8%.[86] Additionally, the variation in stature is significantly higher in those estimated to be male than female.[87] Two males out of 84 and one female out of 65 fell more than two standard deviations below the mean suggesting potential examples of stunted growth.

There were too few adult femora to compare stature from the 18th Dynasty, but values from the Ramesside period tombs TT 290 and TT 298 had no significant difference overall. The mean max femoral length in TT 290 was 435.5 mm (n = 42, S.D. = 27.4) and in TT 298 was 428.9 mm (n = 50; S.D. = 24.8). Even though values in TT 290 are slightly higher than in TT 298, the overall variation is such that the differences are not statistically significant.[88] Despite having different families and extending over different spans of the Ramesside period, stature remained similar between the two tombs.

Overall, these data suggest that physiological stress at Deir el-Medina during childhood and adolescence was relatively similar among women in the village. However, men may have experienced more varied physiological stress at these stages of life, potentially in connection to their changing responsibilities during these critical years in their professional development. As boys who helped with the crew's responsibilities, apprentices to joining the workforce, new members of the crew, and the many who could not secure a place on the crew, men experienced highly varied work responsibilities during this time. These disparities likely extended into adulthood; workmen would have had vastly different labor expected of them even within the crew. Stone cutters,

---

84 These values were calculated using equations from Raxter et al., "Stature Estimation in Ancient Egyptians." Using Robins and Shute, "Predynastic Egyptian Stature and Physical Proportions.", mean male stature was 166.2 cm and mean female stature was 153.0 cm.

85 This difference could suggest health discrepancies between males and females, or, may be a product of univariate metric sex estimation of the femoral head where more gracile males and more robust females are incorrectly classified, thus exaggerating sexual dimorphism.

86 Sonia R. Zakrzewski, Robert A. Foley, and Marta M. Lahr, "Change and Continuity over the Predynastic and Early Dynastic Periods of Ancient Egypt," in *Egyptology at the Dawn of the Twenty-First Century: Proceedings of the Eighth International Congress of Egyptologists, Cairo, 2000*, ed. Zahi A. Hawass and Lyla Pinch Brock, vol. 2 (Cairo; New York: American University in Cairo Press, 2003), 587–597.

87 $F_{1,75}$= 0.204, $p < 0.0001$.

88 In an unpaired t-test: t(90) = 1.21, p = .011.

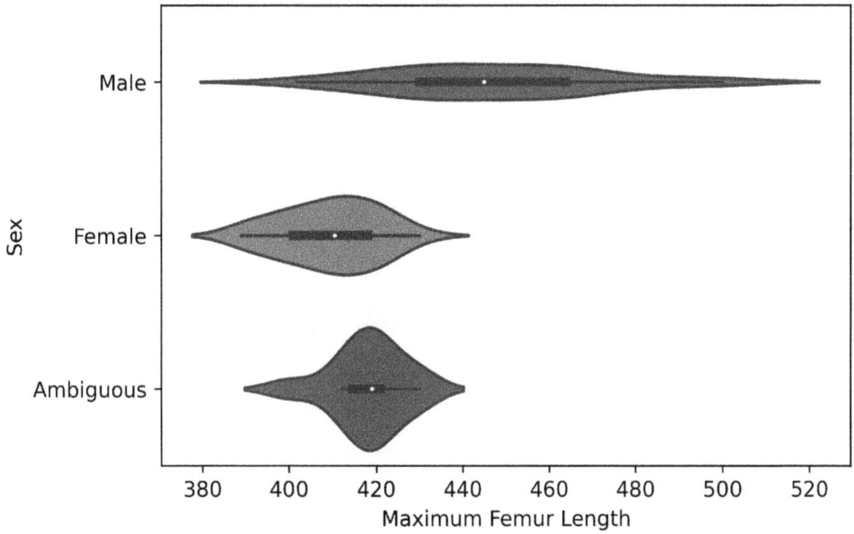

FIGURE 10 Violin chart of maximum femur length by sex estimate

for example, would have experienced more occupational stress than draftsmen, who in turn would have likely experienced more occupational stress than scribes.

Alternatively, these data may reveal differences in how men and women in the village physically responded to the same stressors; in general, males tend to be more sensitive to environmental variation than females, meaning that stressors present during adolescence might only have been severe enough to impact males in the village.[89] Nonetheless, the relatively rare examples of individuals with stature estimates far below the mean suggest stunting was infrequent in the village.

3.1 *Stature in Context*

Comparing stature at Deir el-Medina to other sites in the Nile Valley shows that stature outcomes for Deir el-Medina often fall somewhere between the achieved statures of the most elite groups and other working populations, though in general, stature differences between Deir el-Medina and other sites were insignificant, suggesting that a community's overall stature was impacted only in the most extreme cases of the wealthiest or poorest groups.

89 Sara Stinson, "Sex Differences in Environmental Sensitivity during Growth and Development," *American Journal of Physical Anthropology* 28, no. S6 (1985): 123–147, https://doi.org/10.1002/ajpa.1330280507.

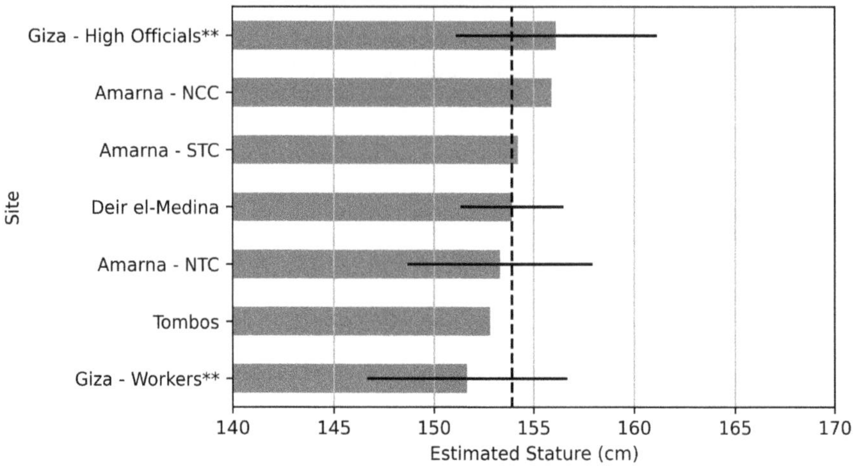

FIGURE 11 Comparison of average stature and its standard deviation by site for those estimated to be female. ** Marks a significant difference with Deir el-Medina

These outcomes varied slightly when comparing females and males across sites. While those estimated to be female at Deir el-Medina had statures that were in the middle of reported values (Figure 11), males at Deir el-Medina were slightly higher than most other New Kingdom sites, positioning them closer to elite cemeteries than those of workers (Figure 12). This is particularly true when comparing stature between Deir el-Medina and the North Tombs Cemetery at Amarna where reported male stature is significantly lower than at Deir el-Medina.[90] Conversely, male stature at Deir el-Medina is significantly lower than Giza high officials, though otherwise, differences in mean are insignificant when compared to other elite and/or non-working populations including New Kingdom pharaohs and men at Tombos.

Comparing stature across sites also reveals that period and region do not sufficiently explain differences in achieved stature. Giza high officials and Giza workers have the most dramatic differences in stature despite being from the same period and location. Similarly, values vary across cemeteries at Amarna for both males and females with females from the NCC having notably higher statures than both the STC and NTC, and males from the NTC having noticeably lower statures than either the NCC or STC. These differences in achieved stature could, instead, be explained by wealth or working conditions, but there are still difficult trends that are hard to explain with these factors alone. For example, stature data for Tombos tend to be lower than many workers' cemeteries.

90 In an unpaired t-test: $t(93) = 2.26$, $p = .026$.

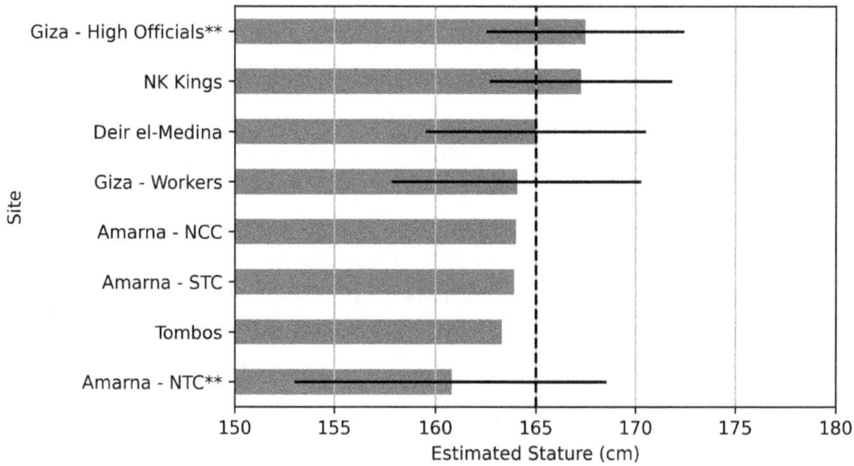

FIGURE 12 Comparison of average stature and its standard deviation by site for those estimated to be male. ** Marks a significant difference with Deir e-Medina

These comparisons are complicated by the fact that genetic differences also impact stature across divergent groups. It is, therefore, useful to also compare groups by their variation in achieved stature. Women at Deir el-Medina have notably less variation than comparable data from other communities in the Nile Valley. The standard deviation of stature estimates is higher in the Amarna NTC, Giza elite, Giza workers, and at Tombos.[91] The relatively lower variation at Deir el-Medina is even more apparent when more broadly comparing the men and women at Deir el-Medina to sites globally. When compared against data from the European module of the *Global History of Health*, those estimated to be female at Deir el-Medina have the lowest standard deviation of all sites.[92] Variation is also relatively lower for those estimated to be male at Deir el-Medina; the standard deviation at Deir el-Medina ranked 28th out of 80 sites from the European module with femoral lengths of 10 or more males. When compared against sites in the Western Hemisphere, both those estimated to be male and female at Deir el-Medina have lower standard deviations than all sites

91 Standard deviations of estimated statures are published for Amarna and Giza in Dabbs, "Bioarchaeology of the Non-Elite North Tombs Cemetery at Amarna"; Hussien, El Banna, and El Din, "Non-Specific Stress Indicators in Ancient Egyptians from Giza and Bahriyah Oasis." At Tombos, standard deviations of femoral lengths are higher than at Deir el-Medina (36.8 for males and 19.4 for females in comparison to 24.4 and 11 for males and females at Deir el-Medina). New Kingdom data from Tombos are published in Buzon, "Tombos during the Napatan Period (~750–660 BC)."

92 Based on samples with at least 10 observations. This is true for both standard deviation and standard error.

in the Western Hemisphere, even when considering variation in sample size.[93] The incredibly low variation at Deir el-Medina and few examples of stunting attest to the similar health outcomes for the community more broadly—that although wealth in some cases correlates to stature at a broader scale for Egyptian populations, within this one village, the wealthiest and poorest are indistinguishable.

Overall, as young children transitioned into adolescent youths at Deir el-Medina, they were buffered from major physiological disruptions that would severely impact their stature. The result is statures that fall between other more elite and working populations in Egypt. Both men and women in the village clearly tended to have less variability than at a wide range of other sites, with women especially exhibiting similar statures to each other. These results suggest that during later childhood and adolescence, the entire community at Deir el-Medina was similarly buffered from major stressors. Further, they suggest that women experienced remarkably similar health outcomes during a period that would have included menarche and possibly marriage and childbirth.

4 Adult Health at Deir el-Medina

Stress markers in adulthood represent the cumulative experiences of individuals throughout their lives. Some of these markers, like trauma, could occur at any point during the life course; others, like degenerative joint disease, tend to manifest in adulthood after a lifetime of physical stress. Skeletal stress markers of adulthood are also more likely to reflect the impact of working conditions on different populations. They, therefore, offer a means to differentiate between the experiences of those who were and were not in the workforce at Deir el-Medina.

4.1 *Trauma*

While trauma could occur at any age, it is included in adult health because traumatic injuries can have a long-term impact on individuals throughout adulthood if those injuries lead to disabling conditions. In addition, traumatic fractures can occur on the job and may reflect different exposures to workplace

93 When comparing both males and females at Deir el-Medina against those estimated to be male and female at sites in the Western Hemisphere with at least 10 observations. It should be noted, however, that many sites do not have femoral lengths for at least ten individuals. Among males, only 10 sites have observations on femoral length for at least 10 individuals. Among females, this value is 44.

injuries during later adolescence and adulthood at Deir el-Medina. Trauma is also often framed within discussions of violence;[94] trauma patterns can be used to reconstruct state-sanctioned violence, interpersonal violence, and warfare in past populations—which often primarily impact adults.[95] However, trauma patterns can also be used as evidence of injuries, impairment, and disabilities.[96]

At Deir el-Medina, data on trauma was gathered by observing the absence or presence of fractures macroscopically on all elements.[97] When a fracture was present, its location on the element, its size, its type,[98] the extent of healing,[99] and the adequacy of alignment[100] were also recorded. Ante- or peri-mortem fractures are differentiated from post-mortem fractures as the former will show evidence of healing, a matching color between the fracture and surrounding bone, and the nature of the fracture itself (e.g., bone tear, plastic deformation, or a break-away notch).[101] While it can be difficult to compare trauma between commingled and complete individuals, some publications report trauma based on individual elements making it possible to compare the proportion of fractures found in the commingled remains at Deir el-Medina to other populations. In some cases, trauma can only be observed in radiographs, and rates for studies that include radiography may therefore be higher. Because of these issues, trauma at Deir el-Medina is only compared to sites in Egypt where methods for scoring trauma and reporting by element/region make it possible.[102]

---

94 Debra L. Martin, Ryan P. Harrod, and Ventura R. Pérez, *The Bioarchaeology of Violence* (Gainesville: University Press of Florida, 2013); Rebecca C. Redfern, *Injury and Trauma in Bioarchaeology: Interpreting Violence in Past Lives* (Cambridge: Cambridge University Press, 2016).

95 Martin, Harrod, and Pérez, *The Bioarchaeology of Violence*.

96 Jennifer F. Byrnes and Jennifer L. Muller, eds., *Bioarchaeology of Impairment and Disability: Theoretical, Ethnohistorical, and Methodological Perspectives*, Bioarchaeology and Social Theory (Cham: Springer, 2017).

97 While some authors include Schmorl's nodes as traumatic injuries, they are here considered separately due to debate over whether they have a traumatic etiology. See Gali Dar et al., "Schmorl's Nodes Distribution in the Human Spine and Its Possible Etiology," *European Spine Journal* 19, no. 4 (April 2010): 670–675, https://doi.org/10.1007/s00586-009-1238-8.

98 Nancy C. Lovell, "Analysis and Interpretation of Skeletal Trauma," in *Biological Anthropology of the Human Skeleton*, ed. Mary Anne Katzenberg and Shelley Rae Saunders, 2nd ed. (Hoboken: Wiley-Liss, 2008), tbl. 11.1.

99 Lovell, tbl. 11.2.

100 Steckel and Rose, *The Backbone of History*, 91.

101 Erin H. Kimmerle and José Pablo Baraybar, eds., *Skeletal Trauma* (Boca Raton: CRC Press, 2008); Markéta Pechníková, Davide Porta, and Cristina Cattaneo, "Distinguishing between Perimortem and Postmortem Fractures: Are Osteons of Any Help?," *International Journal of Legal Medicine* 125, no. 4 (2011): 591–595.

102 While the publications from the *Global History of Health Project* present trauma by region

TABLE 5 Trauma at Deir el-Medina per element

	Sex				Tomb		Region			
	Total	Male	Female	Adult unknown	290	298	Head	Upper limb	Lower limb	Axial
Absent	1326	260	246	820	393	920	142	350	462	151
Present	23	7	5	11	4	16	8	2	8	5
Observable	1349	267	251	831	397	936	150	352	470	156
%Trauma	1.7%	2.6%	2.0%	1.3%	1.0%	1.7%	5.3%	0.6%	1.7%	3.2%

Relatively few incidents of traumatic injuries were noted among the human remains at Deir el-Medina (Table 5).[103] Of the 1,352 elements observed, only 23 show clear evidence of trauma (1.7%).[104] When the sample is reduced only to elements that are 75% or more complete (n = 998), the rate of observed trauma is 2.3% (23/998). Even though these rates are estimated per element rather than per individual, the values would still suggest the overall number of individuals with traumatic injuries is low. In total, Theban Tombs 217, 290, and 298 represent a minimum of 134 individuals, so the trauma rate would be at most 17% (23/134); this value could, however, be lower if multiple injuries belonged to one individual. Traumatic injuries were also evenly distributed between those estimated to be male (2.6%; 7/267) and female (2.0%; 5/252). Given the relatively few examples of trauma, it remains unknown whether these values varied significantly by type or location of the fracture.

Trauma was unevenly distributed in the skeleton, with relatively more trauma observed in the skull and vertebrae (all examples in the axial skeleton) than in the upper or lower limbs. Cranial trauma is more frequently associated with interpersonal violence, especially when the injuries occur in facial bones such as the fully-healed nasal fracture visible on an individual estimated to be 36–50 years old and male from TT 298 (Figure 13).[105] However, cranial trauma

of the body, they do not consistently indicate trauma rates per individual or element. Consequently, these publications are not comparable to Deir el-Medina.

103 Data for TT 217 were recorded per individual and are not included in the breakdown by tomb. Of the 13 individuals studied from TT 217, there were 3 instances of trauma comprised of one nasal fracture and two separate vertebral fractures.

104 Mummified remains were not assessed for trauma because wrappings and preserved soft tissue largely prevent identification of fractures.

105 For example, Margaret A. Judd, "Continuity of Interpersonal Violence between Nubian Communities," *American Journal of Physical Anthropology* 131, no. 3 (2006): 324–333.

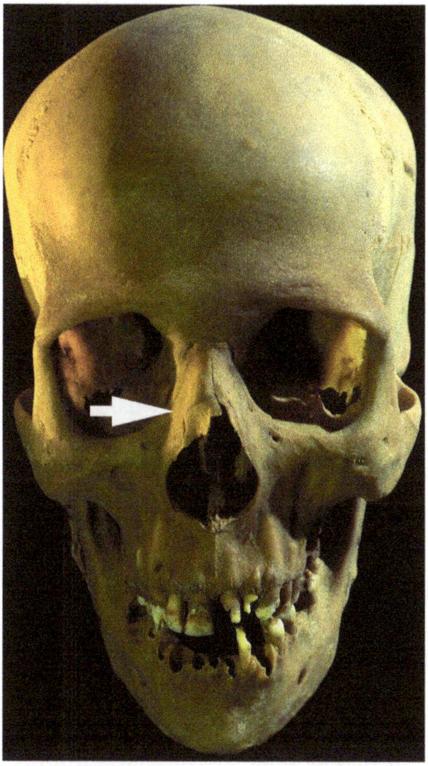

FIGURE 13
Healed nasal fracture (white arrow) on an individual estimated to be 36–50 years old and male from TT 298 (DEM 298.22.088)

could also result from injuries at work—for example, falling debris and rock as the men quarried the royal tombs. Therefore, some researchers separate cranial trauma above and below the "hat brim line" since fractures above this point are more likely to be from interpersonal violence.[106] Considering only examples above the hat-brim line, only 2.9% (2/68) of crania 75% or more complete show evidence for traumatic injuries. Vertebral fractures are more frequently connected to occupational injuries as they are frequently the products of repetitive stress and accidental falls.[107]

Traumatic injuries were also frequently healed; of the 23 fractures, 14 showed evidence of being fully healed. While some fractures would have been potentially debilitating, the limited trauma observed at Deir el-Medina implies that

106 Célia Kremer et al., "Discrimination of Falls and Blows in Blunt Head Trauma: Systematic Study of the Hat Brim Line Rule in Relation to Skull Fractures," *Journal of Forensic Sciences* 53, no. 3 (2008): 716–719, https://doi.org/10.1111/j.1556-4029.2008.00725.x.

107 Nancy C. Lovell, "Trauma Analysis in Paleopathology," *American Journal of Physical Anthropology* 104, no. S25 (1997): 139–170.

the villagers rarely had to deal with violence, accidents, and injuries severe enough to impact the skeleton. This does not, however, preclude the possibility that both state-sanctioned and interpersonal violence were present in the village; rather, it indicates that corporal punishment and fighting in the village were not frequent, were not severe enough to impact bone, or those individuals were not buried in family tombs.

4.1.1 Trauma in Context

Since trauma rates are varyingly reported per element, region of the body, or individual, it can be misleading to place these data visually side-by-side. However, a description of trauma rates at sites across the Nile Valley suggest that trauma is more common in working populations, but that wealth did not necessarily protect individuals from traumatic injuries. In the STC at Amarna, fractures were found in 22% of upper limbs and 11% of lower limbs.[108] In some cases, these fractures may have even resulted from state-sanctioned violence,[109] while others are much more likely the product of rigorous working conditions.[110] In the NCC, traumatic injuries in the arm were present in 25.9% (7/27)[111] of individuals, suggesting that even in this relatively more elite cemetery at Amarna, traumatic injuries were more common than at Deir el-Medina. Similarly, fracture rates were more frequent in male and female workers at Giza, which had a fracture present in 44% and 26% of individuals, respectively.[112]

Even though working populations had higher rates of traumatic injuries, the wealthiest were not necessarily the populations with the least amount of trauma. Among burials of high officials at Giza, 21% of males and 17% of females exhibiting one or more fractures, rates largely driven by osteoporosis.[113] Conversely, at Tombos, only 1.4% (1/72) of crania and 2.3% (19/823) of long bones had fractures.[114] The low overall rates of trauma at Tombos suggest

108 Kemp et al., "Life, Death and beyond in Akhenaten's Egypt," 2013.

109 Gretchen R. Dabbs and Melissa Zabecki, "Slot-Type Fractures of the Scapula at New Kingdom Tell El-Amarna, Egypt," *International Journal of Paleopathology* 11 (December 2015): 12–22, https://doi.org/10.1016/j.ijpp.2015.07.003.

110 At Amarna, researchers have noted especially high degrees of trauma in the spine with many individuals exhibit at least one traumatic lesion Dabbs, "Bioarchaeology of the Non-Elite North Tombs Cemetery at Amarna.". However, this cannot be compared to reported rates for individual, commingled vertebrae at Deir el-Medina.

111 Anna Stevens et al., "Tell El-Amarna, Autumn 2018 to Autumn 2019," *The Journal of Egyptian Archaeology* 106, no. 1–2 (2020): 3–15, https://doi.org/10.1177/0307513320973678.

112 Azza Mohamed Sarry El-Din, "Bone Fractures in Ancient Egyptians from Giza, Old Kingdom," *Egyptian Medical Journal of the National Research Center* 2, no. 2 (2003): 1–13.

113 Sarry El-Din.

114 Michele R. Buzon and Rebecca Richman, "Traumatic Injuries and Imperialism: The Effects

that even though this colonial outpost represented a liminal space between Nubia and Egypt, interpersonal conflict and hazardous workplace injuries were a minor aspect of health status. These values are comparable to Deir el-Medina where 1.7 % (10/591) of mostly complete long bones had fractures.[115]

Trauma related to interpersonal violence also appears relatively low at Deir el-Medina when placed in a broader global context. Cranial trauma, especially above the hat-brim line, was rare at Deir el-Medina and noticeably lower than for all periods prior to the industrial period in the European module of the *Global History of Health Project*.[116]

The relatively low rates of trauma at Deir el-Medina, especially when compared to other sites in Egypt, suggest that despite the potential hazards from cutting into the limestone cliffs, the workforce was generally not experiencing injuries significant enough to affect their skeleton. This is true both when comparing the men to women in the village as well as to broader sites where their injuries more closely paralleled those of non-working populations. We know interpersonal and state-sanctioned violence existed in the village,[117] but skeletal evidence for interpersonal violence is more infrequent than evidence for injuries and accidents at work. When traumatic injuries did occur, villagers frequently recovered from them completely, evidencing survival despite dangerous injuries.

4.2 *Degenerative Joint Disease*

In tandem with trauma, degenerative joint disease (DJD) can also indicate repetitive stress on different joints in the body related to occupation. DJD tends to occur in adulthood after cartilage has eroded with successive joint stress leading to lipping and porosities. The etiology of DJD involves multiple over-

---

of Egyptian Colonial Strategies at Tombos in Upper Nubia," *American Journal of Physical Anthropology* 133, no. 2 (2007): 783–791, https://doi.org/10.1002/ajpa.20585.

115 When including only those long bones that are more than 75 % complete for comparison with Buzon and Richman.

116 Joerg Baten and Richard H. Steckel, "The History of Violence in Europe," in *The Backbone of Europe: Health, Diet, Work and Violence over Two Millennia*, ed. Richard H. Steckel et al., Cambridge Studies in Biological and Evolutionary Anthropology 80 (Cambridge: Cambridge University Press, 2018), fig. 10.3.

117 Christine Hue-Arcé, "The Legal Treatment of Interpersonal Violence in Deir El-Medina," in *Outside the Box: Selected Papers from the Conference "Deir El-Medina and the Theban Necropolis in Contact" Liège, 27–29 2014*, ed. Andreas Dorn and Stéphane Polis, Ægyptiaca Leodiensia (Liège, Belgium: Presses Universitaires de Liège, 2014), 265–279; Christine Hue-Arcé, *La Violence Interpersonnelle En Égypte Au Nouvel Empire et à l'époque Gréco-Romaine* (Wallasey: Abercromby Press, 2020).

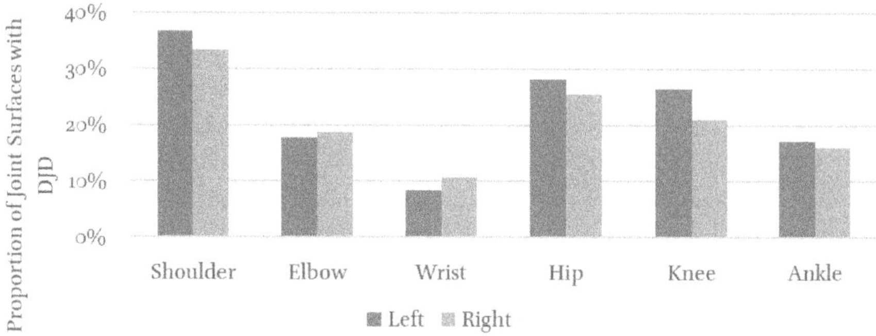

FIGURE 14 Distribution of DJD at Deir el-Medina by joint region and side

lying factors including age, sex, genes, weight, and repetitive use.[118] It is not only difficult to extrapolate how each of these impacts rates of DJD, but it is also difficult to determine how much influence each factor has in the overall chances of developing DJD. Consequently, it is important to evaluate DJD patterns by individual joints as well as by age groups and estimated sex when possible. Regardless of its etiology, DJD can impact occupation either because repetitive stress in work causes DJD or because it creates physical limitations preventing participation in the workforce.

DJD in adults was scored for each of the six major joint regions: shoulder, elbow, wrist, hip, knee, and ankle. Observations for all joints follow scoring criteria used in the *Global History of Health Project*.[119] The presence of DJD was recorded when both marginal osteophytes and changes to the joint surface (i.e., pitting, new bone formation, or change in contour) were visible, as osteophytes alone may not be a reliable indicator of joint destruction.[120] DJD was observed for each joint surface of an element. Overall joint rates are reported instead of individual joint surfaces in order to facilitate comparison with other sites. Additionally, all vertebrae were scored for osteophytosis—bony lipping of the vertebral bodies—following scoring criteria of the *Global History of Health Project*, though these can only be compared by vertebral type since commingled remains do not allow a comparison of the entire vertebral column.

At Deir el-Medina, the overall distribution of average joint scores decreases from the shoulder to the wrist, rising at the hip and then decreasing to the ankle

118 Elizabeth Weiss and Robert Jurmain, "Osteoarthritis Revisited: A Contemporary Review of Aetiology," *International Journal of Osteoarchaeology* 17, no. 5 (2007): 437–450, https://doi.org/10.1002/oa.889.

119 Steckel et al., *The Backbone of Europe*.

120 Juliet Rogers and Tony Waldron, *A Field Guide to Joint Disease in Archaeology* (Chichester: Wiley, 1995), 43–44.

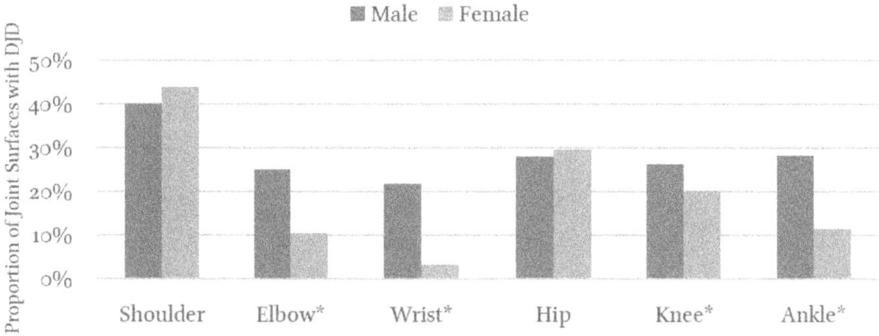

FIGURE 15 DJD distribution by joint and estimated sex. * Marks significant differences between male and female rates.

(Figure 14). These do not vary considerably by side when looking at all individuals. The lower limb has higher average DJD scores than the upper limb, which is to be expected due to increased stress from bearing weight. DJD was observed on 21% (335/1,531) of joint surfaces, but it was very rare to find joints with more excessive degenerative joint disease, such as eburnation—a polished appearance from friction after severe joint destruction—which was present only 1.1% (17/1,531) of the time. These few cases were also distributed throughout a variety of joints and found in elements estimated to be both male and female.

When comparing by estimated sex, rates are similar at the shoulder and hip, but male elements have a higher proportion of DJD in all remaining joint regions (Figure 15).[121] The fact that these differences exist even in non-weight-bearing joints (i.e., the elbow and wrist) suggests that men and women experienced different stressors on their joints in the community, even when differences in DJD due to body size are considered.

The daily stress of the workmen may explain these discrepancies. Movement from Deir el-Medina to the workmen's huts as well as from the huts to and from the royal tombs would have taken its toll on the workforce; the constant climbing up and down would have added increased stress on the knee and ankle specifically.[122] Even though only part of the population at Deir el-Medina were themselves workmen, other male members of the Deir el-Medina community were still expected to travel the Theban cliffs delivering goods to the workforce as either youths or members of the *smd.t*. Similarly, the work of preparing and decorating the rock-cut tomb through stone-cutting and fine chiseling would have placed more stress at the elbow and wrist, and squatting

121 These differences are significant at the elbow: $X^2(1, 293) = 10.77$, $p = 0.001$. They approach significance at the wrist in a Fisher's Exact Test ($p = 0.053$).

122 Austin, "The Cost of a Commute."

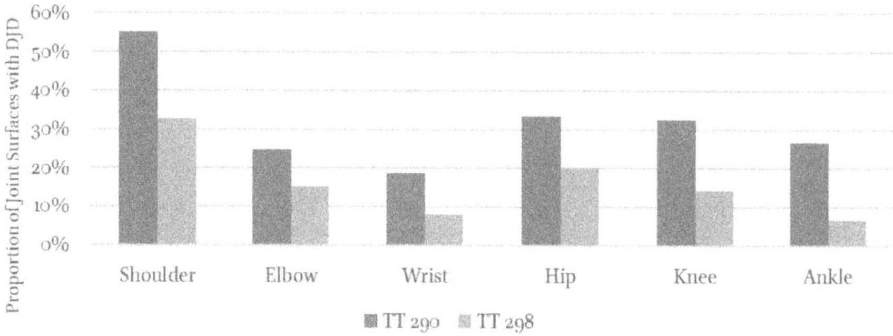

FIGURE 16 Distribution of DJD by joint and tomb

to decorate lower areas of the tomb would have further affected the knees and ankles of the workmen. At its apex, these stressors may have led to such high degrees of joint degeneration that joints eventually fused. Notably, at least two examples of joint fusion at the ankle (between the talus and calcaneus) are present in the human remains at Deir el-Medina, though factors other than degenerative stress could have been the cause.[123]

Unlike the stress indicators discussed thus far, there was a noticeable difference in DJD rates between the two Ramesside era tombs TT 290 and TT 298, perhaps reflecting changes during the broader use of the site or differences between families.[124] DJD rates were higher in TT 290 than in TT 298 across all joints (Figure 16). Conversely, vertebral osteophytosis was lower in TT 290 than in TT 298 with fewer examples of osteophytosis and significantly fewer examples of severe marginal lipping (Figure 17).[125] While differences in osteophytosis could be explained by the presence of more older adults in TT 298, the overall higher rates of non-vertebral DJD suggest that these differences are not only age-related. Since TT 298 was established earlier than TT 290, the divergence in DJD may reflect differences during the Ramesside period with activities related to DJD increasing after the first half of the 19th Dynasty. Alternatively, these differences could represent lived differences between families. While 18th dynasty burials placed TT 217 are too small of a data set to meaning-

123 Fusion between the tarsals (tarsal coalition) has been documented as resulting from degenerative stress, congenital anomaly, traumatic injury, and/or infectious disease. For more information, see Aufderheide, Rodríguez-Martín, and Langsjoen, *The Cambridge Encyclopedia of Human Paleopathology*, 75.

124 These two tombs have similar overall sample sizes (see Chapter 3). The few, complete individuals from the 18th Dynasty currently stored in TT 217 are too limited for comparison, but individual health outcomes including DJD are discussed in more depth in Chapter 7.

125 In a Chi-squared test comparing severe marginal lipping against all other scores: $X^2(1, 277) = 12.86$, $p<.001$.

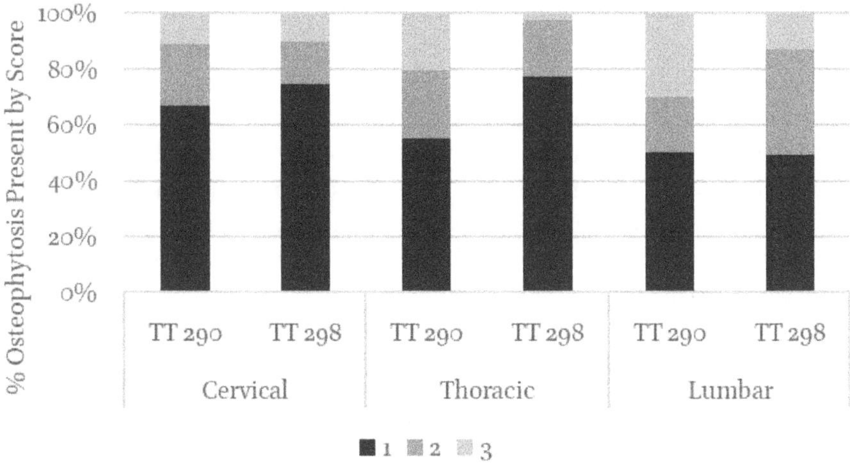

FIGURE 17 Distribution of osteophytosis scores by vertebral type and tomb with severity increasing from 1 to 3

fully compare, it is noteworthy that one man from the 18th Dynasty, *Stȝw*, had some of the most extensive DJD documented at Deir el-Medina to date (see Chapter 7).

4.2.1 Degenerative Joint Disease in Context

Data across the Nile Valley show that DJD rates in ancient Egypt tend to reflect both age- and stress-related changes. These position the people of Deir el-Medina largely with other working populations, though with less evidence of more extreme joint degeneration. In general, rates of DJD at Amarna are higher, especially when comparing rates of eburnation. In the STC at Amarna, DJD was present in 47.7% of the lower limb and 65.9% of the upper limb, with eburnation in 21.6% and 13.7% of the lower and upper limb respectively.[126] Though not broken down by joint region, these rates of DJD are still noticeably higher than rates at Deir el-Medina by joint, and extreme manifestations in the form of eburnation were rarely present at Deir el-Medina. In the STC, there is also a smaller proportion of individuals in the 50+ age category, making the higher rates of DJD even more pronounced as they cannot be explained by age. Kemp and colleagues suggest that the unusually high levels of DJD at Amarna are due to the higher workloads required to build a new capital city in just a few years.[127] The buildings at Amarna were constructed with 70 kg stones, which could be

126 Kemp et al., "Life, Death and beyond in Akhenaten's Egypt," 73.
127 Kemp et al., 2013.

carried by one person at a time, resulting in higher DJD in the upper limb, vertebral column, and lower limb. These same issues were observed in the NTC where DJD was already visible in children as young as 6–8 years old, suggesting child labor was used to build the capital.[128] In the NCC, 63.2% of individuals exhibited some form of non-vertebral DJD, though these examples are comparatively less severe than the other cemeteries at Amarna with less evidence of DJD as a result of extreme workloads. The relatively high rates of DJD even in the NCC suggest that socioeconomic status did not protect people at Amarna from experiencing DJD.

When comparing Deir el-Medina with both populations at Giza,[129] the impact of work for the men at Deir el-Medina becomes clear. Those estimated to be male at Deir el-Medina experienced similar rates of DJD to Giza workers and significantly more DJD than elites (Figure 18).[130] Females at Deir el-Medina had DJD rates that were, in contrast, more similar to Giza elites and significantly lower than Giza workers for both the elbow and knee; in fact, DJD of the elbow at Deir el-Medina was even significantly lower than elite females from Giza. Workers at Giza were organized into crews as at Deir el-Medina, and both workforces would have been required to quarry, remove, and prepare limestone,[131] making the two populations of men much more comparable by occupation. The rich variety of support for women at Deir el-Medina, including forced household labor, may have buffered them from the kinds of joint stress evidenced elsewhere.

Further, the rates of DJD at Deir el-Medina are noticeably higher than non-working populations such as at Tombos where the population most likely did not participate in heavy manual labor like quarrying and/or agriculture until after the New Kingdom.[132] Although DJD at Tombos is reported separately for lipping, porosity, and eburnation,[133] these data were all consistently lower

128 Dabbs, "Bioarchaeology of the Non-Elite North Tombs Cemetery at Amarna."

129 Fawzia H. Hussien et al., "Anthropological Differences between Workers and High Officials from the Old Kingdom at Giza," in *Egyptology at the Dawn of the Twenty-First Century*, ed. Zahi Hawass, vol. 2 (Cairo: American University in Cairo Press, 2003), 324–331.

130 Giza workers had fewer old adults than at Deir el-Medina, so age cannot explain the higher rates of DJD.

131 Ann Macy Roth, *Egyptian Phyles in the Old Kingdom: The Evolution of a System of Social Organization*, Studies in Ancient Oriental Civilization 48 (Chicago: The Oriental Institute of the University of Chicago, 1991).

132 Sarah A. Schrader and Michele R. Buzon, "Everyday Life after Collapse: a Bioarchaeological Examination of Entheseal Change and Accidental Injury in Postcolonial Nubia," *Bioarchaeology International* 1, no. 1–2 (2017): 19–34, https://doi.org/10.5744/bi.2017.1000.

133 Sarah A. Schrader, "Activity Patterns in New Kingdom Nubia: An Examination of Enthe-

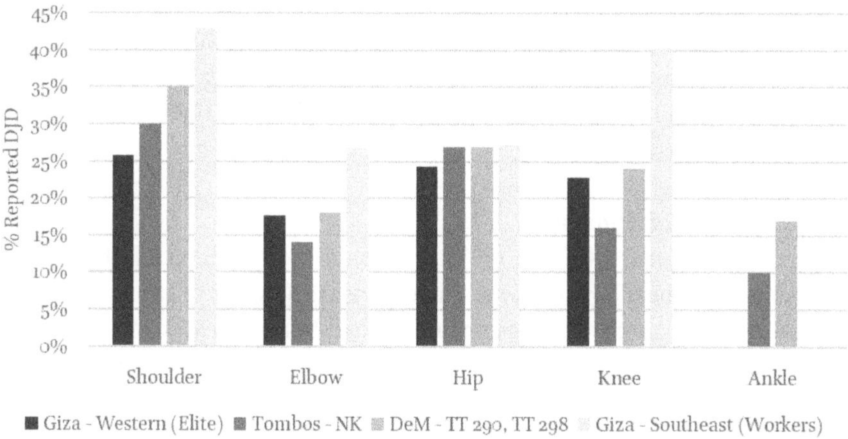

FIGURE 18 DJD by joint region and cemetery

across joints than at Deir el-Medina.[134] Eburnation at Tombos was also rarely observed suggesting that when DJD did occur, it was not extreme. These rates are all lower than those found at Deir el-Medina, and while the differences are not reported by sex, it is of note that the relative difference in rates of DJD by joint between Tombos and Deir el-Medina mirrors the difference between males and females at Deir el-Medina with noticeable differences at the elbow, knee, and ankle. This further supports the possibility that DJD in these regions of the body was driven by the working conditions required of the Deir el-Medina workforce since neither women at Deir el-Medina nor residents at Tombos were required to do such labor.

Comparative rates of DJD in each of these other Egyptian and Nubian populations give context to the potential ways that daily work impacted the villagers at Deir el-Medina. Men had noticeably higher rates of DJD that were more in line with working populations. However, women in the village appear to have had daily life experiences that made their joint stress akin to elite populations. Rates of DJD at Deir el-Medina and working populations in Egypt more broadly appear to have been higher than many sites globally. Of sites with at least 10 observations in the Western Hemisphere, mean DJD rates in the upper limb were 31% and 33% in the lower limb. In the European module, mean DJD rates ranged from 25–34% across the shoulder, elbow, wrist, hips, knee, and ankle.

seal Remodeling and Osteoarthritis at Tombos," *American Journal of Physical Anthropology* 149, no. 1 (September 2012): 60–70, https://doi.org/10.1002/ajpa.22094.

134 The age profiles of the two sites are similar so age cannot account for higher levels of DJD at Deir el-Medina.

These values all trend below workers' cemeteries in ancient Egypt. Researchers looking at distributions in Europe also found consistent differences in mean DJD rates for those estimated to be male vs. female among farmers and craftworkers and similarly point to occupational stress as the driving factor for differences in DJD rates by sex.[135]

4.3 *Periosteal Reactions*

Periosteal reactions[136] refer to the deposition of new bone along the periosteum, the outermost layer of bone, as a response to a variety of stressors including trauma, circulatory disorders, arthritis, blood-borne diseases, infectious disease, and malnutrition.[137] Bisymmetrical periosteal reactions are more likely the result of systemic processes (e.g., infection, malnutrition) rather than local (e.g., trauma).[138] The appearance of periosteal reactions is dictated more by the progression of healing than by a specific underlying etiology,[139] making it another bony lesion that is better suited for evaluating the impact of a variety of stressors rather than one specific infectious disease. Periosteal reactions are thus more indicative of a general immune response to stress.[140] Periosteal reactions that show evidence of healing (e.g., sclerotic or remodeled appearance), in addition, imply survivorship.[141] Consequently, periosteal reactions also can

135 Kimberly D. Williams, Nicholas J. Meinzer, and Clark Spencer Larsen, "History of Degenerative Joint Disease in People Across Europe," in *The Backbone of Europe: Health, Diet, Work and Violence over Two Millennia*, ed. Richard H. Steckel et al., Cambridge Studies in Biological and Evolutionary Anthropology 80 (Cambridge: Cambridge University Press, 2018), 253–299.

136 Periosteal reaction has also been referred to as periostitis, periostosis, periosteal new bone production, and reactive bone formation as discussed in Eric M. Chen et al., "Periosteal Reaction: Review of Various Patterns Associated With Specific Pathology," *Contemporary Diagnostic Radiology* 35, no. 17 (2012): 1–5, https://doi.org/10.1097/01.CDR.0000418464.79923.5c.

137 Darlene A. Weston, "Investigating the Specificity of Periosteal Reactions in Pathology Museum Specimens," *American Journal of Physical Anthropology* 137, no. 1 (2008): 48–59, https://doi.org/10.1002/ajpa.20839.

138 Chen et al., "Periosteal Reaction."

139 Weston, "Investigating the Specificity of Periosteal Reactions in Pathology Museum Specimens."

140 While Weston argues that periosteal reaction is flawed as a stress response because initial stress response inhibits bone production due to glucocorticoids secretion, Klaus argues this only accounts for a partial stress response. For more, see Darlene A. Weston, "Nonspecific Infection in Paleopathology: Interpreting Periosteal Reactions," in *A Companion to Paleopathology*, ed. Anne L. Grauer, Wiley Blackwell Companions to Anthropology (Hoboken: Wiley-Blackwell, 2011), 492–512; Klaus, "Frontiers in the Bioarchaeology of Stress and Disease."

141 Sharon N. DeWitte, "Health in Post-Black Death London (1350–1538): Age Patterns of

TABLE 6 Tibial periosteal reactions at Deir el-Medina

		Sex			Tomb	
	Total	Male	Female	Unknown	290	298
Absent	110	23	33	27	65	45
Present	29	16	7	5	14	15
Observable	139	39	40	32	79	60
% Periosteal Reactions	21%	41%	18%	16%	18%	25%

be correlated with age as older adults are more likely to have experienced and survived stressors leading to a periosteal reaction.[142] Periosteal reactions without evidence of healing are more likely to indicate a response to stressors closer to the time of death. Periosteal reactions can, therefore, be an important indicator of both cumulative stressors impacting individuals through adulthood as well as stressors specific to adulthood.

Scores for periosteal reactions follow the system used in the *Data Collection Codebook* of the *Global History of Health Project*. While periosteal reactions were observed on all long bones, they were most visible on the tibiae. Therefore, comparisons across groups focus on the presence and severity of tibial expressions of periosteal reactions.[143] Comparison by tibiae alone also allows for commingled data to be compared to results from complete individuals.

Overall, periosteal reactions were present on 21% (29/139) of all tibiae and 25% (28/111) of adult tibiae at Deir el-Medina (Table 6).[144] While the rate of periosteal reactions on tibiae did not vary considerably across tombs, there was

Periosteal New Bone Formation in a Post-Epidemic Population," *American Journal of Physical Anthropology* 155, no. 2 (2014): 260–267, https://doi.org/10.1002/ajpa.22510.

142 While DeWitte found an association with age, Marques et al. did not. Sharon N. DeWitte, "Differential Survival among Individuals with Active and Healed Periosteal New Bone Formation," *International Journal of Paleopathology* 7 (2014): 38–44, https://doi.org/10.1016/j.ijpp.2014.06.001; Carina Marques, Vitor Matos, and Nicholas J. Meinzer, "Proliferative Periosteal Reactions," in *The Backbone of Europe*, ed. Clark Spencer Larsen, Charlotte A. Roberts, and Joerg Baten, 2018, 137–174.

143 Klaus, "Frontiers in the Bioarchaeology of Stress and Disease."

144 Additionally, periosteal reactions were observed on juvenile tibia. Out of 28 observable juvenile tibiae, one had periosteal reactions that took the form of a discrete patch of reactive bone. Values are not reported for TT 217 as few tibiae could be observed.

a significant difference when comparing estimated sex where tibiae estimated to be male more frequently exhibited periosteal reactions than those estimated to be female.[145] Additionally, male tibiae dominated more advanced expressions of periosteal reactions; of the 6 tibiae with scores of 4 or higher, 5 were estimated to be male.

4.3.1 Periosteal Reactions in Context

Rates of periosteal reactions are varyingly reported per individual, across all long bones, and specifically for the tibia in other sites from Egyptian and Nubian contexts. As with DJD, this makes it difficult to compare these data side-by-side visually. In some cases, data reflect only individuals where periosteal reactions could be observed symmetrically. In the Tombs of the Nobles, for example, periosteal reactions appear less frequently than other sites (9.5%; 24/229), though this may be because reported rates separate other types of bony inflammation such as osteomyelitis (5.1%; 14/259).[146] These inconsistencies make direct comparison of rates across sites complex, as researchers use varying definitions for the presence of periosteal reactions.

Differences within sites can, nevertheless, help us understand the results at Deir el-Medina in two ways. First, in contrast with Deir el-Medina, many sites report higher rates of periosteal reactions in those estimated to be female than male. At Tombos, periosteal reactions are recorded if observed bilaterally on mostly complete long bones.[147] During the New Kingdom, 19% of individuals overall had periosteal reactions with periosteal reactions present more in females (24%; 4/17) than males (10%; 1/10). Similarly, in the STC at Amarna, females (19%) exhibited tibial periosteal reactions more frequently than males (12%).[148] At Kerma, females also had higher rates of tibial periosteal reactions than males in both sacrificial (61% vs. 44%) and non-sacrificial (55% vs. 44%) contexts.[149]

Second, reported rates of periosteal reactions tend to be consistent within the same site regardless of period or social position. Periosteal reactions are similar across the New Kingdom and Napatan periods at Tombos.[150] They are also similar across both sacrificial and non-sacrificial groups at Kerma.[151] Rates

145 $X^2(1, 79) = 5.29$, $p = .021$.
146 Nerlich and colleagues report periosteal reactions as evidence of scurvy.
147 Buzon, "Tombos during the Napatan Period (~750–660 BC)."
148 Dabbs and Zabecki, "Abandoned Memories. A Cemetery of Forgotten Souls."
149 Buzon and Judd, "Investigating Health at Kerma."
150 Buzon, "Tombos during the Napatan Period (~750–660 BC)."
151 Buzon and Judd, "Investigating Health at Kerma."

in the Tombs of the Nobles are also relatively similar across tombs TT 84, TT 85, and TT 95 for both more modest periosteal bone formation and for more extensive inflammation.[152] These similarities suggest that, unlike other markers of adult health like DJD, periosteal reactions are less likely to be dictated by socioeconomic and/or temporal differences within a site.

When comparing tibial periosteal reactions to the broader findings of the European module of the *Global History of Health Project*, researchers found that 22.2% of individuals exhibited one or more long bones with periosteal reactions. Tibial periosteal reactions were similarly common (22.6%).[153] These values are comparable to the overall rate of periosteal reactions in adults at Deir el-Medina (21%). In the European module, males more frequently exhibited periosteal reactions than females across multiple age groups.[154] The team postulated that these differences could be due to men having higher workloads, trauma risk, and exposure to infectious agents. Research at Deir el-Medina aligns with higher risk due to occupation, given differences in the workload and trauma risk between men and women in the village just discussed.

5 Understanding Stress and Health at Deir el-Medina

This chapter presents a broader picture of health experiences at Deir el-Medina through six skeletal stress indicators. Tracing these from childhood to adulthood, they recount how stressors impacted the men and women at Deir el-Medina throughout their lives. Putting these six skeletal indicators of stress in context with other sites in the Nile Valley offers a bigger picture of the ways social and cultural context impacted ancient Egyptian health outcomes. Thinking of them together and over the life course, they attest to how health was shaped in ancient Egypt in the following ways:

(1) Across ancient Egypt, early childhood health—as measured through enamel hypoplasias—was more correlated to wealth than other factors like period, region, or working conditions. At Deir el-Medina, relatively few individuals experienced severe enough stress during childhood to cause enamel hypoplasias, and rates of enamel hypoplasias were consistent regardless of tomb, period, or sex. The villagers at Deir el-Medina

152 Nerlich et al., "Anthropological and Palaeopathological Analysis of the Human Remains from Three 'Tombs of the Nobles' of the Necropolis of Thebes-West, Upper Egypt."
153 Marques, Matos, and Meinzer, "Proliferative Periosteal Reactions."
154 Marques, Matos, and Meinzer.

were particularly well sheltered from the kinds of early childhood stressors impacting enamel hypoplasias—even when compared to elite populations in Egypt. These benefits were likely true for both children and mothers since maternal health is so closely linked to early childhood outcomes through development during pregnancy and breastfeeding.

(2) Yet, simultaneously, cranial porosities—which also tend to form during childhood—are far less correlated to wealth across the Nile Valley. The people at Deir el-Medina showed no difference by tomb or period and their rates of cranial porosities fell in the middle of reported values. The buffers that protected children and mothers from enamel hypoplasias did not have the same effect on cranial porosities, and infectious diseases like malaria may have had a disproportionate impact on these outcomes.

(3) Achieved stature can be used to assess adolescent health, and this too seems to better correlate to wealth than location, region, or working conditions. The men and women at Deir el-Medina tended to have statures similar to non-working populations. Sparse examples of stunted statures and remarkably low variation in stature at Deir el-Medina suggest that buffers for adolescent health outcomes were shared and consistent for the entire community.

(4) By adulthood, occupational stress takes its toll on working communities in ancient Egypt, including at Deir el-Medina where men had higher rates of DJD. DJD was less severe for women at Deir el-Medina, however, with rates that were comparable to non-working populations. Buffers that may have protected men earlier in their lives did not protect them from the stressors of hiking the Theban hills and working on the royal tombs.

(5) Working conditions may have also largely driven rates of periosteal reactions since they largely do not correlate with wealth, region, or period. Whereas in the Nile Valley, females tend to have periosteal reactions more frequently than males, the reverse is true at Deir el-Medina. Rates at Deir el-Medina may instead reflect the impacts of higher workloads, trauma risk, and exposure to infectious agents for men in the workforce.

(6) In the Nile Valley, trauma rates correlate with working conditions and age at death, with higher rates of trauma occurring in some elite cemeteries due to osteoporosis. Traumatic injuries are sparse at Deir el-Medina and evenly distributed between men and women, with relatively few discernible injuries due to violence. These data suggest that while stressors in adulthood had the most substantial impact on workmen in the village, they were still less likely to experience traumatic injuries, extreme joint degeneration, or periosteal reactions than other working populations in Egypt.

Looking across these six skeletal stress indicators, we can now more clearly assess how period, region, socioeconomic status, and occupation could impact health experiences. Wealthy communities could protect children and adolescents from stressors, as evidenced by enamel hypoplasias and stature, suggesting that wealth did indeed make health in ancient Egypt. However, wealth also carried with it risk into adulthood—especially as aging populations accrued more joint degeneration and trauma.

Infectious diseases—which most clearly impact cranial porosities and periosteal reactions—seem to have impacted populations regardless of their socioeconomic status or working conditions. However, there is also no evidence that they trended by shared regions or periods. This suggests that although environment and technology can impact health, those impacts are not as visible or consistent as social context in influencing ancient Egyptian health outcomes. This makes it clear that wealth made health in ancient Egypt, but these differences within the stress indicators point to the limitations in when and how wealth explains past health outcomes.

This naturally leads to the question: how did ancient Egyptians use their wealth to improve their health? Answering this question at Deir el-Medina is especially important since the data presented in this chapter demonstrate that the people of Deir el-Medina were particularly effective at buffering stress when it was possible. While the village had stress they could not control, like exposure to disease (e.g., malaria) or the physical work required to cut and decorate the royal tombs, they must have had effective ways of buffering stress to allow them even better health outcomes in some cases than non-working elites. This buffering also appeared to help the entire community and not simply its wealthiest members.

This chapter provides the evidence necessary to contextualize health and stress at Deir el-Medina. The following chapters will put these conclusions in context with the *Social Determinants of Health* to evaluate how the people of Deir el-Medina contended with stress so successfully as both individuals and a community. The following three chapters build upon these health patterns by considering the impact of three *Social Determinants of Health* at Deir el-Medina: social support (Chapter 5), access to healthcare (Chapter 6), and economic stability (Chapter 7). In combination, these three *Social Determinants of Health* explain not only *why* the people of Deir el-Medina benefitted from their social position, but also *how* they used their wealth to improve their health.

CHAPTER 5

Forging Social Support

As illustrated in the last chapter, the people of Deir el-Medina evidenced comparatively fewer health interruptions during childhood and adolescence. These differences not only suggest better health experiences during childhood but also pregnancy and breastfeeding when maternal stress can easily impact childhood health outcomes. There are also examples of people living to an incredibly old age both in the human remains and census records from Deir el-Medina, meaning that, though many people died much sooner, it was possible to be an octogenarian in this village. In what ways did social norms, familial expectations, and local laws allow for the villagers at Deir el-Medina to improve childhood and maternal health while also allowing some villagers to survive for so long?

In this chapter, I focus on social support as one mechanism for explaining health patterns at Deir el-Medina and the broader connection between some indicators of stress and wealth in ancient Egypt. I begin the chapter with an overview of previous research on social support as a *Social Determinant of Health* to demonstrate what constitutes social support and how it impacts health in modern populations. I then turn to the texts from Deir el-Medina, identifying if and how social support existed in the village through personal letters documenting interpersonal care. The texts suggest that not only did social support exist in the village, but they also evidence the forms and strategies used to ensure social support was secured in times of illness. I end the chapter reviewing examples of trauma from the human remains to link how social support within the village would impact healing and survival from debilitating conditions. By integrating the evidence from human remains with textual sources documenting social support, it is possible to evaluate the real-life consequences social support would have had on health outcomes at Deir el-Medina.

1 Social Support and its Connection to Improved Health Outcomes

Since the 1970s, researchers in psychology, anthropology, sociology, and public health have sought to explain the connection between stress and the myriad ways our families, partners, and friends take care of us.[1] One way this has been

1 Two widely influential studies are John Cassel, "The Contribution of the Social Environment

 | DOI:10.1163/9789004700871_006

summarized is *social support*, "the provision of assistance or comfort to others, typically to help them cope with biological, psychological, and social stressors."[2] Academic research on social support looks at it both structurally—what are the social structures in place and how does one's social embeddedness connect to health outcomes—and functionally—what forms of social support (e.g., emotional, informational, tangible, and sense of belonging) directly impact health and stress. Researchers further nuance this to differentiate between how structures like social network size and the strength of social ties, as well as the size and distribution of social capital, impact health differently. Studies demonstrate that social support often correlates to improved health outcomes.[3] This correlation operates in a variety of ways:

1. Social support buffers stress so that when people encounter a new stressor, their social support network helps them overcome it. For example, one study found that people with more social ties and more varied social roles were also less likely to get a symptomatic infection when exposed to an infectious dose of the common cold.[4] Social support in the form of both caring for someone's emotional well-being and providing food, money, or other goods during a period of stress can alleviate both the physical and emotional impacts of stressors.[5]
2. Social support creates conditions that prevent people from encountering stressors in the first place. For example, addiction to smoking and alcohol correlates to one's social group, where taking up smoking is socially contagious; similarly, individuals were more likely to quit smoking if a spouse, family member, or close friend also quit.[6]

---

to Host Resistance," *American Journal of Epidemiology* 104, no. 2 (1976): 107–123; Sidney Cobb, "Social Support as a Moderator of Life Stress," *Psychosomatic Medicine* 38, no. 5 (1976): 300–314, https://doi.org/10.1097/00006842-197609000-00003.

2 "APA Dictionary of Psychology," accessed March 8, 2022, https://dictionary.apa.org/.

3 James S. House, Debra Umberson, and K.R. Landis, "Structures and Processes of Social Support," *Annual Review of Sociology* 14, no. 1 (1988): 293–318, https://doi.org/10.1146/annurev.so.14.080188.001453; Bert N. Uchino, John T. Cacioppo, and Janice K. Kiecolt-Glaser, "The Relationship between Social Support and Physiological Processes: A Review with Emphasis on Underlying Mechanisms and Implications for Health.," *Psychological Bulletin* 119, no. 3 (1996): 488–531.

4 Sheldon Cohen et al., "Social Integration and Health: The Case of the Common Cold," *Journal of Social Structure* 1, no. 3 (2000): 1–7.

5 Peggy A. Thoits, "Mechanisms Linking Social Ties and Support to Physical and Mental Health," *Journal of Health and Social Behavior* 52, no. 2 (June 2011): 145–161, https://doi.org/10.1177/0022146510395592.

6 Nicholas A. Christakis and James H. Fowler, "The Collective Dynamics of Smoking in a Large

3. Social support offers a direct health benefit regardless of stressors. For example, the *perception* of social support (the hypothetical expectation for social support regardless of whether it has recently been received) is positively correlated with lower mortality rates—in some cases, even more so than actually receiving support.[7]

These examples illustrate the rich variety of ways health can benefit from social support without needing specialized medical knowledge or providers. In some cases, social support can be sought and received in direct connection with a stressor; for example, if someone were to ask a friend to cover a work shift when they are ill so that they can recover and stay employed. In other cases, social support is indirectly connected to stressors—such as knowing that family members will help you if the need arises. In many situations, social support does not necessitate medical knowledge or effective treatments for symptoms of a disease, yet its outcomes consistently lessen or even prevent illness.

Anthropological research on social support demonstrates the value of comparing it across cultures. For example, Corwin studied how nuns in the midwestern United States use intercessory prayer to ask for divine support for themselves and others.[8] The nuns' petitions include unnecessarily detailed descriptions of the need for social support given their belief in an omniscient God. Corwin argues that these details communicate the need for social support to all those who are present, contributing to the nuns' documented physical and mental well-being. Alternatively, Dressler accomplishes this through cross-cultural studies that identify locally-defined beliefs around social support and health outcomes.[9] For example, Dressler and colleagues described social sup-

Social Network," *New England Journal of Medicine* 358, no. 21 (2008): 2249–2258, https://doi.org/10.1056/NEJMsa0706154.

7 Bert N. Uchino, *Social Support and Physical Health: Understanding the Health Consequences of Relationships* (Yale University Press, 2004), https://doi.org/10.12987/yale/9780300102185.001.0001.

8 Anna I. Corwin, "Lord, Hear Our Prayer: Prayer, Social Support, and Well-Being in a Catholic Convent," *Journal of Linguistic Anthropology* 24, no. 2 (2014): 174–192, https://doi.org/10.1111/jola.12047.

9 William W. Dressler, "Cross-Cultural Differences and Social Influences in Social Support and Cardiovascular Disease," in *Social Support and Cardiovascular Disease*, ed. Sally A. Shumaker and Susan M. Czajkowski, The Springer Series in Behavioral Psychophysiology and Medicine (Boston, MA: Springer US, 1994), 167–192, https://doi.org/10.1007/978-1-4899-2572-5_8; William W. Dressler, Mauro Campos Balieiro, and Jose Ernesto Dos Santos, "The Cultural Construction of Social Support in Brazil: Associations with Health Outcomes," *Culture, Medicine and Psychiatry* 21, no. 3 (September 1, 1997): 303–335, https://doi.org/10.1023/A:1005394416255; William W. Dressler, "Cultural Consonance: Linking Culture, the Individual

port networks in a Central Mexican community and their correlation to blood pressure outcomes.[10] Importantly, they considered not only nuclear families, but also cultural norms around social support from extended families and fictive kin networks (in this case, the *compadrazgo* system, or ritual godparenthood). In both Corwin and Dressler's research, local cultural norms explain how social networks are constructed, the ways social support needs are communicated, and their potential impact on health outcomes.

These studies outlining the benefits of social support also underline how social support is culturally constructed and so must be examined and exemplified within each cultural context. Turning to Deir el-Medina, what kinds of social support were available and how did the villagers sustain, re-enforce, or even transgress them? What do these systems of care tell us about how the people of Deir el-Medina contended with illnesses impacting colleagues, neighbors, and family members?

2 Was Social Support an Emic Concept at Deir el-Medina?

One way to answer these questions is to consider how, when, and why the people of Deir el-Medina write about caring for sick family members or others in the community. Among texts mentioning illnesses at Deir el-Medina, two terms are commonly used to refer to caring for others. The first is the idiomatic expression "You shall pay attention to" (*rdỉ m ḥr*), which uses *ḥr* (𓁷) as a literal representation of the gaze and thus the attention of a person. Among texts related to Deir el-Medina, this phrase is used most frequently in the *Late Ramesside Letters* (LRL). Though the object is primarily people, it can also refer to animals (e.g., LRL 9), orders (e.g., LRL 5), or general actions (e.g., P. BM EA 10185, 3.6). In these broader uses, the phrase connotes the need to be attentive. When used with people, it takes on the added meaning of caretaking. For example, a woman named *Wrnr* writes a letter to the scribe *Ḥy-nfr* (O. DeM 560), where she separately pleads for both *Ḥy-nfr* and *Nfr.t-ḫꜥ* to pay attention to their brother *Ḫꜥy* (i) and not abandon him.[11] In this context, the phrase "pay attention to" is intentionally opposed by the verb *ḫꜣꜥ*, to throw away

and Health," *Preventive Medicine* 55, no. 5 (November 2012): 390–393, https://doi.org/10.1016/j.ypmed.2011.12.022.

10 W.W. Dressler et al., "Social Support and Arterial Pressure in a Central Mexican Community.," *Psychosomatic Medicine* 48, no. 5 (June 1986): 338.

11 The term brother (*sn*) can also be used to describe a husband, making it ambiguous whether *Nfr.t-ḫꜥ* was his wife or sister.

or abandon. The pairing of attention and neglect suggests a norm of regular caretaking, and the pleading requests of *Wrnr* illustrate the broader expectation of brothers and sisters to be attentive to their siblings.[12]

The second term used at Deir el-Medina to refer to caring for others is *nwỉ*. Generally, this term was used in contexts where an individual takes care of possessions on behalf of another person (e.g., P. BM 10509, 3.14 and the Stela of Horemchauef [New York MMA 35.7.55]), but is also used to describe taking care of people more generally or by specifically supplying provisions for someone (e.g., the stele of Seti I for Ramses I in his mortuary temple at Abydos). At Deir el-Medina, it often describes caretaking as provisioning. For example, it can suggest supplying provisions, as in a letter (O. Prague 1826) in which a woman writes to her sister about an argument with her husband. He complains that her family does not take care of her but that other families bring beer and fish daily to their people. Simultaneously, it can describe taking care of a body, such as that of *Ḥr-ms*, which is described in a letter (O. DeM 126) after he is found dead in the house of *Ḥr-m-ḥb*.

Apart from direct references to care, we can see that prayers and wishes for the general health of the recipient are standard and expected in personal letters from Deir el-Medina.[13] Letters often begin with prayers to the gods for the life, prosperity, health, and longevity of the recipient. In closing, letters repeat the wishes for the good health of the recipient. Between these statements, the author often describes their health while also asking for more information about the health of the recipient and their family. These norms can vary based on the author and receiver—letters between family members are more likely to contain reciprocal well wishes; conventionally, those from inferiors to superiors have well wishes, but not vice versa.[14] The need to share both concern and

12 This text may be connected with another ostracon, O. DeM 581—both found in the great pit just two weeks apart in December 1950. *Ḥȝy* (i), writing to *Rʿ-mry* (ii) son of *Mḥ* (i), saying that he is bedridden and sick—he is without fish or vegetables. In this case, he asks *Rʿ-mry* (ii) to provision him.

13 Ben J.J. Haring, "'In Life, Prosperity, Health!' Introductory Formulae in Letters from the Theban Necropolis," in *Texte–Theben–Tonfragmente: Festschrift Für Günter Burkard*, ed. Dieter Kessler et al. (Wiesbaden: Harrassowitz, 2009), 180–191; Kim Ridealgh, "Polite like an Egyptian? Case Studies of Politeness in the Late Ramesside Letters," *Journal of Politeness Research* 12, no. 2 (July 1, 2016): 245–266, https://doi.org/10.1515/pr-2016-0007; Deborah Sweeney, "Idiolects in the Late Ramesside Letters," *Lingua Aegyptia* 4 (1994): 275–324; Deborah Sweeney, *Correspondence and Dialogue: Pragmatic Factors in Late Ramesside Letter Writing*, Ägypten Und Altes Testament 49 (Wiesbaden: Harrassowitz Verlag, 2001).

14 Edward F. Wente, *Letters from Ancient Egypt*, Society of Biblical Literature. Writings from the Ancient World 1 (Atlanta: Scholars Press, 1990), 10.

hope for good health at Deir el-Medina demonstrates that it was normalized as the collective responsibility of friends, family, and colleagues.

The concept of social support was also embedded in wisdom texts—a literary genre that presents maxims, often from father to son, on what he should or should not do to live a good life. These texts appear in a wide range of periods and places in ancient Egypt. However, they are particularly well represented at Deir el-Medina because they were commonly copied and possibly used as exercises to learn to read and write. Some were even composed within the village, such as the *Instruction of Hori* and *Instruction of Amennakht*.[15] Within them, we can see a dedication to taking care of family members, especially a man's mother and children as exhibited in the *Instructions of Any*.[16] Wisdom texts also emphasize supporting the community, as in the *Prohibitions* where the author warns: "You should not ignore your neighbours (on) the days of their need, and they will surround you in [your moment?]."[17] While these texts represent ideals and not always realities, the fact that they were frequently copied and even composed at Deir el-Medina demonstrates the villagers grew up with and reinforced a social expectation to take care of family and community.

Overall, the conventions represented in both personal correspondence and community literature demonstrate how interwoven social health concerns were in ancient Egyptian texts. One's health was not private nor was it an individual responsibility. There was, instead, an expectation to share concerns, prayers, and wishes for good health. Caretaking was embedded into language and conventional wisdom, which dictated that one should offer social support when needed. These well wishes do not guarantee additional acts of social support, but they do make it clear that in New Kingdom Egypt, there was an emic social responsibility for the health and well-being of others.

3 Who Provided and Who Received Social Support

Looking across texts describing illness and care, it is also clear that expectations for social support largely fell on family members; in texts at Deir el-Medina involving both illness and some form of social support, the vast majority occur between nuclear family members who are either of the same generation or one

---

15 Susanne Bickel and Bernard Mathieu, "L'écrivain Amennakht et Son Enseignement," *Bulletin de l'Institut Français d'Archéologie Orientale*, no. 93 (1993): 31–51.

16 Miriam Lichtheim, *Ancient Egyptian Literature: The New Kingdom* (Berkeley: University of California Press, 1976), 141.

17 Fredrik Hagen, "'The Prohibitions': A New Kingdom Didactic Text," *The Journal of Egyptian Archaeology* 91 (2005): 144.

generation apart (i.e., care between siblings, parents, and children). The various texts describing caretaking relationships at Deir el-Medina in this chapter show siblings caring for each other, children caring for their parents, parents caring for their children, and spouses caring for each other. It is noticeable that the nature of who received and provided care is almost always reciprocal, with examples of caretaking across genders and generations. At the same time, the balance of social support falls on men, though this discrepancy might be a matter of evidence rather than reality since their time was accounted for as part of the state bureaucracy.

The administrative texts at Deir el-Medina give us a glimpse into the people workmen took care of when they were away from the royal tomb.[18] Workmen were specifically allowed to be absent because of their daughters, sons, or wives but notably not their siblings or parents. For example, several workmen's absences were explained only by indicating their sons were sick without further information.[19] These recorded absences are rare and brief—examples of absences for sons' illnesses are all only one day. This may, however, be a product of the textual category, which infrequently elucidates *why* workmen were absent in detail. Many more absences, therefore, could connect to caretaking and simply not be recorded. Given the brevity of absence-from-work texts, they also offer little information about what the workmen may have done during these days away from work. However, they do demonstrate the kinds of social relationships that expected some form of social support.

Multiple texts allow workmen to take time off because their daughters and/or wives were menstruating (*ḥzmn*)[20] or giving birth,[21] though whether

18 Specifically, O. BM 5634, O. BTdK 614, O. Cairo 25516–7, O. Cairo 25521, O. Cairo 25531, O. Cairo 25783–4, O. Cairo J. 72452, O. Gardiner AG 032, O. Gardiner 167, O. MMA 14.6.217, and O. Turin N 57388.

19 In O. Cairo 25521 and O. Gardiner AG 032, workmen are out for one day because their sons were sick. These instances use *šri͗* to refer to the son while in O. BTdK 614, a workman is out because his son, *zꜣ*, was sick. The difference in terminology may be more related to the scribe and their preference for a more formal (i.e., *zꜣ*) or informal (i.e., *šri͗*) reference to kinship Hinson, "Coming of Age or an Age of Becoming?".

20 O. BM 5634, O. Cairo CG 25784, O. Gardiner 167, O. MMA 14.6.217, and O. Turin N 57388. While Janssen questions whether *ḥzmn* can refer to menstruation, Frandsen and Wilfong separately demonstrate that this is the most probable meaning for the term. See Jac J. Janssen, "Absence from Work by the Necropolis Workmen of Thebes," *Studien Zur Altägyptischen Kultur* 8 (1980): 141; Paul J. Frandsen, "The Menstrual 'Taboo' in Ancient Egypt," *Journal of Near Eastern Studies* 66, no. 2 (2007): 81–106; Terry G. Wilfong, "Menstrual Synchrony and the 'Place of Women' in Ancient Egypt (OIM 13512)," in *Gold of Praise. Studies on Ancient Egypt in Honor of Edward F. Wente*, ed. Emily Teeter and John A. Larson, Studies in Ancient Oriental Civilization 58 (Chicago: The Oriental Institute of the University of Chicago, 1999), 419–434.

21 O. Cairo CG 25516, O. Cairo CG 25517, O. Cairo CG 25531, and O. Cairo J. 72452.

these absences were due to social support is debatable. Frandsen argues that workmen were absent because a menstrual taboo prevented them from entering the king's tomb,[22] although the nature of their absences makes this explanation less likely. In O. BM 5634, for instance, eight workmen are absent because their wives or daughters (or both) were menstruating, but always for a single day. If these absences were related to impurity, then we might expect workmen to be absent for the duration of a woman's menstruation. If workmen required one day to perform purification rites to accommodate their absence, then we might alternatively question why these rites required a full day's absence. We might also expect workmen to be absent due to the menstruation of other women in the community with whom they interacted, including their sisters and mothers.[23] Absences due to menstruation may have, however, been directly connected to close family members living in the same house, since siblings likely had their own households by the time a workman joined the workforce and his sister reached menarche. Finally, as Hudson points out, while the concept of male contamination via contact with menstrual blood has cultural parallels, there are no explicit prohibitions in ancient Egyptian texts.[24]

Instead, these absences could be because workmen were expected to provision their wives and daughters as part of their social support responsibilities. Looking at other references to menstruation at Deir el-Medina, we see that food and other objects were given to menstruating women in O. OIM 19208 and O. Berlin P 10631. This kind of provisioning may have been necessary if menstruating women were socially separated from their community; O. OIM 13512 mentions eight menstruating women leaving from "the place of women," which may suggest that the people of Deir el-Medina practiced menstrual seclusion.[25] Alternatively, it could relate to provisioning for feasts and parties celebrating menarche.[26]

22 "The Menstrual 'Taboo' in Ancient Egypt."

23 Toivari-Viitala suggests that mothers may have been excluded because they had already reached menopause. Toivari-Viitala, *Women at Deir El-Medina.*

24 "Ashmolean HO 774 and Ashmolean HO 804: New Light on Accounting Texts from Deir El-Medina," *Chronique d'Egypte* 89, no. 178 (July 2014): 236–247, https://doi.org/10.1484/J.CDE.5.103550.

25 For more explanation of the "place of women," see Wilfong, "Menstrual Synchrony and the 'Place of Women' in Ancient Egypt (OIM 13512)." and Toivari-Viitala, *Women at Deir El-Medina.*

26 These are discussed in more detail in section 5 of this chapter.

Relatedly, we see that workmen could be absent when their wives give birth[27] and that these absences could last up to three days,[28] though examples are relatively rare. Perhaps these absences were for deliveries that were exceptionally difficult and necessitated the husband to be present.[29] Alternatively, these absences could connect to issues of purification and impurity in specific circumstances,[30] though it remains unknown why some births required such absences while others did not; in an extreme case recorded on O. Cairo J 72452, the entire crew was absent due to one childbirth.[31] As with menstruation, we do not have clear prohibitions connecting childbirth with impurity in the ancient Egyptian textual record. Of the four cases mentioning childbirth, three occur in years 1 and 2 of the reign of Siptah, and this may owe more to differences in scribal practice—with some scribes not recording the detail of childbirth in their bureaucratic records—than anything else. With menstruation and childbirth, the permission for workmen to be absent demonstrates that men were included in at least some traditions around these health events, underlining their responsibilities toward caretaking for their daughters and wives.

Outside of family members, we also see examples where workmen could be absent to take care of their colleagues, though in some cases, this is clearly connected to their role as physician or perhaps their responsibilities toward their superiors.[32] As mentioned, standard opening and closing salutations in letters tend to include wishes for good health when writing to a superior, but not to an inferior. Here, too, absences from work show a potential disparity of social support. When *Nfr-ḥtp* (ii) was too sick to work (O. Cairo CG 25783 and 25784), one or two workmen also took those days off to be with him.[33] However, we

---

27 As evidenced in O. Cairo CG 25516, 25517, 25521, and O Cairo J. 72452 Toivari-Viitala, *Women at Deir El-Medina*, 172.

28 This may also be connected to post-partum rituals and offerings which include a three-day ritual period Marie Lys Arnette, "Purification Du Post-Partum et Rites Des Relevailles Dans l'Égypte Ancienne," *Bulletin de l'Institut Français d'Archéologie Orientale*, no. 114 (2015): 19–72.

29 Toivari-Viitala, *Women at Deir El-Medina*, 172.

30 Arnette, "Purification Du Post-Partum et Rites Des Relevailles Dans l'Égypte Ancienne," 26.

31 Toivari-Viitala *Women at Deir El-Medina*, 277. indicates this, though also notes that she was confused about the reference. Given that the line is broken and missing just after the childbirth is mentioned, it is alternatively possible that this only accounted for one reason for non-work among multiple.

32 This is more thoroughly discussed in the next chapter.

33 These absences list specific workman as "with their superior." While in some cases, their superior is ambiguous and could refer to either a foreman or the scribe, several absences specify they are with *Nfr-ḥtp* on the days he is ill (e.g., Year 4, 3rd month of *šm.w*, days 16, 17, 18 and 21).

rarely see other instances of workmen listed as off work to be with a sick colleague, and in the cases where care does come up, the workman who is off is most likely the designated doctor (*zwn.w*).

Conversely, in at least one example from the *Late Ramesside Letters*, the scribe *Ḏḥwty-ms*, who is in a near-constant state of illness, indicates that his supervisor made sure that he was properly provisioned in order to become well. This appears to be an especially generous act since it was at his supervisor's expense who provided "a *mḏḳ.t*-jar for five days, five of bread provisions daily, and one *nw* jar, while he receives 5 *hnw* of beer daily in his rations" (P. BM 10326, recto 11–12). *Ḏḥwty-ms* wrote this letter during his participation in the Nubian campaign in year 10 of the *wḥm-msw.t*. At this point, he was far removed from Deir el-Medina and his family, meaning he had little access to the kinds of social support upon which he may have normally relied. Under these circumstances, his supervisor ensured *Ḏḥwty-ms* could recover from his illness by providing him with beer and daily provisions, potentially even from his own allotment since *Ḏḥwty-ms* writes that "it," referencing his supervisor's beer, "removed the illness that was in me." While the text does not use the phrases "pay attention to" or "care" (*nwi͗*), both are implied by the supervisor's lack of idleness or neglect. This may have been unusual if supervisors were expected to receive, but not give, social support to their subordinates.

4 Provisioning

While absence records offer examples of social support for and from the workmen, they provide less evidence for the kinds of social support occurring within the village. Personal letters and legal texts offer more substantive information about the social support that women, the elderly, and children received at Deir el-Medina, demonstrating both the forms of social support that people could expect and the social pressure to provide care for family members. As the texts reveal, social support often took the form of provisioning parents, children, and siblings, and individuals expected reciprocation one way or another.

Looking across the examples of social support from Deir el-Medina, many records focus on provisioning a variety of necessities including food, clothing, and medical ingredients. These practical and direct examples of social support appear both in times of illness as well as more generally. For example, in O. Prague 1826, a woman's husband berates her into asking for help with provisions from her family members:

Transliteration:[34]
|[1] *ḏd.n Tꜣ-ḫnty.t-šps.t n sn.t=s:* |[2] *ꞽIi m ꜥnḫ wḏꜣ snb ḥnꜥ ḏd r ntt: iw=i r di(.t) in.tw n=t nꜣ it mtw=t di.t sḥm=w* |[3] *n=i mtw=t di.t bd.t ḥr=sn mtw=t ir=w n=i m ꜥḳ.w* |[4] *pꜣ-wn tw=i ḥr ṯwṯw*[35] *ḥnꜥ Mry-Mꜣꜥ.t ḫꜣꜥ=(i) tw r-bnr* |[5] *ḫr=f mi.nꜣ iw=f ḥr ṯw(ṯw) m-di(=i) tꜣy=i mw.t ḥr nḏ ḫr.t it n* |[6] *t ḫr bw jr tꜣy=t mw.t ir.t n=t nkt ḫr=f n=i ḥr dd ḥr* |[7] *wn m.di=t sn.w ḫr bw ir=w nw r=t ḫft iw=f ḥr nr* |[8] *m-di=i m-mn.t ḫr ptr pꜣy i.ir=t r=i m-šꜣꜥ* |[9] *n-ḏr ḥms=(i) di iw rmṯ nb ḥr fꜣ t, ḥnḳ.t,* |[10] *rm.w m-mn.t nꜣy=sn rmṯ*

Translation:
|[1] What *Tꜣ-ḫnty.t-šps.t* said to her sister: |[2] *ꞽIi* in life, prosperity, and health, and regarding the matter: I will send you the barley and you will have it ground |[3] for me and you will add emmer to it. And you shall make them for me as provisions |[4] because I am quarreling with *Mry-Mꜣꜥ.t*. "(I) will throw you out,"[36] |[5] he says when he quarrels with me (over) my mother asking the amount of barley for |[6] bread. "Now, your mother does nothing for you" he says to me, saying "Even though |[7] you have siblings, they do not take care of you," so he says, yelling |[8] at me daily. "Now look, this is what you have done to me ever |[9] since (I) resided here while everyone is bringing bread, beer, |[10] and fish daily (to) their people."

This text suggests that immediate family members were expected to support each other by providing both the food and labor required to process ingredients. The husband's frustration with his wife and her mother demonstrates his expectation that they provision him with his in-laws' extra fish and beer, as this was common practice as evidenced by everyone else bringing beer and fish to "their people" (*nꜣy=sn rmṯ*). This phrase, which separates *Mry-Mꜣꜥ.t* and his wife, shows that families were immediately responsible for their relatives. The strength of one's social support network was, therefore, directly related to

34 Transliteration and translation based on Břetislav Vachala, "Der Brief Einer Gescholtenen Ehefrau an Ihre Schwester (o Prag 1826)," in *Times, Signs and Pyramids: Studies in Honour of Miroslav Verner on the Occasion of His Seventieth Birthday*, ed. Vivienne G. Callender et al. (Faculty of Arts, Charles University, 2011), 423–427; Wente, *Letters from Ancient Egypt*, 147–148.

35 Variant on *ṯṯṯ* (Wb 5, 413.6–8) as also seen in line 5.

36 The phrase "to throw out" (*ḫꜣꜥ*) at Deir el-Medina is often translated as "to divorce" since the concepts of marriage and divorce are directly connected to cohabitation. See Leonard H. Lesko and Barbara S. Lesko, *A Dictionary of Late Egyptian*, vol. I–V (Berkeley: B.C. Scribe Publications, 1982), 159; Pieter W. Pestman, *Marriage and Matrimonial Property in Ancient Egypt*, Papyrologica Lugduno-Batava 9 (Leiden: Brill, 1961), 60.

family context; close family members were expected to reliably share their food and labor more so than other members of the community.

Similarly, people at Deir el-Medina turned to their family members to provide medical ingredients. For example, in O. Berlin 11247, a man asks for eye treatment from his son:[37]

> |[v1] *ḏd.t.n sš-qd Pꜣy n zꜣ⸗f Pꜣ-Rꜥ-[ḥtp]* |[v2] *m ꞽrꞽ ḫꜣꜥ ḥꜣ⸗k r⸗ꞽ nn tw⸗ꞽ m-šs m ꞽrꞽ g[rḥ(?)] [...]* |[v3] *m rmꞽ.t n⸗ꞽ pꜣ-wn tw⸗ꞽ m pꜣ [...]* |[v4] *nb⸗ꞽ ꞽImn ḥꜣ⸗f r⸗ꞽ* |[r1] *ꞽnꞽ.tw⸗k(?) n⸗ꞽ m nkt bꞽ.t n ꞽr.tꞽ⸗ꞽ m-mꞽt.t stꞽ* |[r2] *ꞽw⸗f m sḫt wꜣḏ* |[r3] *msdm.t mꜣꜥ.t* |[r4] *[...] sp 2 sp 2 tw n⸗k(?) sp 2 sp 2* |[r5] *ꞽs-bn ꞽnk pꜣꞽ⸗k ꞽt* |[r6] *ḫr tw⸗ꞽ gbꞽ* |[r7] *tw⸗ꞽ ḥr wḫꜣ ꞽr.tꞽ⸗ꞽ nn sw*
>
> |[v1] That which the draftsman *Pꜣy* (i) said to his son *Pꜣ-Rꜥ-[ḥtp]* |[v2] Do not turn your back on me, I am not well [...]. [Do not stop] |[v3] weeping for me because I am in [darkness] |[v4] My lord Amun (has turned) his back against me. |[r1] You shall bring for me some honey for my eyes and likewise ochre |[r2] That is freshly molded. |[r3] And real black eye paint |[r4] [...]! And [...]! |[r5] Am I not your father? |[r6] I am damaged |[r7] And searching for my sight, but it is gone.

While the draftsman feels abandoned by Amun in his appeals to have his vision restored, he still believes that his son can acquire the necessary medical ingredients to assist him. In rhetorically asking, "Am I not your father?" the workman appeals to his son's duty to provide him with care. The father appeals to his specific need for social support during times of illness by emphasizing that his son should not abandon him when he is unwell. Indeed, he now sees more hope in getting the help he needs to cure his blindness from his son than even from the god Amun.

This social expectation to provide and care for immediate family—particularly children—was so strong that, even in cases where villagers could not have biological children, they were expected to adopt so they could fulfill their role as caregivers. Not doing so was a moral failure, as outlined in O. Berlin P 10627. The author of this letter admonishes the scribe *Nḫw-m-Mw.t*, questions his masculinity for failing to impregnate his wife, and chastises him for not sharing his wealth. Then, the author tells him: *ꞽr pꜣ nty ꞽw mn m-dꞽ⸗f ꜥḏd ḫr-ꞽn⸗f n⸗f ky nmḥ sḫpr⸗f mnt⸗f dꞽ.t mw r ḏr.t⸗f tw⸗k m šrꞽ ꜥꜣ n ḥꜥt⸗f* "As for someone who has no

37 This is based on the transliteration provided via Deir el-Medine Online (2009) at: http://dem-online.gwi.uni-muenchen.de/fragment.php?id = 209, accessed August 22, 2022.

children, he gets for himself another, an orphan, to raise (him) so he may place water on his hand. You are like a big child on his own."[38] By calling *Nḫw-m-Mw.t* a youth, the author makes it clear that adult men were expected to be fathers—by blood or adoption—and care for their children by sharing their wealth.

While these cases demonstrate that social support was expected from family, it was not always offered freely and could carry expectations of returning or providing in-kind support in the future. In O. Cairo 25725, *Qn-ḥr-ḫpš⸗f* accuses his daughter of keeping a garment (*dꜣỉ.w*) he gave to her while she was sick. After she recovered, he told her to return it. The text continues with a variety of exchanges in goods between the two, none of which *Qn-ḥr-ḫpš⸗f* ultimately deemed sufficient to reimburse him for the cost of the original *dꜣỉ.w*-cloth. *Qn-ḥr-ḫpš⸗f* places this fight before the *qnb.t*, a legal court, and thus publicly denounces his daughter for not returning his garment. This action also demonstrates that *Qn-ḥr-ḫpš⸗f* firmly believes that he is due the garment or something equivalent. This exchange demonstrates that, at least in the mind of *Qn-ḥr-ḫpš⸗f*, it is appropriate to borrow items while sick, but these items are only loaned temporarily, even among immediate family members. His decision to go before the legal court further demonstrates that he believes this is the social norm and contract, and the focus on economic exchange shows us that this fight is not about a beloved garment, but rather the quantification of social support and the expectation for equal reciprocation. In this sense, social support is transformed into an economically quantifiable commodity requiring equal future compensation.

5 The Principle of Reciprocal Giving

The case of *Qn-ḥr-ḫpš⸗f* most obviously reflects the theme of reciprocation from Deir el-Medina, but among the texts discussed so far, there is a noticeable symmetry in who gives and receives some form of social support regardless of generation, gender, or position. Parents and children reciprocate care, though perhaps at different times in their lives. Brothers reciprocate care with

38 Lines 10–13, translation and transliteration based on transcription in Kenneth A. Kitchen, *Ramesside Inscriptions*, vol. VI (Oxford: B.H. Blackwell, 1983), 155–156. For the significance of "so he may place water on his hand," see additional discussion in Max Guilmot, "Une Lettre de Remontrances, l'Ostracon Berlin P. 10627," *Chronique d'Egypte* 40, no. 80 (1965): n. 18, https://doi.org/10.1484/J.CDE.2.308019. This phrase is alternatively translated as "It is he who (thus) provides himself with offspring" in Kenneth A. Kitchen, *Ramesside Inscriptions. Translated & Annotated.*, vol. 6 (Oxford: Wiley-Blackwell, 2012), 126.

their sisters, and husbands reciprocate care with their wives. Even workmen reciprocate care with their superiors, though this may have been unequally distributed. This entangled network of social support, therefore, meant that when one person failed to provide care—either due to neglect or inability—others could be relied on.

The concept of reciprocity was further reinforced outside of these individual examples of social support through communal provisioning as part of large feasts or parties. Indeed, the *Prohibitions* warn that, "You should not celebrate your festival without your neighbours,"[39] which is further evidenced in a small corpus of texts that list specific goods given by members of the community.[40] These lists were not necessarily public nor official; they do not include witnesses and rarely offer more information about the event, not even its date. They sometimes include the occasion in question, indicating that members in the community all gave at the same time for events related to drinking, which both men and women attended.[41]

The objects listed in these texts most frequently include small quantities of food, such as varied loaves of bread. However, the number of people who give is usually quite large making the total quantity of donated food enormous. For example, in O. DeM 222, at least 28 people bring various food items with well over 60 loaves of bread along with many other foods all given for the same occasion on the same day.[42] What each individual gives can vary considerably—there are examples where a guest brings just one loaf/cake whereas another guest brings over 30 different foods. But the quantity an individual brings does not seem to be entirely linked to either status or kinship, since scribes are documented bringing some of the lowest quantities of food, and siblings could bring vastly different quantities as well.[43]

The combined traits of these texts suggest that they served as aide-mémoires, possibly for the person hosting the event who would need to remember

39 Hagen, "The Prohibitions," 144.

40 Most notably studied by Jac J. Janssen, "Gift-Giving in Ancient Egypt as an Economic Feature," *The Journal of Egyptian Archaeology* 68 (1982): 253–258, https://doi.org/10.2307/3821641; Janssen, *Village Varia*, 1997, 55–86; See also Heidi Jauhiainen, "'Do Not Celebrate Your Feast without Your Neighbours': A Study of References to Feasts and Festivals in Non-Literary Documents from Ramesside Period Deir El-Medina" (Ph.D. Dissertation, University of Helsinki, 2009), 258–264.

41 Jac J. Janssen, *Village Varia: Ten Studies on the History and Administration of Deir El-Medina* (Leiden: Nederlands Instituut voor het Nabije Oosten, 1997), 84.

42 Janssen, 61–64.

43 Koenraad Donker van Heel, *Mrs. Naunakhte & Family: The Women of Ramesside Deir al-Medina* (Cairo: American University in Cairo Press, 2016), 142; Janssen, *Village Varia*, 1997, 66–67.

and reciprocate with similar quantities or types of food at a future party. While these texts do not suggest community gift-giving in times of illness, they do point to the broader communal responsibility toward reciprocal social support; they demonstrate the need to remember who exactly gave what in anticipation of future reciprocity. Moreover, they demonstrate the broader, intertwined social networks of some of the people at Deir el-Medina where parties tangibly created social connections.

These parties also show the sheer force of communal contributions toward social support and may have been an important part of re-enforcing these networks during transitional and stressful moments for a household like childbirth, marriage, coming-of-age, or death. Indeed, some texts show gift-giving during these moments of transition, though attested examples do not have the sheer volume of gift-givers and so likely operate somewhat differently. O. DeM 952, for example, documents a man receiving gifts on four occasions related to the birth of his daughter: the day of her birth, three days later, 14 days after birth, and at a drinking party on an unspecified date.[44] These dates correlate to the critical post-birth period when both mother and child faced uncertain futures as they contend with the variety of complications that can come after birth. This period included both rituals and goods given to a new mother in the weeks after childbirth to ensure her and her child's health and survival.[45] There could be related goods given in contexts where menstruation carries with it extra significance (e.g., menarche), which may explain the variety of goods given when women "come into menstruation" (*ỉw m ḥzmn*) (e.g., O. Berlin P 10631, O. Brussels E 6311, O. OIC 9, O. Turin 57356,[46] and HO 804).[47] These examples fit into the broader acts of reciprocal gift-giving, but demonstrate that among the events warranting such communal reciprocation were childbirth and possibly menarche. They re-enforce that the health of women and children during these critical transitions was not just individual responsibility. Rather, they involved both gifts and celebrations from the men and women in their social networks.

5.1 *Reciprocation across Generations*

Gift-giving at important life stages also relates to the changing needs of those who provide and receive social support across generations. Some members of

44 Pierre Grandet, *Catalogue des ostraca hieratiques non litteraires de Deir el-Medineh Tome IX* (Cairo: Institut français d'archéologie orientale, 2003), 124–126 and 395–398.

45 Arnette, "Purification Du Post-Partum et Rites Des Relevailles Dans l'Égypte Ancienne."

46 These first four texts are discussed by Toivari-Viitala in *Women at Deir El-Medina*, 165.

47 Hudson, "Ashmolean HO 774 and Ashmolean HO 804."

the Deir el-Medina community lived to be octogenarians, and many individuals reached an age where they had adult children and grandchildren.[48] In these later decades, when it would have become impossible for men to continue traversing the valley as workmen, the principle of reciprocal giving allowed them to retire and still receive social support when they could no longer earn rations. Similarly, widowed women, who were less likely to earn independent incomes, relied on reciprocation of their maternal care to receive social support from their adult children.

At Deir el-Medina, the principle of reciprocation re-enforced that adult children should support elderly female family members. This aspect of care is attested as part of a son's duty to his mother in the *Instruction of Any*, a wisdom text found at Deir el-Medina but more completely attested from the 22nd Dynasty P. Boulaq IV. The following translation reconstructs the text based on these two sources:[49]

> Double the food your mother gave you,
> Support her as she supported you;
> She had a heavy load in you,
> But she did not abandon you.
> When you were born after your months,
> She was yet yoked (to you),
> Her breast in your mouth for three years.
> As you grew and your excrement disgusted,
> She was not disgusted, saying: "What shall I do!"
> When she sent you to school,
> And you were taught to write,
> She kept watching over you daily,
> With bread and beer in her house.
> When as a youth you take a wife,
> And you are settled in your house,

---

48 Morris L. Bierbrier, *The Late New Kingdom in Egypt (c. 1300–664 B.C.): A Genealogical and Chronological Investigation*, Liverpool Monographs in Archaeology and Oriental Studies (Warminster: Aris & Phillips Ltd., 1975), 115–116; Davies, *Who's Who at Deir El-Medina*; Andrea G. McDowell, "Legal Aspects of Care of the Elderly in Egypt to the End of the New Kingdom," in *The Care of the Elderly in the Ancient Near East*, ed. Marten Stol and S.P. Vleeming, Studies in the History and Culture of the Ancient Near East 14 (Leiden: Brill, 1998), 199–221; Deborah Sweeney, "Women Growing Older at Deir El-Medina," in *Living and Writing in Deir El-Medine: Socio-Historical Embodiment of Deir El-Medine Texts*, ed. Andreas Dorn and Tobias Hofmann (Basel: Schwabe, 2006), 135–154.

49 Translation from Lichtheim, *Ancient Egyptian Literature*, 141.

> Pay attention to your offspring,
> Bring him up as did your mother.
> Do not give her cause to blame you.

The instruction offers clear examples of the effort involved in caring for children, all of which emphasize that a mother is due caretaking in old age for the years of support she provided her children. This act of reciprocation then cycles forward with the next generation when a man is expected to care for his own offspring as his mother cared for him. At Deir el-Medina, reciprocation took the form of giving a mother monthly provisions[50] or having her live in a son's household, as evidenced in census records.[51]

Fathers, on the other hand, do not appear in wisdom texts as someone to be looked after, nor are they recorded in census records as living with their adult children, perhaps because, as McDowell points out, there was "a disinclination to present the father as a dependent."[52] Instead, elderly elite men could keep a salary without necessarily working by appointing their son to share their position as their "Staff of Old Age." For example, *ʾImn-nḫt* shared his position on the workforce with his son, yet maintained the same salary after his son took on the office.[53] Both the father and son were given a wage, though the son likely shouldered many of the responsibilities formerly held by his father. Another option for elderly men was that workmen would pay their father's stipends (*dỉ.w*[54]) out of their own salaries. For example, *Wsḫt-nmt.t* paid his father a monthly wage immediately after his father's name disappears from the ration texts, suggesting that this was meant to provision his father after retiring.[55] Women could also receive similar stipends, though it is ambiguous who qualified for such payments: divorced women who were no longer living with their former husbands, widows, or the elderly.[56]

---

50 See discussion of the Will of *Nỉw.t-nḫt.tỉ* below for one such example.

51 Robert J. Demarée and Dominique Valbelle, *Les registres de recensement du village de Deir el-Médineh* (*le "Stato Civile"*) (Leuven: Peeters, 2011).

52 McDowell, "Legal Aspects of Care of the Elderly in Egypt to the End of the New Kingdom," 200.

53 McDowell, 208.

54 Mandeville in Richard Mandeville, "Wage Accounting in Deir El-Medina" (PhD Dissertation, University of Liverpool, 2010), 14.

55 McDowell, "Legal Aspects of Care of the Elderly in Egypt to the End of the New Kingdom," 211.

56 McDowell, 213.

6 Securing Social Support through the Legal System

Records created at Deir el-Medina often signal that someone was acting in opposition to the status quo, rather than in line with it. In cases of social support, villagers used the legal system to ensure that there were social and fiscal ramifications when family members neglected loved ones.

Legal texts demonstrate that when family members were negligent at Deir el-Medina, they could be publicly shamed and fiscally punished. We see this most clearly in P. Ashmolean Museum 1945.97, the famous will of *Nꞽw.t-nḫt.tꞽ*[57] —a relatively wealthy woman having inherited multiple generations of accumulated wealth. She was solely in control of property from both her father and her first husband, the scribe *Qn-ḥr-ḫpš⸗f* (i) who would have also inherited from his adoptive father, the scribe *Rꜥ-ms* (i). Furthermore, she was in control of one-third of the property shared with her second husband *Ḫꜥ-m-Nwn*,[58] with whom she had at least eight children. In her will, *Nꞽw.t-nḫt.tꞽ* divides up this property unevenly among her children, cutting several out entirely. She justifies her decision by saying:

> Transliteration[59]
> |[2.1] *ꞽr ꞽnk ꞽnk nmḥy n pꜣ tꜣ n Pr ꜥꜣ ꜥ.w.s.* |[2.2] *ꞽrwy.ꞽ sḫpr.w pꜣy 8 bꜣkꞽw tn myw* |[2.3] *ꞽw.ꞽ ḥr dꞽt n.sn grg pr m ꜣḫt nb nty tw.tw ḥr ꞽr.f* |[2.4] *n nꜣ nty mꞽ ḳd.w ḫr ptrꞽ tw.ꞽ ꞽꜣwt.kꞽ* |[2.5] *ḫr ptrꞽ bn st ḥr ꞽrt ḫrt.ꞽ gr ꞽnk* |[2.6] *ꞽr pꜣ wꜣḥ nb drt.f ḥr drt.ꞽ ꞽm.w ꞽw.ꞽ r dꞽ n.f ꜣḫt.ꞽ* |[2.7] *ꞽr pꜣ nty bwpw.f dꞽt n.ꞽ bn ꞽw[.ꞽ] r dꞽ n.f m ꜣḫt.ꞽ* |
>
> Translation[60]
> [2.1] "As for me, I am a free woman of the land of Pharaoh (LPH). [2.2] I brought up these eight servants[61] of yours and [2.3] gave them an outfit of everything

57 Jaroslav Černý, "The Will of Naunakhte and the Related Documents," *The Journal of Egyptian Archaeology* 31 (1945): 29–53, https://doi.org/10.2307/3855381.

58 In cases of divorce, property is divided into thirds. In many cases, women receive one-third of the property while men receive the other two-thirds. This decision may in fact be due to the obligation for men, in many cases, to take care of their children. O. DeM 764 indicates that when a couple with young children divorce, the parent who takes care of the children will receive two-thirds of the shared property. Jaana Toivari-Viitala, "O. DeM 764: A Note Concerning Property Rights.," *Göttinger Miszellen: Beiträge Zur Ägyptologischen Diskussion*, no. 195 (2003): 87–96.

59 Transliteration based on Arlette David, *The Legal Register of Ramesside Private Law Instruments*, Göttinger Orientforschungen IV. Reihe Ägypten 38 (Wiesbaden: Harrassowitz Verlag, 2010), 62.

60 Translation from Černý, "The Will of Naunakhte and the Related Documents," 31.

61 As Černý argues, this term may have been used in a legal setting to indicate her chil-

> (such) as is usually made [2.4] for those in their station. But see, I am grown old. [2.5] And see, they are not looking after me in my turn. [2.6] Whoever of them has aided me, to him I will give ⟨of⟩ my property, [2.7] (but) he who has not given to me, to him I will not give of my property"

The document then lists the children to whom she gave property; she rewards *Mꜣꜣ.n=i͗-nḫt=f* (iii), *ʾImn-nḫt* (xxvi), *Wꜣs.t-nḫt.ti͗*, and *Qn-ḥr-ḫpš=f* (iv). The text goes on to explain that these children contributed to a regular ration to their parents consisting of an oipe of emmer and a hin of fat. The will specifies that *Qn-ḥr-ḫpš=f* (iv) receives an extra reward in the form of a washbowl. In reality, *Ḫʿ-m-Nwn* and *Ni͗w.t-nḫt.ti͗* already transferred the washbowl in a legal proceeding dated weeks earlier (P. Ashmolean Museum 1945.95), but this document also elucidates why *Qn-ḥr-ḫpš=f* (iv) received more than his siblings. In this text, *Qn-ḥr-ḫpš=f* (iv) swears to give his father, *Ḫʿ-m-Nwn*, a regular grain ration. In exchange, he receives the washbowl valued at 13 deben of copper. While this evidences reciprocal giving for elderly men, it also may reflect *Ni͗w.t-nḫt.ti͗*'s concern about how to ensure that her husband is cared for after her death since only her children would inherit her property.

One daughter, *Mnʿ.t-nḫt.ti͗* (i), stands out for occurring both among those children who receive and do not receive property in *Ni͗w.t-nḫt.ti͗*'s will. The document specifies that because she never contributed to the regular rations for her aging parents, *Mnʿ.t-nḫt.ti͗* (i) will not inherit any portion of those rations after *Ni͗w.t-nḫt.ti͗*'s death. She will, however, participate in the much more substantial items that remain of *Ni͗w.t-nḫt.ti͗*'s property. This small detail suggests that if children were only expected to care for their parents through provisioning, *Mnʿ.t-nḫt.ti͗*(i) would be excluded in the will entirely. Instead, whatever other forms of social support she gave to *Ni͗w.t-nḫt.ti͗* were sufficient to warrant her receiving an inheritance.

Ni͗w.t-nḫt.ti͗'s three remaining children—*Nfr-ḥtp* (xvi), *Ḥnw.t-šn.w*, and *Ḫʿ-tꜣ-nbw*—are excluded from provisions as well as her property, though they would receive from the two-thirds owned by their father. After describing this division, *Ni͗w.t-nḫt.ti͗* makes a separate statement about her son, *Nfr-ḥtp* (xvi).[62] She lists 40 deben worth of objects she had previously given to him so that he could

dren were "the obedient servants" of the village leaders leading the court proceedings. See Černý, 45.

62 While he is not named, the context and content of this portion of the text makes the identification of *Nfr-ḥtp* (xvi) clear. See Černý, "The Will of Naunakhte and the Related Documents."

purchase food for himself and indicates that those constitute his portion of her property, he shall not receive any more.

This will demonstrates several ways in which *Nỉw.t-nḫt.tỉ* used the legal system to secure social support for and from her family:

1. The washbowl she gives to her son *Qn-ḥr-ḫpš⸗f* (iv) guarantees her husband's care after her death. This condition may have been necessary if the couple relied in some part on the wealth that she inherited from her family and first husband, all of which would be inherited by her children.
2. When she disinherits several of her children, she indicates it is because they were not reciprocating the expected care in her old age. David describes this as the retributive principle, a legal principle found more commonly in wills and other legal texts, which demonstrates that the concept of reciprocal care was a widely held belief that carried with it legal weight.[63] *Nỉw.t-nḫt.tỉ* emphasizes this social and legal contract further by listing all the objects she had given to *Nfr-ḥtp* (xvi) to allow him to take care of himself into adulthood, quantifying social support similar to how *Ḳn-ḥr-ḫpš⸗f* quantified the value of the shirt he lent to his daughter.
3. She makes her statement in front of 14 witnesses, an unusually high number, which includes the most senior members of the community. By publicly calling out those members of the family who were negligent and by rewarding those who took care of her, *Nỉw.t-nḫt.tỉ* uses her notable position in the community to coerce her children into providing social support.

Bruyère's excavations at Deir el-Medina revealed two additional documents (P. DeM 23 and 25) that shed light on *Nỉw.t-nḫt.tỉ*'s will by indicating the actual division of *Nỉw.t-nḫt.tỉ*'s property after her death, confirming her will was executed as it was written. Indeed, the three excluded children—*Nfr-ḥtp* (xvi), *Ḥnw.t-šn.w*, and *Ḫꜥ-tꜣ-nbw*—received none of the items listed in these two documents. Furthermore, an addendum a year later to *Nỉw.t-nḫt.tỉ*'s will indicates that the family returned to court, making *Nfr-ḥtp* (xvi) swear an oath that he would not receive any of *Nỉw.t-nḫt.tỉ*'s possessions or risk 100 blows.[64] Clearly, the will was upheld, even after *Nfr-ḥtp* (xvi) attempted to contest it. These legal documents demonstrate how effective *Nỉw.t-nḫt.tỉ* was at fiscally punishing and shaming her children who did not take care of her. She uses this strategy to not only maintain social support for herself, but also her husband, maintaining social support as they aged beyond working years.

63 David, *The Legal Register of Ramesside Private Law Instruments*, 67.
64 Černý, "The Will of Naunakhte and the Related Documents," 32.

Whereas in the case of *Nỉw.t-nḫt.tỉ*, punishment was meted out against her children after they did not reciprocate care in her old age, *ꞽImn-Pꜣ-Ḥꜥpy* used this same principle to punish his wife after one specific incident related to illness (O. UC 39619/O. Petrie 18).[65] He writes that while he was sick, his wife neglected him for a month, taking the *dꜣỉ.w*-cloth given to him as part of the payments made by the king to the workforce. He then indicates that while his wife did not take care of him, the workman *ꞽImn-wꜥ* (ii), possibly *ꞽImn-Pꜣ-Ḥꜥpy*'s son, did.[66] *ꞽImn-Pꜣ-Ḥꜥpy* ends the text indicating that his possessions and tomb are to be awarded to *Nḫw-m-Mw.t* (iv), his grandson.

ꞽImn-Pꜣ-Ḥꜥpy's accusations carry weight because there is an expectation that husbands and wives take care of each other, especially in times of illness. Further, he indicates that his wife stole a *dꜣỉ.w*-cloth (the same kind of garment *Ḳn-ḥr-ḫpš⸗f* lent his daughter), something given from the state and potentially state property. While the text does not specify divorce ("throwing out," *ḫꜣꜥ* [*r bnr*][67]), it demonstrates that his wife was legally wrong to abandon him during his illness and this could justify divorce and disinheritance. Instead, it is most likely his son and grandson who took on these responsibilities, resulting in *ꞽImn-Pꜣ-Ḥꜥpy* awarding his belongings to his grandson.

Though it is unclear whether *ꞽImn-Pꜣ-Ḥꜥpy* and his wife divorced, or more importantly, how that divorce may have impacted social support for each of them, we do have two texts demonstrating that when women were thrown out of their home, others in their social network intervened to house and feed them. In O. Ashmolean Museum 1945.39,[68] *H̱nmw-ms* describes supporting *Rt*'s wife after he threw her out/divorced her.[69] *H̱nmw-ms* housed her for 40 days, providing emmer and bread loaves. He goes on to write that when *Rt* threw

65 It is unclear if this legal text dates to just after this incident, or if these details were provided at a later date as a justification for disinheritance in front of the court.

66 The workman *ꞽImn-wꜥ*, who offers care instead, has been identified as *ꞽImn-Pꜣ-Ḥꜥpy*'s son, but from this text alone: Davies, *Who's Who at Deir El-Medina*, 172. This ostracon is heavily worn and in particular the passage identifying *ꞽImn-wꜥ* is incomplete, making this transcription possible, but we should also consider that the text uses *šrỉ* to differentiate *ꞽImn-wꜥ* from another workman (e.g., *ꞽImn-wꜥ* [i]) who may have been active simultaneously.

67 This phrase, which more literally means to abandon or throw out, has more widely been translated as divorce when used between married couples since the act of throwing a spouse out is used in legal texts to indicate when a husband and wife no longer live together and need to divide their assets. See Jaana Toivari-Viitala, "Marriage and Divorce," UCLA *Encyclopedia of Egyptology* 1, no. 1 (2013), https://escholarship.org/uc/item/68f6w5gw; Valbelle, *Les ouvriers de la Tombe*, 236–238.

68 Also numbered O. Ashmolean Museum 1199.

69 This summary of the text is based on the transcription in Kenneth A. Kitchen, *Ramesside Inscriptions*, vol. V (Oxford: B.H. Blackwell, 1983), 587.

his wife out a second time, she stayed 20 more days in the house of *Mnnꜣ*, but *Ḫnmw-ms* continued to support her by providing emmer, an *ỉn.t*-cloth, a *stỉ*-cloth, and likely more items since the text is incomplete.

This passage follows *Ḫnmw-ms*'s description of the variety of objects he has given to *Rt* in exchange for a sarcophagus, as well as the work he and his son have done on *Rt*'s storehouse and tomb. Consequently, it reads as a favor or exchange done for *Rt* more than support for his (ex)-wife. *Ḫnmw-ms* ensures that *Rt*'s wife has housing, clothing, and food, keeping track of the time she has spent in his home and the food and clothing he has provided. Given the detailed record keeping of this text and the fact that *Ḫnmw-ms* documented this exchange over at least 60 days, it seems likely this text fits into a legal or economic dispute between the two men.

The text further indicates that *Rt* and his wife temporarily reconcile, at least to the extent that she lives with him again until he throws her out a second time, at which point she stays in the home of *Mnnꜣ*. So, who were *Ḫnmw-ms* and *Mnnꜣ* to this woman, and why did she stay in their households? Unfortunately, both names are common at Deir el-Medina and the text does not name *Rt*'s (ex)-wife. The text also does not mention the two men's wives, who could have been related to the woman. Donker Van Heel suggests *Ḫnmw-ms* may have been the woman's father,[70] but acknowledges that this is speculative. We might find additional support for this theory in O. UC 39656, when *Ḥr-m-wỉꜣ* (i) declares that if *Bꜣki* (ii) divorces his wife, *Ḥr-m-wỉꜣ* will provide his storehouse for her. This text is particularly interesting because *Ḥr-m-wỉꜣ* is likely the father of *Bꜣki*, and therefore offering to take care of his daughter-in-law in the event his own son divorces her.[71] The implication in these varied texts is that the broader network of people supporting each other at Deir el-Medina clearly extends beyond immediate blood relatives to include those related by marriage.

Before we interpret these examples of neglect and divorce as evidence for a lack of social support, we need to recognize that each text demonstrates how the broader network of family and friends helped individuals contend with their life stressors—whether illness, old age, or marital strife. The strength of one's social support is, in these examples, not reliant on one person, but rather built into the network of family, friends, and colleagues present at Deir el-Medina, catching those who might otherwise fall through the cracks.

---

70 Donker van Heel, *Mrs. Naunakhte & Family*, 198–199.

71 Davies, *Who's Who at Deir El-Medina*, 11; Donker van Heel, *Mrs. Naunakhte & Family*, 199; Toivari-Viitala, *Women at Deir El-Medina*, 91.

7 Forms and Strategies of Social Support at Deir el-Medina and their Connection to Stress

The snapshots of life evidenced in the texts illustrate both the forms of social support as well as the variety of strategies individuals at Deir el-Medina used to ensure they received support when they needed it (Figure 19). In these texts, social support took the form of provisioning food, clothing, medicine, labor, and general caretaking. To ensure social support was available, members of this community appealed to family relationships, practiced a communal principle of reciprocity, and resorted to fiscal rewards and public shaming through the legal system. These examples reflect the nature of the texts—personal letters, legal documents, and private lists—where the transactions of goods needed to be recorded. Other acts like emotional support are less attested, yet their absence is most likely a product of the archaeological record in which such conversations are unlikely to be recorded and preserved. While this captures only what we can infer from the written record, it demonstrates substantive ways people received and benefitted from social support within their community, especially in times of illness.

Figure 19 also illustrates how social support at Deir el-Medina depended on the strength and stability of one's family and community. Even when family members neglected their sick and aging relatives, other community members took on those caretaking responsibilities. In research on social support, scholars have used the term *social cohesion* to describe this sense of connectedness and solidarity within a group. One way social cohesion is more clearly defined is as "(1) the absence of latent social conflict—whether in the form of income/wealth inequality; racial/ethnic tensions; disparities in political participation; or other forms of polarization; and (2) the presence of strong social bonds—measured by levels of trust and norms of reciprocity."[72] Communities with strong social cohesion also tend to have better health outcomes.[73] The positive effects of social relationships on health can begin in childhood and accumulate throughout a lifetime, impacting health through biological, social, and psychological pathways.[74] These cumulative effects would then be

---

72 Ichiro Kawachi and Lisa F. Berkman, "Social Epidemiology," in *Social Capital, Social Cohesion, and Health*, ed. Lisa F. Berkman, Ichiro Kawachi, and M. Maria Glymour, 2nd ed. (Oxford University Press, 2014), 175, https://oxfordmedicine.com/view/10.1093/med/9780195377903.001.0001/med-9780195377903-chapter-8.

73 Julianne Holt-Lunstad, Timothy B. Smith, and J. Bradley Layton, "Social Relationships and Mortality Risk: A Meta-Analytic Review," *PLOS Medicine* 7, no. 7 (2010): e1000316, https://doi.org/10.1371/journal.pmed.1000316.

74 Debra Umberson and Jennifer Karas Montez, "Social Relationships and Health: A Flash-

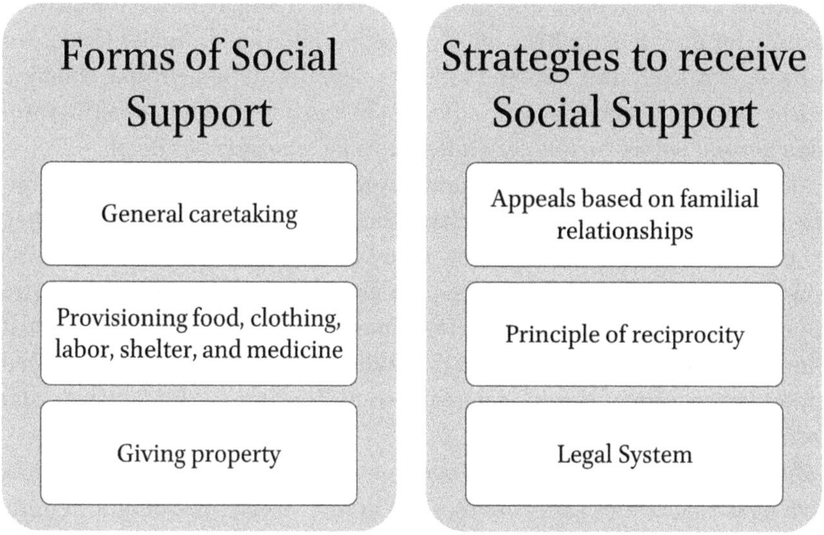

FIGURE 19 Forms and Strategies of Social Support at Deir el-Medina

visible in a person's physiological responses to stress where they would both encounter fewer stressors and be better equipped to fight stressors from childhood on.

The nature of the community enabled Deir el-Medina to have high levels of social cohesion because of the web of interrelationships within the village, including extended families that intermarried, lived near each other, and worked side-by-side. The community's physical and social boundaries clearly defined its membership, and the state support for the villagers meant that many social conflicts could be largely avoided. Parties and feasts emphasized the importance of reciprocity and made public the value and quantity of social ties individuals had and recorded in their gift-giving texts. Indeed, this makes tangible why the *Prohibitions* warn, "You should not celebrate your festival without your neighbours."[75] The need to secure social bonds through feasting was a strong, communal principle that acted as a glue for social cohesion at Deir el-Medina.

Social support at Deir el-Medina was further strengthened when individuals could leverage their family wealth and social ties to get support when they needed it by emphasizing familial duties and what might be lost if those tasks went unfulfilled. Wealth accumulated over multiple generations among

point for Health Policy," *Journal of Health and Social Behavior* 51, no. Suppl (2010): S54–66, https://doi.org/10.1177/0022146510383501.

75 Hagen, "The Prohibitions," 144.

families at Deir el-Medina, and people relied on intergenerational wealth to advocate for their health. *Nỉw.t-nḫt.tỉ*'s wealth—inherited from her father, her husband, and likely her husband's father—went on to benefit her children. Even her son *Nfr-ḥtp* (xvi) benefitted from *Nỉw.t-nḫt.tỉ*'s inherited wealth to provision himself before he was cut off from this income after her death.

Social cohesion and inherited family wealth at Deir el-Medina likely improved the villagers' health by stabilizing their access to food, clothing, shelter, and medicine. As people aged, they were buffered from occupational stress by having the means to retire, live in their children's household, and get extra support from their adult children. They may even have indirectly benefitted from the system by feeling confident in the continued existence of future social support in the form of communal emphasis on feasting, the legal system, and wisdom texts.

These factors translate to ways a community like Deir el-Medina evidences better health outcomes than communities in short-term, state-building efforts like those buried at the North Tombs Cemetery at Amarna or the workers buried in Giza. In these shorter-term settlements, where many residents may have been separated from their families, there was little opportunity for the community to generate intergenerational wealth and insufficient time to create a strong sense of social cohesion. Even if these communities shared similar values, like an emphasis on reciprocity, they may not have had the material wealth to enact the substantial social support they needed.

8 Physical Limitations and Social Support at Deir el-Medina

This chapter ends by looking at several examples of individuals at Deir el-Medina whose more extreme conditions do not appear in the texts but who would require the forms of social support described above. Topics like death are rarely discussed at Deir el-Medina, and debilitating injuries were not recorded in administrative records, perhaps because they did not serve a bureaucratic purpose. When a workman's injury was severe enough that they could never work again on the royal tombs, they would likely disappear from administrative records. Alternatively, if an individual was unable to join the workforce, their name might only come up in the smaller corpus of texts from daily life in the village outside of work.

Indeed, for these reasons, we need case studies from the human remains to identify physical limitations among the villagers. Deir el-Medina's location, nestled at the base of the Theban hills and relatively far from the Nile, meant that any form of walking impairment would be severely limiting. Yet, bioarchaeological evidence demonstrates several people at Deir el-Medina who had such impairments, in some cases since they were children. The following three examples are all from commingled remains found in TT 290 and TT 298 and thus represent experiences during or shortly after the Ramesside occupation of the site. All three examples are isolated, adult femora, making it difficult to estimate how old they were when they died. Even as isolated bones, however, these examples illustrate how the people of Deir el-Medina would have required social support for survival after a possibly fatal injury, with an injury leading to permanent disability, and with an impairment that began during childhood.

The first example involves a leg fracture of an adult male who died while the injury was still healing. The oblique fracture is located in the shaft of the proximal third of femur DEM 290.14.058 (Figure 20).[76] This femur was found in TT 290 and could consequently date anytime between the reign of Ramesses II and the early 21st Dynasty. The fracture is beveled and its color matches surrounding bone, suggesting a peri-mortem (i.e., around time of death) rather than post-mortem injury. There is no evidence of an attempted union with the proximal shaft, though there is increased irregularity in reactive bone formation at the posterior edge of the fracture and signs of rounding along the superior edge of the fracture. This active bony response further suggests the break was prior to death and the body had sufficient time to begin healing. The fracture edges are smooth, placing the injury at least one week before death or longer, as there are also extensive periosteal reactions covering the entire shaft which can slow down the healing response time.[77] Separately, there is osteoarthritis, evidenced through lipping and porosity, on both the medial and lateral condyles.

The extent of periosteal new bone formation on the femoral shaft despite the lack of healing at the fracture site also indicates that this individual may have been suffering from a disease before completely fracturing their femur. Most likely, within weeks or months of this break—which clearly prevented this individual from walking—he would have died. This complete fracture of the femur could have been pathological (i.e., a fracture occurring where the

---

76 Sex estimation for this element is based on distal epiphyseal breadth (86 mm) following univariate sexing criteria in Gretchen R. Dabbs, "Estimating the Sex of Ancient Egyptian Skeletal Remains: Methods from Tell El-Amarna," *Bioarchaeology of the Near East* 14 (2020): 11–26. Epiphyseal fusion suggests an adult, but age can otherwise not be determined.

77 Norman J. Sauer, "The Timing of Injuries and Manner of Death: Distinguishing among Antemortem, Perimortem and Postmortem Trauma," ed. Kathy Reichs, *Forensic Osteology: Advances in the Identification of Human Remains* 2 (1998): 321–331.

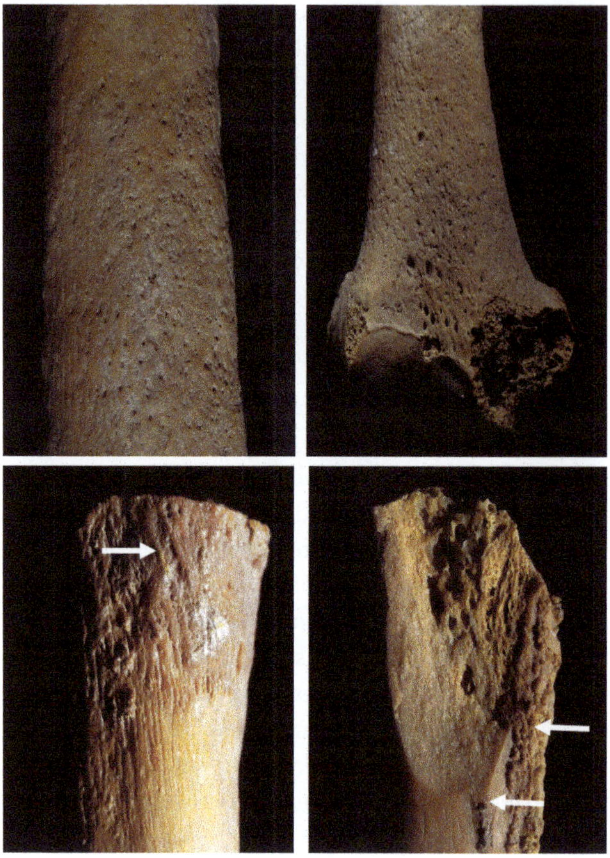

FIGURE 20 Peri-mortem fracture on femur DEM 290.14.058. Note the extensive periosteal reactions along the shaft (upper left and right) and near the anterior and posterior edges of the oblique fracture (lower left and right).

bone was already weakened by another disease) or the fracture could have been open (i.e., breaking through the skin) leading to extensive infection during the attempted healing process. In either case, the man would have been visibly impaired, never fully recovering from this injury.

Though this individual did not survive long after such a devastating injury, the extensive periosteal reactions present along the femur indicate some period of survival where he must have relied on social support from his community. This was a time when the individual could no longer work, and he would have relied on provisions, labor, and medicine from family and his community, mirroring the circumstances of *Pꜣy*, who relied on his son for medicine after losing some or all of his eyesight. Given the completeness of the fracture, this man may have also realized that he would never work again on the royal tombs. If he was a workman, he might have taken advantage of the social support of a son for regular rations just as the father of *Wsḫt-nmt.t* received a salary out of his son's rations after leaving the workforce.

Our second example is from an individual who survived long enough to fully heal from a severe leg fracture that was misaligned when it healed. Femur DEM 298.20.193, estimated to be that of an adult female,[78] exhibits a fully-healed fracture of the femoral shaft 12 cm below the femoral neck (Figure 21). The healed fracture is 6 cm long and contains three cloacae—openings that served as drainage channels during healing—located along the anterior, inferior, and medial edges of the femoral shaft. The fracture was misaligned when it healed, resulting in an abnormal angle in the femoral shaft below the fracture and transversely rotating the distal two-thirds of the femur. The result was that she had a noticeably different gait as her leg was bent and rotated along the middle of her thigh; the multiple cloacae would have led to visible swelling and possibly soft tissue lesions surrounding her leg. While she survived the fracture, she lived with this impairment for the rest of her life.

A woman with a severe fracture that permanently impacted her gait would likely need support with any tasks requiring extensive walking, though in this case, it would have been clear this support was required for the rest of her lifetime. We know women would turn to their family in times of need, just as *Tꜣ-ḫnty.t-šps.t* turned to her sister asking for help with getting and grinding grain after being berated by her husband. We also see how women who have had and raised children may have had an advantage, relying on the reciprocal care from their children for regular rations in their old age, just as *Nỉw.t-nḫt.tỉ* relied on the regular contributes of emmer and fat from her children.

These two examples rely on reciprocation from adult children to their parents. The final example focuses on an impairment that began in childhood or adolescence, necessitating care for most or all of the individual's life. The right femur DEM 291.14.013 of an individual estimated to be an adult male exhibits *coxa valga*, a condition describing an abnormally obtuse angle between the shaft and the femoral head[79] that is typical when "partial to complete paralysis

78 Sex estimation for this element is based on distal epiphyseal breadth (63 mm) and femoral head diameter (34 mm) following univariate sexing criteria in Dabbs, "Estimating the Sex of Ancient Egyptian Skeletal Remains: Methods from Tell El-Amarna"; Michelle H. Raxter, "Metric Sex Estimation in an Ancient Egyptian Skeletal Sample," *SAS Bulletin: Newsletter of the Society for Archaeological Sciences* 30, no. 4 (2007): 9–12. Epiphyseal fusion suggests an adult, but age can otherwise not be determined.

79 Tony Waldron, *Palaeopathology* (Cambridge: Cambridge University Press, 2008), 109.

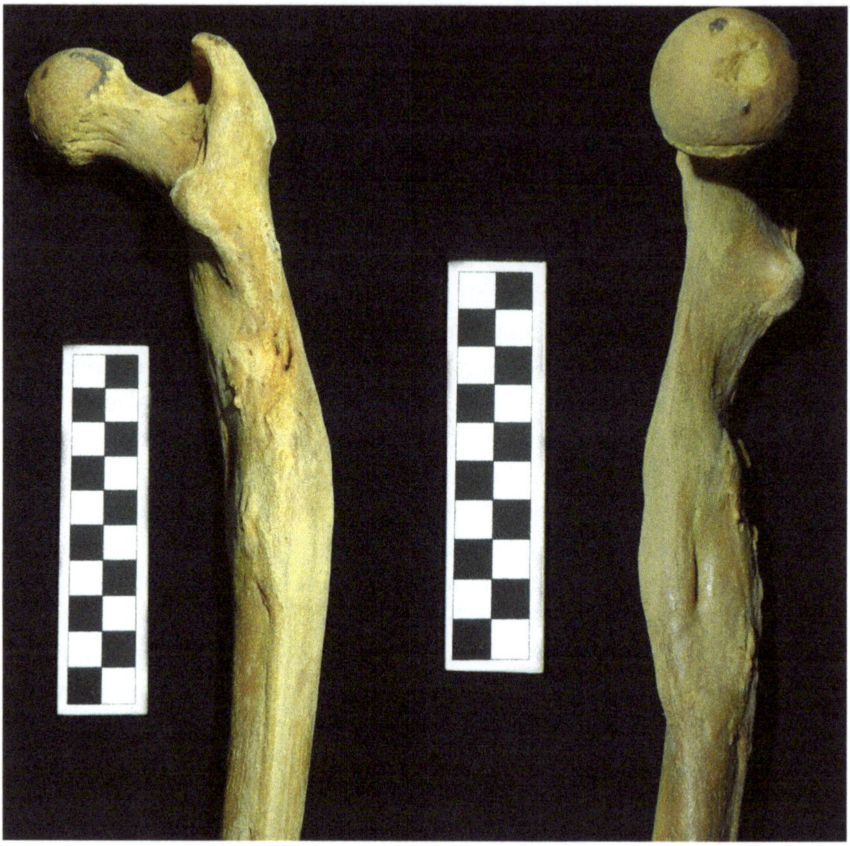

FIGURE 21 Fully-healed fracture of the femoral shaft on DEM 298.20.193, estimated to be the femur of an adult woman

of the limb occurs during the growth phase."[80] The right femur DEM 290.14.013 (Figure 22) has an angle between the femoral shaft and head exceeding 145°, the greater trochanters is elongated, and its surface surrounding the insertion site for the *gluteus medius* muscle shows microporosity and irregular growth and flattening when compared to a normally developed femur.[81] The plane of the greater trochanter also shifts from an angle that would normally be perpendicular to the acetabulum, to one that is nearly vertical. Additionally, there is an anterolateral bend in the shaft—a condition that more commonly occurs

80 Donald J. Ortner, *Identification of Pathological Conditions in Human Skeletal Remains*, 2nd ed. (San Diego: Academic Press, 2003), 291.

81 This description mirrors an example of postparalytic *coxa valga* as a result of poliomyelitis in Ortner, 477.

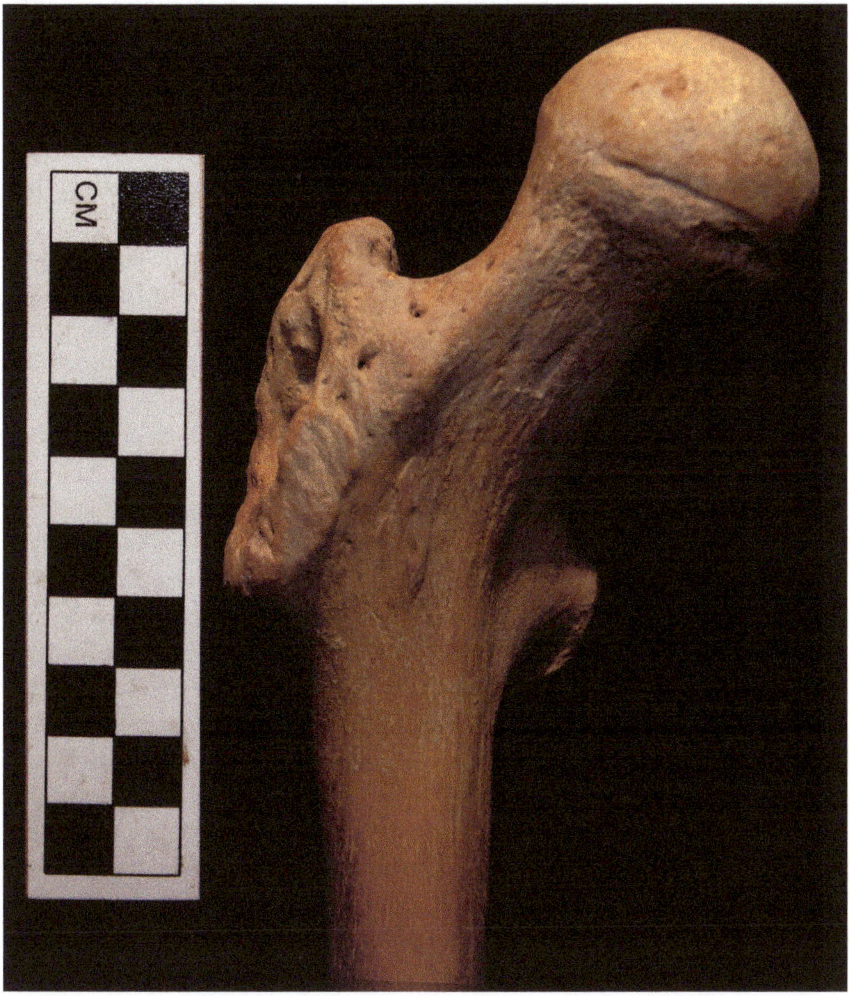

FIGURE 22 Coxa Valga present on DeM 291.14.013 estimated to belong to an adult male

if the leg was not weight-bearing during development. There is also little evidence of consistent muscle use in the lower limb. There is no evidence of joint degeneration, and the *intertrochanteric line* and *linea aspera* are both faint with relatively little rugosity. In combination, the lack of visible use and presence of *coxa valga* make it clear that this leg was not used for weight-bearing.

Coxa valga can occur in neuromuscular disorders, infectious diseases, metabolic conditions, or any disease that results in paralysis of the lower limb.[82]

82 Ortner, *Identification of Pathological Conditions in Human Skeletal Remains*, p. 261.

Coxa valga is not only more likely to manifest after paralysis of the leg, but afterward impairs adduction,[83] leading to a lifetime of limited mobility. It develops because paralysis reduces stimulation of growth along the trochanteric growth plate and femoral neck, causing the femoral neck to continue to lengthen along an axis more parallel with the femoral shaft.[84] It is consequently a deformity that must occur due to paralysis in childhood or early adolescence rather than adulthood.

One of the most common disorders associated with *coxa valga* is poliomyelitis. Globally, the earliest evidence for the poliovirus comes from Thebes in the New Kingdom; the stela of Roma shows a depiction of Roma with a shortened and atrophied leg that has elsewhere been conjectured as poliomyelitis.[85] The 19th Dynasty king Siptah had a shortened and atrophied right leg, which was suggested to be the result of poliomyelitis,[86] though both of these examples are circumstantial.

Regardless of whether the etiology of this case of *coxa valga* was poliomyelitis or another disorder, its presence suggests that this individual had paralysis in the lower limb and that this condition started when he was a teenager or younger. With at least one paralyzed leg, he would not have been able to hike outside of the village and, therefore, would never have been able to participate in work on the tombs even though this was the *raison-d'être* of the Deir el-Medina community. He could have contributed to the commissioned work completed within the village but would still need support acquiring such work from outside the village. From an early age, his family would have known that he would have regularly required such social support to get provisions, but without the benefit of the examples above where the individuals could have already invested the time and wealth into family necessary in order to have their care reciprocated. Despite this limitation, he was included in the family tomb and buried as a member of the community, suggesting that social support can extend far beyond reciprocation.

These physical limitations, therefore, would have made it difficult for these three people from Deir el-Medina to survive without the kinds of social support referenced in the texts. A man with *coxa valga*, who would have been unable

---

83 E. Barnes, *Atlas of Developmental Field Anomalies of the Human Skeleton: A Paleopathology Perspective*, (John Wiley & Sons, 2012), p. 168.

84 Resnick, *Bone and joint imaging*, p. 918.

85 Harold V. Wyatt, "Poliomyelitis," in *The Cambridge World History of Human Disease*, ed. Kenneth F. Kiple (New York: Cambridge University Press, 1993), 947.

86 James E. Harris and Kent R. Weeks, *X-Raying the Pharaohs* (New York: Charles Scribner's Sons, 1973).

to provide for himself economically, would have regularly relied on provisions from family or friends, just as *Nfr-ḥtp* (xvi) relied on his mother to support him even as an adult. A woman with such a severe fracture that she could no longer walk the same again would similarly need support with preparing and getting food, just as *Tꜣ-ḫnty.t-šps.t* wrote to her sister asking for help preparing bread. And a man who died with a fracture that never fully healed would have been suddenly unable to work. He likely would have searched for both medical relief and economic support with such an acute and severe injury, just as the father *Pꜣy* asked his son for medicine and just as the father of *Wsḫt-nmt.t* received a salary out of his son's rations after leaving the workforce.

The three osteological examples demonstrate the kind of debilitating injuries and conditions that could prevent men and women at Deir el-Medina from hiking in the Theban cliffs or walking to the river, places they would need to access if they were to participate in the royal workforce or buy and sell goods at the local market. For men, this was particularly disastrous because these physical impairments were also economic ones, making it difficult, if not impossible, for them to independently earn a living. Women may have fared better with these physical limitations since they spent considerably more time within the village, and they could still partake in many time-consuming household tasks[87] such as making cloth and may have even been able to sell some goods locally.[88] Any impaired individual may have needed extra support, especially around preparing food like bread and beer or planting and harvesting in the agricultural fields outside the village (see Chapter 7). The state support for the village, however, meant they did not have to complete some common household tasks, like laundering clothing in the Nile, that would have been more difficult with such physical impairments.

9 Social Support and Health Outcomes at Deir el-Medina

Textual evidence of social support and traumatic injuries in human remains demonstrate concrete ways social support benefitted health at Deir el-Medina. Research on social support in modern populations suggests that the kinds of support offered at Deir el-Medina—including caretaking, provisioning of necessities, and giving property—as well as the strong social cohesion within

87 For a more comprehensive review of the kinds of tasks women might perform at Deir el-Medina as well as their potential physical requirements, see Sweeney, "Women Growing Older at Deir El-Medina."

88 Toivari-Viitala, *Women at Deir El-Medina*, 233.

the community affected the health of the residents of Deir el-Medina in many of the same ways modern people benefit from social support. Modern health studies indicate that social support buffers stress by helping individuals overcome new stressors, creating conditions that prevent people from encountering stressors, and lessening the impact of stressors through stronger emotionally sustaining behaviors. At Deir el-Medina, we see examples of social support that mirror each of these buffering mechanisms. When a father was ill, he asked his son to get him medical ingredients, buffering the negative impacts of his perceived blindness. When *Nỉw.t-nḫt.tỉ*'s husband *Ḫꜥ-m-Nwn* retired, he did not even encounter the stress of a lost income because his wife had already secured a regular stipend from their son, *Ḳn-ḥr-ḫpš⸗f* (iv). New parents could rely on expectations of gift-giving feasts soon after childbirth to assure them that their community would offer social support during this tenuous period.

Social support can thus be used to explain several health patterns seen in Chapter 4. Strong social cohesion explains why at Deir el-Medina, enamel hypoplasias are so low and why there is so little variation in stature across tombs. This social cohesion allowed villagers to support new families and those outside of the workforce with regular meals, clothing, and even housing. Simultaneously, the use of intergenerational wealth to promote social support also explains why wealth could create health in ancient Egypt more broadly. Intergenerational wealth ensured social support was offered through giving or withholding property in wills.

This chapter does not, however, explain two broader trends identified in Chapter 4. First, it remains ambiguous whether social support at Deir el-Medina would be stronger than for those buried in elite cemeteries. These individuals had more intergenerational wealth to rely on, though perhaps not as strong a sense of community as the residents of Deir el-Medina. So how can we otherwise explain why those at Deir el-Medina sometimes had better health outcomes than their elite counterparts? Second, this chapter offers little to explain why and how health discrepancies grew in adulthood as men joined the workforce.

To address these two trends, the next chapter focuses on healthcare access by discussing working conditions and access to medical care at Deir el-Medina. While this chapter focuses on the role of the community, the next chapter demonstrates how the Egyptian state's investment in the Deir el-Medina community unusually benefitted their health outcomes.

CHAPTER 6

Accessing Healthcare

The people of Deir el-Medina buffered stress equitably, especially during adolescence, as their low variation in stature evidenced (see Chapter 4). Additionally, many members of the community were able to successfully recover from significant injuries, given that the vast majority of fractures were fully healed, including one example of a fully healed complete fracture in the femur of a woman from the last chapter. Together, these attributes suggest that the people of Deir el-Medina show remarkable similarities and equity when it comes to certain measurable health outcomes and that they had the knowledge, skill, and resources to treat potentially life-threatening injuries successfully. This chapter focuses on how equitable healthcare access offers insights into both equitable health outcomes and successful medical interventions in the village.

I begin this chapter by explaining how healthcare access impacts health across populations. While this connection may seem straightforward, it is complicated by cross-cultural definitions of medicine and the factors influencing healthcare access. Identifying the forms of healthcare professionals present in the village makes it possible to evaluate the structures of healthcare access at Deir el-Medina. Equally important to healthcare professionals is evidence for medical literacy at Deir el-Medina, since it predicts when and how often people can access healthcare and their personal actions to manage health issues. My sources include the papyri and ostraca mentioning illnesses and treatments, which clarify the actual forms of medical care sought and provided at Deir el-Medina. The chapter ends with three case studies from the human remains to complement the textual evidence for medical care. These three examples illustrate cases where ancient Egyptian medical knowledge reflects the successful and unsuccessful health outcomes seen in human remains. Across the chapter, evidence for healthcare access demonstrates that the villagers at Deir el-Medina maintained their health by using both state resources and private knowledge to tailor treatments and care to the kinds of injuries and illnesses common in the village.

1 Linking Healthcare Access to Community Health Outcomes

To understand healthcare access at Deir el-Medina, it is necessary to understand what kind of healthcare system existed for the villagers, if any at all.

 | DOI:10.1163/9789004700871_007

Medical anthropologists approach this task by defining healthcare as the myriad ways a society treats illnesses. Kleinman has grouped these into three relevant sectors: popular, professional, and folk care.[1] In this framework, popular care constitutes the ways individuals seek out treatments for illnesses within their support networks (i.e., caretaking in Chapter 5). Professional healthcare, instead, constitutes treatments from those specially trained in medicine. Finally, individuals may seek treatments from folk care-practitioners who function as healers without requiring formal medical training. Healthcare, by this definition, requires designated providers, specialized knowledge, and a systematic means for ensuring access to these resources.

While the quality of medical care people receive can clearly impact health outcomes, equitable *access* to these services is another key *Social Determinant of Health* used to explain health patterns across cultures. Equitable healthcare access may hinge on culturally-specific criteria such as whether or not an individual is insured or whether specific healthcare providers offer services to a community.[2] Access may also be limited due to biases in treatment where groups are systematically denied relevant or equal treatment in medical contexts.[3] Equitable access includes whether healthcare services are equally available, of similar quality, and financially accessible—but also whether issues of access are related to healthcare needs, utilization, or both. Essentially, healthcare access can be limited because people may not be aware of when to seek assistance, and when they do, providers may not offer the same treatments to all their patients.

The impacts of healthcare access on health outcomes are not just a byproduct of the efficacy of healthcare interventions but also the relationship between healthcare professionals and their patients, as well as the patient's own awareness and ability to seek healthcare when needed. In a 25-year study comparing insured and uninsured adults in the U.S., the mortality rate for adults without insurance was almost double those who were insured, and the higher mortality rate of the uninsured persisted even after considering related factors such

1 Arthur Kleinman, *Patients and Healers in the Context of Culture: An Exploration of the Borderland Between Anthropology, Medicine, and Psychiatry* (Berkeley: University of California Press, 1980).

2 Maria Goddard and Peter Smith, "Equity of Access to Health Care Services: Theory and Evidence from the UK," *Social Science & Medicine* 53, no. 9 (2001): 1149–1162, https://doi.org/10.1016/S0277-9536(00)00415-9.

3 Brian D. Smedley, Adrienne Y. Stith, and Alan R. Nelson, eds., *Unequal Treatment: Confronting Racial and Ethnic Disparities in Health Care* (Washington, D.C.: National Academies Press, 2003).

as age, income, education, and perceived health.[4] Regardless of insurance status, the indirect costs of receiving healthcare (e.g., lost wages, transportation costs, lack of employer sick days)[5] are another barrier that prevents people from seeking healthcare when they have an illness.[6] When individuals from rural communities have to travel further to receive appropriate care, they also experience negative health outcomes including higher rates of hospitalizations because they did not receive earlier interventions.[7] These impacts have been found in a variety of cultural contexts and not just in the United States.[8]

Literacy also mediates healthcare access because individuals with more health literacy can navigate healthcare more successfully. Health literacy includes the ability to read, write, and understand healthcare information as well as the "infrastructure, policies, processes, materials and relationships" necessary to navigate, understand, and use health information to improve health.[9] Understanding medical literacy requires culturally-specific definitions of medicine. Consequently, researchers on modern populations must integrate local medicine and biomedicine when evaluating what constitutes health literacy.[10] Barriers to health literacy can ultimately become barriers to healthcare

4 Peter Franks, Carolyn M. Clancy, and Marthe R. Gold, "Health Insurance and Mortality. Evidence from a National Cohort," *Journal of the American Medical Association* 270, no. 6 (1993): 737–741, https://doi.org/10.1001/jama.1993.03510060083037.

5 Robyn Panther Gleason and Shawn M. Kneipp, "Employment-Related Constraints: Determinants of Primary Health Care Access?," *Policy, Politics, & Nursing Practice* 5, no. 2 (May 2004): 73–83, https://doi.org/10.1177/1527154404263265; Samina T. Syed, Ben S. Gerber, and Lisa K. Sharp, "Traveling Towards Disease: Transportation Barriers to Health Care Access," *Journal of Community Health* 38, no. 5 (October 2013): 976–993, https://doi.org/10.1007/s10900-013-9681-1.

6 Kirsty B. Hill et al., "Adult Dental Health Survey 2009: Relationships between Dental Attendance, Patterns Oral Health Behaviour and the Current Barriers to Dental Care," *British Dental Journal* 214, no. 1 (2013): 25–32, https://doi.org/10.1038/sj.bdj.2012.1176.

7 Nathan Douthit et al., "Exposing Some Important Barriers to Health Care Access in the Rural USA," *Public Health* 129, no. 6 (June 2015): 611–620, https://doi.org/10.1016/j.puhe.2015.04.001.

8 For example, Margaret S. Winchester and Brian King, "Decentralization, Healthcare Access, and Inequality in Mpumalanga, South Africa," *Health & Place* 51 (2018): 200–207, https://doi.org/10.1016/j.healthplace.2018.02.009; Xufan Zhang et al., "Urban-Rural Differences in the Association between Access to Healthcare and Health Outcomes among Older Adults in China," *BMC Geriatrics* 17, no. 1 (2017): 151, https://doi.org/10.1186/s12877-017-0538-9.

9 Orkan Okan et al., eds., *International Handbook of Health Literacy: Research, Practice and Policy across the Lifespan* (Bristol: Policy Press, 2019), 13.

10 Zhiyi Qian et al., "Understanding Health Literacy from a Traditional Chinese Medicine Perspective," *Journal of Integrative Medicine* 21, no. 3 (2023): 215–220, https://doi.org/10.1016/j.joim.2023.03.001.

because they impact how and whether individuals advocate for healthcare, both in conversations with providers and through home interventions. Medical literacy includes cross-cultural differences in communication, with immigrants facing both language and cultural communication barriers to healthcare access.[11] Communities with lower abilities to read and write to healthcare professionals also have lower self-perceived health and more physical impairments,[12] demonstrating that medical literacy also impacts health outcomes.

Equitable healthcare access is a useful way for researchers to understand *hidden heterogeneity in frailty* because it offers a causal explanation for underlying patterns in health outcomes within larger populations. Differences in health outcomes by race, ethnicity, indigeneity, socioeconomic status, and employment can be linked to barriers in access to healthcare. While these patterns relate to the quality and nature of the care patients receive, they also relate to the direct benefits of participating in a therapeutic encounter, which can reduce pain, stress, and anxiety.[13] Therefore, these benefits can persist even if medical treatments are otherwise ineffective. In ancient Egypt, where healthcare often required close, direct interactions between a patient and practitioner, one might expect these same kinds of benefits. Assessing both the structure of healthcare and healthcare access, therefore, offers a useful way to explain patterns in health outcomes in past populations, where one might expect benefits from both therapeutic interactions and the kinds of treatments and pharmacological ingredients used.

2 Healthcare Professionals at Deir el-Medina

In order to understand healthcare access at Deir el-Medina, it is important to establish what healthcare existed in the village—how did the people of Deir el-Medina treat illnesses? This includes the forms of treatment, providers, and healers whom people in the village sought when they were ill. Administrative, medical, and personal texts that mention individuals who treated illnesses sug-

11 Lenore Manderson and Pascale Allotey, "Cultural Politics and Clinical Competence in Australian Health Services," *Anthropology & Medicine* 10, no. 1 (2003): 71–85, https://doi.org/10.1080/13648470301266.

12 Miranda R. Andrus and Mary T. Roth, "Health Literacy: A Review," *Pharmacotherapy: The Journal of Human Pharmacology and Drug Therapy* 22, no. 3 (2002): 282–302, https://doi.org/10.1592/phco.22.5.282.33191.

13 Franklin G. Miller, Luana Colloca, and Ted J. Kaptchuk, "The Placebo Effect: Illness and Interpersonal Healing," *Perspectives in Biology and Medicine* 52, no. 4 (2009): 518, https://doi.org/10.1353/pbm.0.0115.

gest that professional, folk, and popular healthcare all existed in the village. These texts identify several individuals within the village who were mentioned multiple times in the context of healthcare and who likely served the professional and folk sectors of healthcare at the site. By evaluating where these individuals are mentioned, whom they treated, and their modalities of treatment, it is possible to partially reconstruct the forms of healthcare available more broadly at Deir el-Medina.

2.1 *Finding the* zwn.w *at Deir el-Medina*

Dozens of texts from Deir el-Medina[14] mention a *zwn.w*, referring to a formal, professional practitioner who used magical, surgical, and pharmacological skills to treat illness. The title *zwn.w* was in use throughout Pharaonic history,[15] and has generally been translated as "doctor" or "physician" based on its association with healing and medicine.[16] The *zwn.w* were associated with the applications of topical remedies and prescriptions, usually denoted as *pẖr.t* or *zp.w*,[17] though they also can perform surgical interventions.[18] They also used magical recitations side-by-side with these others healing acts.[19] Their specialized knowledge was treated as a secret of their training.[20] Treatments by the *zwn.w*

---

14 Gabler has published a comprehensive table of texts from Deir el-Medina referencing the *zwn.w*. See Gabler, *Who's Who around Deir el-Medina*, tbl. 19b.

15 An initial catalog of individuals with the title *zwn.w* was published in Frans Jonckheere, *Les Médecins de l'Egypte Pharaonique: Essai de Prosopographie*, La Médecine Égyptienne 3 (Bruxelles: Fondation égyptologique reine Élisabeth, 1958). This was then expanded upon by other scholars and included in a tabulated compendium in John F. Nunn, *Ancient Egyptian Medicine* (Norman: University of Oklahoma Press, 1996), 211–214.

16 Paul Ghalioungui, *La Médecine Des Pharaons: Magie et science medicale dans l'Egypte ancienne* (Paris: Robert Laffont, 1983); Bruno Halioua, Bernard Ziskind, and M.B. DeBevoise, *Medicine in the Days of the Pharaohs* (Cambridge: Belknap Press of Harvard University Press, 2005); Jonckheere, *Les Médecins de l'Egypte Pharaonique*; Nunn, *Ancient Egyptian Medicine*.

17 P. Ebers 156 suggests that these remedies (*pẖr.t*) were the specific "craft of the *zwn.w*" (*ḥmw.t zwn.w*).

18 The *zwn.w* is mentioned in cases involving surgical procedures (P. Ebers 501, 69.9) and bandaging wounds (P. Edwin Smith 9, 5.4).

19 As evidenced by recitations specified within a treatment (e.g., P. Edwin Smith, case 9), or by the integration of recitations more generally as discussed in: Hans-Werner Fischer-Elfert, ed., "Pap. Ebers Nr. 1–3—Reflexionen eines altägyptischen Heilers über seine Initiation?," in *Papyrus Ebers und die antike Heilkunde: Akten der Tagung vom 15.–16. 3. 2002 in der Albertina/UB der Universität Leipzig*, Marburger altertumskundliche Abhandlungen 7 (Wiesbaden: Harrassowitz Verlag, 2005), 133–148.

20 Further, P. Ebers 188 and 206 both suggest that the *zwn.w* specifically possessed the knowledge necessary to compose these remedies: *ỉrỉ.ḫr=k zp n sštꜣ n sm.yt jrr.w zwn.w*, "Then you should make a secret herbal remedy which the *zwn.w* makes" (P. Ebers 188, 36.10);

were made more effective through speech inspired by the divine, as in P. Ebers 1.8–1.9:[21] *ỉw⸗f dỉ⸗f mdwỉ.t drf ỉrỉ⸗f dmḏ.t ḏỉ⸗f ꜣḫ n rḫ.w-(ỉ)ḫ.t n zwn.w* "He (Thoth) is the one who caused writing to be spoken, he makes a collection, he gives efficacy to the knowledgeable,[22] to the *zwn.w*." Consequently, individuals sought the special knowledge of the *zwn.w* to treat their illnesses through remedies, recitations, and surgery, though notably, these treatments did not differentiate between religion, magic, and medicine.[23]

At Deir el-Medina, eight individuals held the title *zwn.w*: *Pꜣ-ḥr.y-pḏ.t* (iii), *Pꜣ-ꜥn*, *Knr*, *Ḥr-s.t-ỉt⸗f*, *Mnw-ḫꜥ*, *Pwr/Pw-rꜥ* (i) or *Nwr/Nw-rꜣ* (using the otherwise unattested version of the title *wr zwn.w*[24]), *Dỉ-ꞽImn-wꜣs.t*, and *Jmn-ḥtp* (xiv).[25] It was typical to identify the *zwn.w* without name, and even among these eight instances, not all are explicitly given this title.[26] Those identified as *zwn.w* lived between the reign of Ramesses II and the 21st Dynasty, with no clear overlap between individuals. Additionally, ration texts frequently mention only the title without a name using the definite article (*pꜣ*), suggesting that there would have only been one person appointed at a time as the village *zwn.w*.[27] The lack of overlapping men carrying the title suggests the role was successive throughout the Ramesside period with one *zwn.w* for the workforce.[28] Finally, the *zwn.w* are most frequently mentioned in the context of bureaucratic texts for the workforce, such as absence lists and grain rations, indicating they were usually a member of the workforce.

ỉrỉ.ḫr⸗k n⸗f zp.w n.w s(š)tꜣ r ẖr zwn.w wpw-r sꜣ.t⸗k ḏs⸗k, "Then you should make for him a remedy (that is even) a secret from an assistant of the *zwn.w* except for your own daughter" (P. Ebers 206, 42.5–42.6). This may lend authority to both the *zwn.w* and the texts, increasing their value as specialized knowledge.

21 A parallel passage exists in P. Hearst 78, 6 and 9–10.

22 Literally translated as "the one who knows things," which Ritner takes to indicate secret and sacred knowledge with specifically religious and magical overtones. See Robert K. Ritner, *The Mechanics of Ancient Egyptian Magical Practice*, Studies in Ancient Oriental Civilization 54 (Chicago: The Oriental Institute of the University of Chicago, 1993), 229–230.

23 James Allen, *The Art of Medicine in Ancient Egypt* (New York: Metropolitan Museum of Art, 2005), 102. For further information on the blurring between these professional titles, see Halioua, Ziskind, and DeBevoise, *Medicine in the Days of the Pharaohs*, 11–12.

24 Gabler, *Who's Who around Deir el-Medina*, 400.

25 For a list of attestations of each name, see Gabler, tbl. 19a; Janssen, *Village Varia*, 1997, 26–27.

26 See discussion of *Pꜣ-ḥr.y-pḏ.t* (iii) below.

27 Gabler, *Who's Who around Deir el-Medina*, 399.

28 One text, O. Berlin P 14264, has been interpreted as indicating the *zwn.w* was from outside the community, but Gabler and McDowell effectively argue that this is meant to indicate the *zwn.w*, in this instance, was not present rather than from another town. For further discussion, see Gabler, 402. Additionally, Gabler notes that the *zwn.w* was frequently listed from the left-side of the crew, though not invariably.

Texts mentioning the *zwn.w* at Deir el-Medina document his ration distributions but are only partially illustrative of his role in the village. Of ostraca and papyri relating to the title *zwn.w*, the plurality are grain ration texts. Of the remaining texts, three are too fragmentary for analysis leaving only eight non-ration texts explicitly mentioning the *zwn.w* with contents we can reconstruct. These include letters, absence records,[29] and one legal text.

These texts demonstrate that the Egyptian state fiscally supported the services of the *zwn.w* and his expertise through supplementary rations. Grain rations mentioning the *zwn.w* present a much smaller payment than that given out to workmen, the scribe, or the foremen; Janssen has, however, interpreted this amount as an additional payment on top of a pre-existing salary as a workman,[30] thus making the pay for the *zwn.w* more than an average workman but less than foremen and scribes. Given mentions of the *zwn.w* in ration distributions, it is likely he was a member of the village and a workman who was permitted absences from work to prepare remedies and treat other members of the community.[31]

As well as excused time from working on the tomb, the *zwn.w* also had an assistant to prepare medications and treat illnesses. Ironically, the text that gives us the most insight into the *zwn.w* at Deir el-Medina does not explicitly use the title. O. BM 5634 contains several absences by the workman *Pꜣ-ḥr.y-pḏ.t* (iii) related to caretaking and the production of medicine (*pḫr.t*), though he is never given the title *zwn.w* nor is this title ever attributed to him in other texts.[32] Scholars have, nonetheless, assumed *Pꜣ-ḥr.y-pḏ.t* (iii) was the village *zwn.w* based on his absences from work.[33] In some cases, he was even allowed the help of another workman to assist with producing these remedies (e.g., *Ḫnsw* in O. BM 5634).[34] Given how literate a *zwn.w* must have been to use and acquire medical texts, it may have been an attractive alternative to other exclusive positions for the literate such as the scribe.

29 O. BM 5634 is included in this list, under the assumption that *Pꜣ-ḥr.y-pḏ.t* (iii) was the village *zwn.w* during year 40 of Ramesses II, a point discussed in more detail below.

30 Janssen, *Commodity Prices from the Ramessid Period*, 460.

31 For more discussion of the position of the zwn.w within the workforce, see Gabler, *Who's Who around Deir el-Medina*, 398–407.

32 No other published texts link *Pꜣ-ḥr.y-pḏ.t* (iii) with the title *zwn.w*. The following unpublished texts require further examination: O. IFAO 181, O. IFAO 449, O. IFAO 488, O. IFAO 901, O. IFAO 1461, and O. IFAO 1467.

33 Janssen, "Absence from Work by the Necropolis Workmen of Thebes."

34 The assistant could have also been in an apprenticeship to become a *zwn.w*, though the lack of references to the names of individuals with this title makes this impossible to test.

The absences in O. BM 5634 further suggest that the *zwn.w* could treat both the workmen and their families. In O. BM 5634, *Pꜣ-ḥr.y-pḏ.t* (iii)'s longest consecutive absence for preparing medicine is from I *šm.w* 25 to II *šm.w* 8, a period of 13 days, to prepare remedies for the scribe's wife. This extended absence might have been necessary if the ingredients for the remedies had to be acquired outside of the community, if *Pꜣ-ḥr.y-pḏ.t* (iii) had to consult medical compendia unavailable at Deir el-Medina, or if his absences included the time for treatment. As the *zwn.w* was given rations and days off to attend to the workmen and their families, being a member of the community of Deir el-Medina was itself a prerequisite for healthcare access.

The broader use of *zwn.w* is further supported by O. Wente, which offers insight into who was able to access services of the community specifically in cases of illness.[35] In this text, the author demands that *Mnṯw-ms* acquire a goat for his wife who is sick. He ends the letter arguing, "I'm not aware that I have been removed from the necropolis community!" (*bw rḫ=ỉ r-ḏd jṯꜣ.tw=⟨ỉ⟩ ⟨m⟩ pꜣ ḫr*).[36] If Wente's reconstruction of this line is correct, it suggests that the workman is emphasizing that the benefits he receives as a member of the necropolis community include the services of the police captain to assist in getting a goat for his sick wife. This fits into the broader roles of support staff in servicing not just the workmen, but their families as part of the village community. These benefits thus likely extended to include other positions compensated with regular rations.

In O. BM 5634, *Pꜣ-ḥr.y-pḏ.t* (iii) was also excused from work to care for sick colleagues and prepare their medicinal treatments. He was absent from III *ꜣḫ.t* 21 to IV *ꜣḫ.t* 17, nearly an entire month, to take care of *ꜥꜣ-pḥ.t.y*, who was sick at this time. His shorter absences on III *šm.w* 3 and III *pr.t* 25–27, in contrast, show that some remedies could be prepared in a day or two.[37] In several other instances, workmen were sick for extended periods, and *Pꜣ-ḥr.y-pḏ.t* (iii) was not a caretaker. Other workmen could be out to care for sick colleagues and family members for shorter periods such as *Pn-nbw* (i) who was caring for his sick mother on IV *pr.t* 24–25. These examples reinforce that the professional care of the *zwn.w* was simply one component of the broader village healthcare

35 Translation from Wente, *Letters from Ancient Egypt*, 143; Edward F. Wente, "A Goat for an Ailing Woman (Ostracon Wente)," in *Studies in Honor of William Kelly Simpson*, ed. Peter Der Manuelian, vol. 2 (Boston: Boston Museum of Fine Arts, 1996), 855–867.

36 The final line reads: *bw rḫ=ỉ r-ḏd jṯꜣ=tw pꜣ ḫr*. Wente suggests the following alterations to make sense of the text: *bw rḫ=ỉ r-ḏd jṯꜣ.tw=⟨ỉ⟩ ⟨m⟩ pꜣ ḫr*, "I did not know that I was removed from the necropolis" in Wente, "A Goat for an Ailing Woman (Ostracon Wente)."

37 In both of these examples, he prepares the remedies with his fellow workman *Ḫnsw*.

and that others in the community could be sought as caretakers or specialists when colleagues and family members were ill (Chapter 5).

The *zwn.w* may also have benefited from private payments on top of their additional rations since certain texts mention items privately delivered to the *zwn.w*, though they often lack information about why and from whom the items were distributed. In O. DEM 788, the *zwn.w Knr* receives *nḥḥ*-oil[38] and fat (*ꜥḏ*) from an unknown sender. These items could have been part of a normal distribution to the workforce, in which case the government would still have made the payment.[39] Alternatively, these could have been a previously agreed upon private payment from an individual to the *zwn.w*.[40] The oil and fat also could have been a transaction between the *zwn.w* and the sender based on a separate agreement, unrelated to medicine. As a final option, these could have been given to the *zwn.w* to be used for medical purposes, perhaps because the sender required the *zwn.w* to use them to treat himself/herself, or a sick friend or relative. The use of fat (*ꜥḏ*) in medical texts is well attested,[41] while the use of *nḥḥ*-oil is relatively rare.[42] *Knr* is also involved in other exchanges of commodities such as bread (e.g., O. Berlin P 14254), and such exchanges could be unrelated to his role as *zwn.w*.

The Turin Strike Papyrus (P. Turin Cat. 1880)[43] offers clearer evidence for private payments to the *zwn.w*,[44] though it is similarly unclear why the *zwn.w*

---

38 By the reign of Ramesses III, *nḥḥ*-oil was used to describe a high-quality oil that likely often was olive oil, but could also refer to high-quality sesame oil. See Jose Alba Gomez, "Some Oils in Ancient Egypt: Debate between Moringa, Olive and Sesame Oils," in *Olive Oil and Wine Production in Eastern Mediterranean during Antiquity: International Symposium Proceedings, 17–19 November 2011, Urla–Turkey*, ed. Adnan Diler, Ahmet Kaan Şenol, and Ümit Aydınoğlu (İzmir: Ege Üniversitesi Basımevi, 2015), 209–220.

39 The presence of administrative records documenting the distribution of sesame oil (e.g., P. Turin 1894) and fat (e.g., P. Turin Cat 2044, recto 3.9) indicate these were part of normal administrative distributions.

40 The lack of a specified amount suggests that, if used as payment, the amount of oil and fat were already known to the doctor and did not need to be specified.

41 Hermann Grapow, Wolfhart Westendorf, and Hildegard von Deines, *Grundriss der Medizin der alten Ägypter*, vol. 6 (Berlin: Akademie-Verlag, 1959), 115–121.

42 Grapow, Westendorf, and Deines, 6:311.

43 Translation and transliteration based on transcription in Alan H. Gardiner, *Ramesside Administrative Documents* (Oxford: Oxford University Press, 1948), 47–48.

44 The practice of using one's specialized skills and even work days for private commissions was common at Deir el-Medina, and well-attested in the commissioning of private funerary arts, see Kathlyn M. Cooney, *The Cost of Death: The Social and Economic Value of Ancient Egyptian Funerary Art in the Rameside Period*, Egyptologische Uitgaven 22 (Leiden: Nederlands Instituut voor het Nabije Oosten, 2007). Even though the *zwn.w* was paid only a supplementary ration, his title and status may have afforded him additional profitable

needed to be paid. The *zwn.w* is allocated a variety of items from *Wsr-ḥ3.t* with a total value of 20 deben.[45] The payment for the *zwn.w* was equivalent to slightly less than two months' grain rations.[46] While some scholars have conjectured that this payment represents a very high sum,[47] the lack of supplementary information makes this claim impossible to assess. After these two distributions are detailed, the text continues with an oath made in front of the court (verso 6.4–6.5): *w3ḥ ʾImn w3ḥ p3 ḥḳ3 ʿ.w.s bn i͗.i͗n.tw t3y=i͗ 3 ẖrd.w ḥr.r=i͗ bn i͗.i͗n.tw=i͗ ḥr.r=w* "As Amun endures and as the king, L.P.H., endures, my three daughters shall not be taken from me and I shall not be taken from them."[48] The nature of these payments seems to be related to *Wsr-ḥ3.t*'s oath, and McDowell suggested that, "it is perhaps not too fanciful to conjecture that Weser-hat's wife had died in childbirth, leaving the widower to care for their three children."[49] If these payments were indeed for a doctor's services, it would be difficult to determine why, in this solitary instance, *Wsr-ḥ3.t* was required to make payments. It is possible that this was required if *Wsr-ḥ3.t* was not a workman at all nor a current member of the Deir el-Medina community.[50] Alternatively, this text could involve a private property settlement unrelated to the responsibilities of a physician.[51] These few and ambiguous payments to the *zwn.w* suggest that they were rarely, if ever, paid by members of the community to provide healthcare at Deir el-Medina.

In addition to understanding how and when the *zwn.w* were paid, it is also important to establish how long they could treat any single person. O. OIM 16973 is another ambiguous example where the *zwn.w* may have spent

opportunities outside of the village. Thus, if he was given private payments, these would have increased his total income from his role as a *zwn.w*.

45 While in verso 5.12, the total given is 22 deben, the actual sum of the items is 19 ½ deben and the final total given in verso 5.20 is 20 deben.

46 If we assume that one *ḫ3r* of grain equates to two deben for this text (Janssen, Commodity Prices, 124), and that workmen were paid a total of 5 ½ *ḫ3r* in grain rations per month (Janssen, Commodity Prices, 460; Černý, Prices and Wages, 917).

47 Barbara S. Lesko, "Rank, Roles, and Rights," in *Pharaoh's Workers: The Villagers of Deir El Medina*, ed. Leonard Lesko (Ithaca: Cornell University Press, 1994), 21.

48 Gardiner, *Ramesside Administrative Documents*, 48.

49 McDowell, *Village Life in Ancient Egypt*, 36.

50 Davies identifies at least nine individuals with this name, several living during this time period. Davies suggests that the *zwn.w* in this text is named *Wsr-ḥ3.t*; however, the preposition "*i͗n*," suggests the payment was to the physician *by Wsr-ḥ3.t*, rather than to the physician, *Wsr-ḥ3.t*. See Davies, *Who's Who at Deir El-Medina*, 43.

51 Allam suggests it is a private property settlement. This is discussed further in Gabler, *Who's Who around Deir el-Medina*, 403–404.

multiple months treating the same patient.[52] This document contains charges against a workman who was away for five months because his wife was with the *zwn.w*. Janssen speculates that, "the unknown workman did not turn up at work, being out of himself because his wife had eloped with another workman who acted as the doctor."[53] This reasoning does not explain why the man was referred to by the title *zwn.w*, rather than being named as the adulterer.[54] Alternatively, this text could reference a workman who remained absent from work in order to take care of his sick wife, even though the *zwn.w* was already attending to her. The charges (*sḫꜣ-r*) in the text indicate the workman's absences were legally unacceptable, most likely due to their extensive duration. If the absences were completely unacceptable, we would expect him to have been punished and forced to return to work much sooner. Given the delay, this accusation could have come at the heels of other social and professional pressures, such as an unsatisfactory report on tomb progress or a complaint filed by a fellow workman.[55]

2.2 *The* ḫrp-Srq.t *as a Medical Professional*

The title *ḫrp-Srq.t* is less common than *zwn.w*, though it is still associated with medical care that was likely predicated on specialized knowledge. Gardiner identified this title fourteen times throughout Egyptian history, two of which simultaneously use the title *zwn.w*,[56] suggesting that while these roles may be related, they did not entirely overlap. The title, "the controller of the goddess Serqet" (represented by a scorpion 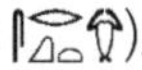), is religiously charged and carries with it connotations of protection against scorpions and similar dangers such as venomous snakes. Consequently, this title is often translated as "scorpion charmer" to address this individual's role in protecting against scorpions and other dangerous creatures. In a detailed discussion of texts mentioning the *ḫrp-Srq.t*, however, Gardiner convincingly demonstrates—mostly through texts from Deir el-Medina—that they would have specialized in medical treatments related to venomous bites and stings but may also have acted as an intermediary with the divine to treat illnesses.

---

52 Only lines 1–2 of this text are published and no transliteration is available. See Janssen, *Village Varia*, 1997, 91; Toivari-Viitala, *Women at Deir El-Medina*, 214.

53 Janssen, *Village Varia*, 1997, 91.

54 Other cases of adultery directly name the adulterer (e.g., O. Ashmolean 186; P. BM 10055; P. BM 10416).

55 Both complaints filed against individual workmen (e.g., O. BM EA 66408) and inspection reports (e.g., O. Florence 2621) have been documented among the texts from Deir el-Medina.

56 Alan H. Gardiner, "Professional Magicians in Ancient Egypt," *Proceedings of the Society of Biblical Archaeology* 39 (1917): 34–44.

The title *ḫrp-Srq.t* occurs in at least 12 ostraca and papyri from Deir el-Medina (Table 7)[57] as well as graffiti belonging to *Ptḥ-šd* (i) and *Nfr-ḥtp*.[58] There are five individuals named as *ḫrp-Srq.t*,[59] ranging from the 19th to the end of the 20th Dynasty and, like the *zwn.w*, some of these individuals were also workmen, suggesting that the role of *ḫrp-Srq.t* was fulfilled by someone from the workforce. Ration payments allocated to the *ḫrp-Srq.t* are the same amount as those for the *zwn.w*. This indicates both roles are given a supplementary wage.[60] P. Turin Cat. 1929 and 2062 mention both the *ḫrp-Srq.t* and the *zwn.w*, also demonstrating that these positions would have existed at the village concurrently. This means the two roles must have fulfilled different functions for the workforce. One possibility is that the *zwn.w* focused on treatments requiring prescriptions, while the *ḫrp-Srq.t* managed treatments requiring a divine intermediary, though texts suggest that either role could use incantations and medical ingredients in healing.

Only two texts referring to the *ḫrp-Srq.t* offer further insight into their role, and both reference a *ḫrp-Srq.t* named *ỉmn-ms*. In O. UCL 3/O. UC 31933, *ỉmn-ms* writes to request several items for a sick priest including one measure of grain (*npỉ/npr*), one jar of syrup (*ds ḫwwy*),[61] and one festival date juice (*bnr ḥb*).[62] In this context, the *ḫrp-Srq.t* is prescribing treatment for an individual, though we do not have enough context to understand the nature of the illness other than to say that the priest is ill, perhaps to the point where they were

57 Additionally, Gabler lists O. BTdK 547, O. Gardiner AG 129, and O. DeM 10248. Gabler, *Who's Who around Deir el-Medina*, 408.

58 Janssen, *Village Varia*, 1997, 29.

59 *Ptḥ-šd* (i) and a *Nfr-ḥtp* are both attested with the title *ḫrp-Srq.t* in graffiti, but this title does not appear in other texts connected to these names. *ỉmn-ḫʿ* is noted as a *ḫrp-Srq.t* in the Tomb Robbery Papyri. The name *ỉmn-ms* is connected to the title in multiple texts ranging from late Dynasty 19 to the reign of Ramesses V which suggests two different men with the same name and title. *ỉmn-ms* (i), owner of TT 9, is most likely the *ḫrp-Srq.t* described in O. UCL 3/O. UC 31933. A later *ỉmn-ms* is described in multiple 20th Dynasty texts such as O. IFAO 1296. While it is possible these men were related, the relative popularity of the name *ỉmn-ms* makes this unverifiable. For more information, see Davies, *Who's Who at Deir El-Medina*, 7–8; Janssen, *Village Varia*, 1997, 27–29; Frédérique von Känel, *Les prêtres-ouâb de Sekhmet et les conjurateurs de Serket*, Bibliothèque de l'École des hautes études. Sciences religieuses 87 (Paris: Presses Universitaires de France, 1984).

60 Janssen, *Village Varia*, 1997, 29. Also, see Richard Mandeville, *Wage Accounting in Deir El-Medina* (Wallasey: Abercromby Press, 2014).

61 For full information about the translation "jar of syrup," see further discussion by Battiscombe Gunn, "The Decree of Amonrasonthēr for Neskhons," *The Journal of Egyptian Archaeology* 41 (December 1955): 94, note 3.

62 Based on the transcription in Kenneth A. Kitchen, *Ramesside Inscriptions*, vol. VII (Oxford: B.H. Blackwell, 1989), 214.

TABLE 7 Texts from Deir el-Medina relating to the ḫrp-Srq.t

Accession number	Summary of contents	Date
O. Ashmolean 4	Divine intermediary in legal accusation	Dyn 20 (Year 5, Ramesses IV)
O. Ashmolean 21	Grain rations	Unknown
O. Berlin P 11249	Grain rations	Dyn 20
O. Cairo CG 25660 + JE 37649	Feasting/Gift-giving list	Dyn 20 (Ramesses IV)
O. DEM 200	Beer rations	Dyn 20 (Ramesses III)
O. DEM 388	Grain and beer rations	Dyn 20
O. DEM 10045	Too fragmentary	Dyn 20 (Ramesses III, year 16)
O. Toronto ROM 906.20.6	Vinegar rations	Dyn 20 (Ramesses IV or V)
O. UCL 3/O. UC 31933	Request for medical ingredients	Dyn 19 or 20
P. Turin Cat 1929	Name list (possibly for rations)	Unknown
P. Turin Cat 2062	Grain rations	Dyn 20 (Year 2, Ramesses V)
O. IFAO 1296*	Private letter from a *ḫrp-Srq.t* to the scribe *Ḥr.y* complaining about late rations (*di͗.w*)	Dyn 20

*This text is unpublished, but is described in Janssen, Village Varia, 1997, 28.

worried he would die.[63] The second text, O. Ashmolean 4, mentions the *ḫrp-Srq.t* in a capacity unrelated to medicine. Here, the chisel-bearer *Qḥ* (iv) uses *’Imn-ms* as an intermediary to communicate with the deified Amenhotep I during a public accusation against the daughter of the scribe *’Imn-nḫt*. The fact that the *ḫrp-Srq.t* would have been used in this capacity, while the *zwn.w* is not attested at Deir el-Medina as a divine intermediary, suggests the *ḫrp-Srq.t* had more specialized knowledge to do with divine forces.

When compared to the *zwn.w*, the *ḫrp-Srq.t* is less attested with fewer mentions in grain ration texts and no examples of private payments. These differences could be due to chance preservation given the similarly long attestation of men with this title during the village's occupation.[64] Their relative absence from the written record may, however, also suggest that the role of the *ḫrp-Srq.t* was less integrated into the state support system for the workforce than the *zwn.w*. The fewer grain ration texts citing the *ḫrp-Srq.t* could underline

63 The author uses the general term for sickness (*mr*), though it is written with the dead man determinative, , perhaps indicating the severity of the illness.

64 Gabler, *Who's Who around Deir el-Medina*, 409.

that the role was only formally integrated into the workforce rosters at some point during the 20th Dynasty, from which time the majority of our attestations emerge. Regardless, by the end of Deir el-Medina's occupation, both the roles of *zwn.w* and *ḫrp-Srq.t* were allotted extra rations by the state to support the workforce. The formal payment for these two roles and the state support for absences meant that healthcare was readily accessible to the workforce.

2.3 *The Wise Woman as a Folk Practitioner*

Unlike the professional roles of the *ḫrp-Srq.t* and *zwn.w*, the wise woman, *tꜣ rḫ.t*, fits more in line with the role of a folk practitioner in treating illnesses. The wise woman acted as an intermediary to explain illnesses and deaths caused by divine forces. Her services were specifically required when an individual was unaware of the wrong they committed or to whom they should supplicate. Individuals sought her out in several cases of illness or even death because of her ability to interact with the divine. She, therefore, served as a kind of folk practitioner for the villagers, offering her unique ability to interact with the divine and using this ability to address illnesses in some cases.

Six texts mention the wise woman from Deir el-Medina, though some of them may be related to the same individuals or circumstances (Table 8).[65] None of these texts mention a personal name written in conjunction with the title *tꜣ rḫ.t*. It is also of note that in O. DEM 1690, the author uses the indefinite article, requesting the recipient see *a* wise woman, suggesting that there may be more than one woman with this title. The Metternich Stela refers to Isis as "a wise woman in her town,"[66] perhaps indicating that each community would have had a wise woman, and within the context of O. DEM 1690, an individual could seek the services of a wise woman outside of their community. The more consistent use of the definite article, *tꜣ rḫ.t*, would suggest that normally the workmen and their families would consult the local wise woman for Deir el-Medina.

Whether or not the wise woman was part of the village remains speculative. Texts mentioning *tꜣ rḫ.t* specify that individuals should go to her, suggesting she was located outside the village.[67] These few mentions of the wise woman occur

---

65 Doris Karl, "Funktion Und Bedeutung Einer Weisen Frau Im Alten Ägypten," *Studien Zur Altägyptischen Kultur* 28 (2000): 131–160; Toivari-Viitala, *Women at Deir El-Medina*, 228–231.

66 Joris F. Borghouts, "Divine Intervention in Ancient Egypt and Its Manifestation (B3w)," in *Gleanings from Deir El-Medina*, ed. Robert J. Demarée and Jac J. Janssen (Leiden: Nederlands Instituut voor het Nabije Oosten, 1982), 26, note 123.

67 For texts referencing "going to" the wise woman, see Toivari-Viitala, *Women at Deir El-Medina*, 288, note 11.

TABLE 8 Texts from Deir el-Medina relating to the wise woman

Accession number	Summary of contents	Date
O. Cairo CG 25674	A broken text that mentions going to the wise woman where she cites the *bꜣ.w* of Taweret	Dyn 19 or 20
O. DEM 1688	The male author goes to the wise woman to determine the *bꜣ.w* affecting the eyes of a woman (potentially related to O. DeM 1690)	Dyn 19 or 20
O. DEM 1690	The author urges a man to seek out a wise woman about the *bꜣ.w* affecting a woman, mentioning Taweret. The author further asks about the *bꜣ.w* affecting the eyes (potentially related to O. DeM 1688)	Dyn 19 or 20
O. Gardiner 149	The female author asks the wise woman to determine the *bꜣw* affecting her and the Wise Woman mentions the *bꜣw* of Ptah.	Unknown
O. Letellier	*Qn-ḥr-ḫpš⸗f* requests a woman to see the wise woman to understand why two youths have died (potentially related to O. Nelson 8)	Late Dyn 19
O. Nelson 8/O. OIM 16974	The male author went to the wise woman about two children (potentially related to O. Letellier) and said their illness is from an unnamed god.	Late Dyn 19

in private letters with no texts explicitly mentioning paying the wise woman. Such a small corpus may not include private payments if they were communicated orally.

The textual records of the *zwn.w* and the *ḫrp-Srq.t* were dominated by administrative texts and more specifically, grain rations. In contrast, the complete lack of any mention of the wise woman in these ration texts implies that she was not part of the formal administration of the village. Her presence as a folk practitioner is significant, however, since even very literate members of the village would turn to the wise woman for help with illness. These examples may be in cases where the *zwn.w* or *ḫrp-Srq.t* could not treat illnesses successfully.

All of our references call for an individual to go to the wise woman in order to identify how a recent incident was influenced by various *bꜣ.w*—aspects of the divine representing both their power and their visible manifestations.[68] While

68 Jan Assmann, *The Search for God in Ancient Egypt* (Ithaca: Cornell University Press, 2001), 239–240.

both men and women consult the wise woman, the few attestations may indicate that the wise woman's abilities to treat illnesses were more focused on women and children. The sources also refer to the *bꜣ.w* of divine beings connected with protections for mothers and children (e.g., Taweret), though other divine beings such as Ptah are also mentioned.

In the Metternich Stela, dating to the 30th Dynasty, the wise woman was consulted to determine divine causes for illnesses but not necessarily treat them.[69] However, her role at Deir el-Medina may have served both to act as a "seer" and "healer."[70] The text which most clearly addresses the wise woman's role in treating illness is O. DEM 1690.[71] In this text, a man is told to consult the wise woman about the *bꜣ.w* causing a woman blindness or a related problem with her eyes. Here, the author specifically cited the *bꜣ.w* of Taweret as the culprits, though in other examples, people sought the wise woman to know which divinity could be causing an illness.

As a village situated in the midst of the Theban hills, Deir el-Medina was surrounded by necropolises and temples, placing them in a particularly precarious position for interactions with the dead. While the wise woman's knowledge of the divine could assist in diagnosis, so too could her ability to communicate with the spirits of the dead. This role can be tentatively reconstructed in O. DEM 1688:[72] *tw=ỉ ḥn n tꜣ rḫ.(t) n mwt ỉw Pꜣ-šd pr n=ỉ ỉw=f ḥr ḏd n=ỉ bꜣw n Ptḥ ꜥnḫ m*[*wt*] "I went to the wise woman because of the death and *Pꜣ-šd* came to me and said to me, '{It is} the *bꜣ.w* of Ptah. The dead live.'" This enigmatic text suggests that there was a death for which the author needed more information. *Pꜣ-šd* may refer to the dead individual himself who communicated through the wise woman to tell the author that his death was because of the manifestations of Ptah.

The need to consult with the wise woman after a death occurs as well in O. Letellier,[73] when *Qn-ḥr-ḫpš=f* requests a woman go to the wise woman after

69 Borghouts, "Divine Intervention in Ancient Egypt and Its Manifestation (B3w)," 26.

70 Karl, "Funktion Und Bedeutung Einer Weisen Frau Im Alten Ägypten," 159.

71 Karl, 134–135; Bernard Mathieu, "Sur Quelques Ostraca Hiératiques Littéraires Récemment Publiés," *Bulletin de l'Institut Français d'Archéologie Orientale* 93 (1994): 335–336; Toivari-Viitala, *Women at Deir El-Medina*, 229.

72 Translation based on the transliteration and commentary provided by Karl, "Funktion Und Bedeutung Einer Weisen Frau Im Alten Ägypten," 135–136; Toivari-Viitala, *Women at Deir El-Medina*, 229.

73 Published originally by Bernadette Letellier, "La Destinée de Deux Enfants, Un Ostracon Ramesside Inédit," in *IFAO Livre Du Centenaire, 1880–1980*, ed. Jean Vercoutter, Mémoires Publiés Par Les Membres de l'Institut Français d'archéologie Orientale Du Caire 104 (Cairo: Institut français d'archéologie orientale, 1980), 127–133. Translation based on additional

the death of two boys to determine if this was their destinies (*šꜣ.yt*) or fortunes (*rnn.t*). If this text is related to O. Nelson 8/O. OIM 16974, their death may have occurred after an illness. O. Nelson 8/O. OIM 16974 mentions two youths whose illness (*hk*)[74] was caused by an unnamed god.[75] Additionally, Taweret is mentioned later in the text, though it is too fragmentary to determine whether the two are connected. In O. Letellier, *Qn-ḥr-ḫpš=f* writes to a woman telling her not only to ask about the two youths, but also to inquire on his behalf and on behalf of the boys' mother to see their lives. He tells this woman to write to him about the identities of the gods related to the deaths of these children, indicating that he needed to appease the *bꜣ.w* in fear of potential retributions against his life and the mother's.[76] The wise woman thus serves to resolve the deaths of these two youths, while also providing information for the future protection of *Qn-ḥr-ḫpš=f* and their mother.

2.4 *Missing Medical Professionals*

While the *zwn.w*, *ḫrp-Srq.t*, and *rḫ.t* were documented practitioners that people sought to treat illnesses at Deir el-Medina, several other practitioners mentioned outside Deir el-Medina appear to be wholly absent from the village. Neither the *zꜣ.w* (amulet maker[77]) nor the *wꜥb* priests of Sekhmet are mentioned in any letters to or from the village. The *zꜣ.w* would have acted as a divine intermediary and likely would have been sought for preventative medicine given their role of producing apotropaic amulets. The role of the *zꜣ.w* thus parallels the role of the *ḫrp-Srq.t* in intervening with the divine prior to illness. This func-

published commentary in Karl, "Funktion Und Bedeutung Einer Weisen Frau Im Alten Ägypten," 134.

74 The only other cited attestations in TLA (lemma 859894) comes from P. BM EA 10685, v. 6.5–8.12 in which the illness comes amidst remedies for illnesses of the head and has been assumed to reference migraines/headaches. See Alan H. Gardiner, ed., *Hieratic Papyri in the British Museum*, vol. 1, Third Series Chester Beatty Gift (London: British Museum Press, 1935), 51–52; Hildegard von Deines and Wolfhart Westendorf, *Wörterbuch der medizinischen Texte*, vol. VII, 2, Grundriss der Medizin der Alten Ägypter (Berlin: Akademie-Verlag, 1962), 573.

75 Mohamed A. Nassar, "The Wise Woman and the Healing Practice (O. OIM 16974)," *Journal of Ancient Egyptian Interconnections* 24, no. 1 (2019), http://journals.librarypublishing.arizona.edu/jaei/article/id/1396/.

76 Toivari-Viitala suggests that this may also indicate that he is their father. See Toivari-Viitala, *Women at Deir El-Medina*, 229.

77 The term *zꜣ.w* derives from the noun for both protection and amulet and refers to those who produced amulets for protection and who likely had other magical abilities that were used as part of a medical profession. See Ritner, *The Mechanics of Ancient Egyptian Magical Practice*, 51–53.

tion may have been subsumed by the *ḫrp-Srq.t* at Deir el-Medina, especially as the latter would have been able to specialize in amulets protecting against bites and stings, a well-documented concern for the villagers.[78] The physical presence of such protective amulets at Deir el-Medina indicates that they were one way people managed illnesses, but the high degree of literacy in the village and access to medical texts might have allowed residents to create these amulets themselves, bypassing the need for a specialist. If so, protective amulets would have been part of broader popular healthcare in the village.

The *wꜥb* priests of Sekhmet are also mentioned in the medical papyri with duties specifically associated with maintaining hygiene through ritual washing, pacifying Sekhmet to stop the spread of infectious disease, and using the pulse to diagnose illnesses.[79] Frequently, individuals with this title were also *zwn.w*. *Wꜥb* priests of Sekhmet were clearly present in Thebes during the New Kingdom (e.g., *ꞽImn-wꜣḥ-sw*, TT 111, whose tomb dates to Ramesses II), and thus it is possible that the villagers accessed these individuals as part of their interaction with the broader Theban community if they were not part of the village.

Finally, it should be noted that in Pharaonic Egypt in general, we do not see textual references to individuals who specialized in assistance during childbirth, even though there are medical papyri that directly address gynecological issues (e.g., UC 32057 from Kahun and P. Leiden I 348). These texts offer treatments to determine pregnancy, increase lactation, and make contraceptives,[80] but offer no specific mention of a "midwife" and relatively little discussion of issues in childbirth. Most research supplements this relative lack of information on childbirth with evidence from the Westcar papyrus,[81] a text that references divine births. Even the very moment of birth is rarely mentioned at Deir el-Medina, though it sometimes validated absences when a workman's wife was in labor.[82]

78 As evidenced in both absences related to scorpion stings and treatments for stings and bites in medical texts.

79 Heinz Engelmann and Jochen Hallof, "Der Sachmetpriester, Ein Früher Repräsentant Der Hygiene Und Des Seuchenschutzes," *Studien Zur Altägyptischen Kultur* 23 (1996): 103–146; Núria Torras Benezet, "The Pure Priest of Sekhmet, Between Health and Disease," in *Pharmacy and Medicine in Ancient Egypt: Proceedings of the Conference Held in Barcelona (2018)*, ed. Rosa Dinarès Solà, Mikel Fernàndez Georges, and Maria Rosa Guasch-Jané (Oxford: Archaeopress, 2021), 116–124, https://doi.org/10.2307/j.ctv1r2xx81.

80 Erika Feucht, *Das Kind im Alten Ägypten: die Stellung des Kindes in Familie und Gesellschaft nach altägyptischen Texten und Darstellungen* (Frankfurt: Campus, 1995), 97–103.

81 e.g., Geoffrey Chamberlain, "Historical Perspectives on Health: Childbirth in Ancient Egypt," *The Journal of the Royal Society for the Promotion of Health* 124, no. 6 (November 1, 2004): 284–286, https://doi.org/10.1177/146642400412400618.

82 Toivari-Viitala, *Women at Deir El-Medina*, 172–173. Also, see Chapter 5, section 3.

Texts and artifacts from Deir el-Medina, however, demonstrate multiple ways that the community sought for successful childbirth and the health of mother and child in the weeks after birth. This suggests that some form of healthcare for childbirth existed at the site and these forms of care were either popular or had practitioners that were not recorded in the site's texts. Amulets for childbirth that most likely originated from Deir el-Medina suggest that childbirth could have been within the purview of a *zꜣ.w* or *ḫrp-Srq.t*.[83] Additionally, fertility figures used to ensure pregnancy[84] and post-partum rituals[85] suggest specific rites that could benefit women in childbirth, but still leave unknown which if any specialists aided in the success of childbirth. Since women could act as divine intermediaries and female goddesses served as midwives in Papyrus Westcar, it is plausible that women also acted as midwives at Deir el-Medina, but these roles did not need to be recorded in the administrative texts at the site because they were not paid for their services. While the wise woman was known to interact with the divine, other women may have also had divine connections to gods associated with protecting the health of women and children (i.e., Hathor and Bes/Beset) at Deir el-Medina given the presence of women's tattoos associated with these divinities at the site.[86] The very nature of midwifery may have also been treated as different from medicine given that gynecological texts focus on treating pain, evaluating fertility, determining a child's sex, contraception, and abortion. If childbirth was not viewed as something to be treated with mixed remedies, it would not be documented in most medical texts.

The evidence of various types of healthcare practitioners at Deir el-Medina thus indicates that some, but not all, professionals used to treat illnesses in Egypt were documented in the village. It also gives some indication of how the roles of these professionals were separated, with the *zwn.w* and *ḫrp-Srq.t* likely occupying specific duties for professional healthcare, while the wise woman

83 Janssen, *Commodity Prices from the Ramessid Period*, 310–311.

84 Geraldine Pinch, "Childbirth and Female Figurines at Deir El-Medina and El-ʿAmarna," *Orientalia* 52, no. 3 (1983): 405–414.

85 Arnette, "Purification Du Post-Partum et Rites Des Relevailles Dans l'Égypte Ancienne."

86 Anne E. Austin and Marie-Lys Arnette, "Of Ink and Clay: Tattooed Mummified Human Remains and Female Figurines from Deir El-Medina," *The Journal of Egyptian Archaeology* 108, no. 1–2 (2022): 63–80, https://doi.org/10.1177/03075133221130089; Anne E. Austin and Cédric Gobeil, "Embodying the Divine: A Tattooed Female Mummy from Deir El-Medina," *Bulletin de l'Institut Français d'Archéologie Orientale*, no. 116 (2017): 23–46. For additional discussion on the possible connections between tattooing and midwifery, see Vittoria Rapisidara, "'Indossare' i Tatuaggi: Studio Del Tatuaggio Nell'Antico Egitto Sui Resti Umani, Archeologici e Iconografici" (MA Thesis, Pisa, Università di Pisa, 2020).

TABLE 9 Distribution of medical ingredients to members of the workforce (O. Gardiner 246)

Workman	Incense (*sntr*)	*sfṯ*-oil	*ḥḥ*-oil	Honey	Fat (*ʿḏ*)
Wsḫt-nmt.t (right)	x		x		
Bw-qn.tw=f	x		x		
ʾImn-nḫt (ix) son of *Ks* (vi)		x			
Mnṯw-Pꜣ-Ḥʿpy (i)		x			
Ḥr-šrỉ				x	x
Nb-nfr				x*	x**

**It was given in place of fat (ʿḏ)*
***It was given in place of grease (mrḥ), to satisfy the entire workforce* [...]
Note: Grease (mrḥ) was also distributed, but the text is broken and so excluded.

was more connected to the folk sector. Both the roles of *zwn.w* and *ḫrp-Srq.t* appear to be integral to the workforce with members of the crew taking on these responsibilities and specialized knowledge consistently across the documented periods from the 19th to the end of the 20th Dynasties. Their services were supported through regular rations and, at least in the case of the *zwn.w*, time off from work and an assistant.

2.5 *State Support for Medical Ingredients*

In addition to receiving support for access to medical care, there is also evidence that the state distributed ingredients common in basic medical treatments to the workforce. O. Gardiner 246 begins "Regnal year 2, month 4 of *ꜣḫ.t*, day 15: portion of medicine (*pḫr.t*) for the crew on this day."[87] The text then lists specific workmen and their provisions (Table 9).

While several of these ingredients are common and used for various purposes, their portioning as specifically medicine (*pḫr.t*) in the beginning of the text suggests they were meant to treat illnesses rather than be used for other reasons. The fact that *Wsḫt-nmt.t* is listed as "right" (*wnmy*) and the distribution of each ingredient was to two workmen suggests that these medical ingredients were distributed to each side of the crew. The statement that *Nb-nfr* received grease in place of fat to satisfy[88] the entire workforce further corroborates this

87 The transliteration of this text is based on its transcription in a scan of Černý Notebook 31.46 provided by the Griffith Institute of Oxford University.

88 Helck uses the verb erfüllen, though this may be based on the generic Egyptian verb *ỉrỉ* which has a multitude of meanings. Regardless, the reference to the broader workforce suggests that this was not for private use. See W. Helck, *Die datierten und datierbaren Ostraka, Papyri und Graffiti von Deir el-Medineh*, (Otto Harrassowitz Verlag, 2002), p. 375.

reading. One would expect that the members of the crew receiving medical provisions would be the foremen or scribes, as their level of literacy would have given them the most access to medical texts. Alternatively, of course, one might expect to see the *zwn.w* or *ḫrp-Srq.t* listed, such as *Pꜣ-ʿn* who was a *zwn.w* in Deir el-Medina during the reign of Ramesses IV.[89] None of the individuals mentioned in this text, however, had titles associated with either medicine or leadership in the workforce.[90] Instead, the provisioning of these particular medical ingredients, especially honey and fat, to workmen may have been because they could be used without the assistance of a professional physician, given their common applications. It is, therefore, possible that fellow workmen could offer some level of medical care for illnesses requiring basic medical knowledge for the use of honey, oil, and fat, rather than the more specific ingredients and knowledge found in longer medical texts.

3 Medical Literacy

The use of medical ingredients by the workforce attests to a broader degree of medical literacy within the community. Even with access to medical professionals and ingredients, family medical texts suggest that people within the village sometimes sought their own solutions independent of the medical professionals. These not only attest to unusually high degrees of medical literacy, but also the kinds of illnesses that concerned the community.

Here, medical texts include any treatment used to cure, ameliorate, or prevent an illness, a definition that avoids differentiating between medicine and magic[91] and instead follows recent scholarship, which has consistently argued that from an Egyptian worldview, treatments would have included both ap-

89 Mentioned in O. DeM 617, dated by Kitchen broadly to Ramesses IV.

90 Based on Helck's date for the text of year 2 of Ramesses IV. *Ḥr-šri͗*, referenced in Davies as Harshire (i), was a draftsman at this time and had not yet been promoted to scribe nor yet acted as assistant to the senior scribe. For further discussion, see Davies, *Who's Who at Deir El-Medina*, 114–116.

91 For examples of previous scholarship arguing for a differentiation between medicine and magic on the basis of rationality, see Chauncey Depew Leake, *The Old Egyptian Medical Papyri* (Lawrence: University of Kansas Press, 1952); Serge Sauneron, *Les prêtres de l'ancienne Égypte*, Le temps qui court 5 (Paris: Éditions du Seuil, 1957). However, Egyptian texts demonstrate fluidity across these categories. For example, in case nine of P. Edwin Smith, the treatment fluidly transitions from prescribing a medical bandage wrapped around a poultice for the wound to a magical incantation to cleanse the blood effectively and protect it from getting infected.

proaches.[92] Texts addressing illnesses with a wide variety of treatments (e.g., pharmacological and amuletic) are, therefore, applicable.

3.1 *Who was Medically Literate?*

The most abundant information on medical care from Deir el-Medina comes from the Chester Beatty Papyri,[93] a set of papyri that had been maintained within one family over multiple generations as evidenced by the multiple hands augmenting the texts as well as colophons added to the papyri.[94] They were owned at one point by *Qn-ḥr-ḫpš=f* (i) and subsequently passed down via his wife *Nỉw.t-nḫt.tỉ* to her second husband and their children. Based on analysis of the handwriting, the medical portions of the Chester Beatty papyri were compiled and copied by four or more individuals,[95] with more than one author contributing to the same papyrus in some instances (e.g., Chester Beatty 6). Additionally, as seen in the recto of Chester Beatty 6, a scribe at some point went through and corrected the text,[96] indicating that they were not only able to copy these texts, but also read them fluently. Various members of this family could thus access and add to the medical compendia.

Many of the papyri recovered in this collection include preventative or reactive medical text (see Table 10), offering insights into how one family treated illnesses. Several medical ostraca from Deir el-Medina show similar concerns with medical treatments, for instance, against scorpion stings (O. DeM 1213, O. DeM 1263), against a dead man or dead woman entering the eyes (O. DeM 1062), or for stomach issues (O. DeM 1216). Amuletic texts from the site (e.g., P. Berlin 15749, P. DEM 36, P. DEM 40, P. DEM 44) offer other specific examples where an amulet was made to treat an illness including several involving fevers from female and male dead, spirits, enemies, and adversaries. These ostraca and papyri suggest that the illnesses mentioned in the Chester Beatty papyri were broader concerns within the village and not just specific to one individual.

Despite high degrees of medical literacy, neither *Qn-ḥr-ḫpš=f* (i) nor other family members were ever attested to serve as the crew's *zwn.w* or *ḫrp-Srq.t*.

---

92 For example, see Philippa Lang, *Medicine and Society in Ptolemaic Egypt* (Leiden: Brill, 2013); Ritner, *The Mechanics of Ancient Egyptian Magical Practice*.

93 Gardiner, *Hieratic Papyri in the British Museum*.

94 Pieter W. Pestman, "Who Were the Owners, in the 'Community of Workmen', of the Chester Beatty Papyri," in *Gleanings from Deir El-Medîna*, ed. Robert J. Demarée and Jac. J. Janseen, Egyptologische Uitgaven 1 (Leiden: Nederlands Instituut voor het Nabije Oosten, 1982), 155–172.

95 Gardiner, *Hieratic Papyri in the British Museum*.

96 Gardiner, 1:53.

TABLE 10 Medical texts in the Chester Beatty Collection

Chester Beatty #	BM #	Description of medical contents
5	10685	Amuletic recitations for removing headaches and scorpion stings
6	10686	Incantation against a *nsy/nsy.t* demon
		Topical remedy for removing injury
		Remedies for the anus and bladder
7	10687	Recitations for removing the venom of scorpions
		Recitation against fever
8	10688	Oral remedy for removing venom of a god, dead man, or dead woman
		Recitation for protection of each part of the body, organized head-to-toe as a means of purification
		Amuletic recitation to protect from dead, demons, and the magic of enemies
9	10689	Fumigation to remove an illness
15	10695	Oral remedy against a dead man or woman
		Protection against an "enemy who is in the tooth of N"
16	10696	Recitations of purification
18	10698	Very fragmentary medical texts

Yet, the family-owned medical texts including treatments that are specifically for the use of a *zwn.w* (P. BM 10686, 6.8–6.10). The entire corpus of medical texts from Deir el-Medina indicate that they could be privately owned by individuals with levels of literacy that were high enough to understand them. Medical knowledge was not, in fact, the exclusive purview of paid medical professionals.

These various medical texts would have been more accessible at Deir el-Medina than in many ancient Egyptian villages because of the higher degrees of literacy in the community.[97] These would have included scribes like *Qn-ḥr-ḫpš=f*

97 Baines and Eyre argue that literacy at Deir el-Medina was higher than the general population in John Baines and Christopher J. Eyre, "Four Notes on Literacy," *Göttinger Miszellen* 61 (1983): 65–96. Additionally, the estimate of literacy at Deir el-Medina is likely higher than initially proposed by Baines and Eyre. See Jac J. Janssen, "Literacy and Letters at Deir El-Medîna," in *Village Voices: Proceedings of the Symposium "Texts from Deir El-Medîna and Their Interpretation", Leiden, May 31-June 1, 1991*, ed. Robert J. Demarée and A. Egberts, CNWS Publications 13 (Leiden: Centre of Non-Western Studies, Leiden University, 1992), 81–94.

(i), but also men holding the basic positions on the crew such as *ʾImn-nḫt* (xxvi), who inherited the papyri and included his own colophon. While we have more evidence of literacy among men at Deir el-Medina, some women may also have been literate.[98] The exact proportion of the village who had enough literacy to read medical texts remains ambiguous, but the texts demonstrate that it would have included more than the designated scribes and medical professionals on the village rosters.

The degree of medical literacy necessary to use these texts sometimes required knowledge normally inaccessible outside of the elite. While many of the ingredients mentioned were common household items (e.g., beer, honey, fat, oil), some ingredients also existed at distant locations and would likely have been rare or expensive. For example, one treatment calls for plants from the oases and fish from the sea, using the Semitic loan word, *ym* (P. Chester Beatty 6, 4.1–4.10). Winand argues that for the people of Deir el-Medina, "the sea was a very remote reality that had little chance to be a relevant topic in their texts" and that the term *ym* was only found in texts belonging to "high culture."[99] This further suggests that the owners of the Chester Beatty papyri had an unusual degree of medical literacy normally exclusively found in elite circles.

Additionally, the inclusion of longer texts describing symptoms in the Chester Beatty papyri suggests the owners were not only able to read these texts, but also aware of the processes of how to diagnose illnesses, determine a prognosis, and treat them. In Chester Beatty 6, 6.2–6.6, an enema composed of fat, honey, and milk is used to treat a man with symptoms of infection including swelling or sores on the bladder (*bn.wt ḥr špy.t*), fever, painful urination, and diarrhea.[100] While most medical treatments described in the medical texts from Deir el-Medina dealing with pharmacological ingredients focus simply on a short, rubricized title and the list of relevant ingredients, this example includes both a detailed description of symptoms used in the diagnosis and prognosis for the illness.[101]

---

98 Deborah Sweeney, "Women's Correspondence from Deir El-Medineh," in *Acts of the Sixth International Conference of Egyptology*, vol. 2, Sesto Congresso Internazionale Di Egittologia. Atti, 1993, 523–529; Toivari-Viitala, *Women at Deir El-Medina*, 187–193.

99 Jean Winand, "Identifying Semitic Loanwords in Late Egyptian," in *Greek Influence on Egyptian-Coptic: Contact-Induced Change in an Ancient African Language*, ed. Eitan Grossman et al. (Hamburg: Widmaier, 2017), 492.

100 Since these symptoms are focused on the bladder and anus, they seem most in line with a urinary tract or kidney infection, but this remains speculative.

101 This more systematic approach is used in the earlier attested P. Edwin Smith, but more rarely found in similar pharmacological papyri such as P. Ebers.

While anyone with enough literacy could be medically literate, access to these medical texts may have been limited. P. Geneva MAH 15274 + P. Turin CGT 54063 verso documents the transfer of a spell to seize venom/poison (*r n ṯꜣy tꜣ mt.wt*) between the scribe *Pꜣ-ḥm-nṯr* and the scribe *Pꜣ-nfr-m-ḏd.w* (i) in the house of *ꜣb-ʾImn.t.t.*[102] This text explicitly documents the transfer of an individual medical treatment. Further, this transfer was likely overseen and witnessed by an outside party, *ꜣb-ʾImn.t.t.* While one can only speculate exactly why this transfer was made, its documentation suggests that the transfer of medical knowledge—even in small, individual increments—was both valued and carefully monitored. Access to these texts was, therefore, not something to be taken for granted.

Those engaging with medical texts like the Chester Beatty Papyri were able to understand the medical processes of diagnosis and prognosis, read and correct the texts, evaluate the efficacy of treatments, and know the terminology for unusual ingredients. This exclusive access in both the maintenance and use of medical knowledge would have given the highly literate an upper hand in their medical care. Even at Deir el-Medina, where medical professionals were expected to provide care to the broader community, the long-term maintenance of the Chester Beatty papyri reveal there was an incentive to invest in private medical documents and care.

3.2 *Customizing Healthcare through Medical Literacy*

In addition to what these papyri tell us about who could and could not use medical texts, they also tell us about the kinds of treatments provided at Deir el-Medina and the illnesses that most concerned the community. This is because the medical papyri most likely were constructed over time rather than copied in their entirety. This process explains why some segments of the Chester Beatty papyri also share the same texts as found in the medical ostraca (e.g., Chester Beatty V, vs. 3.1–3.2 = O. DEM 1213 1–2[103]). The varieties of illnesses and treatments most commonly found in medical texts, therefore, reflect the needs of the community and the ingredients necessary for medical care.

P. Chester Beatty 6 contains 41 different legible texts, and at least 32 of them deal with digestive disorders, particularly those affecting the anus (*pḥ.wyt*). These disorders include remedies for removing the *ʿn*, "turning around" in the anus, and a *dns* "heaviness" of the anus. Treatments for digestive disorders often

102 Adhémar Massart, "The Egyptian Geneva Papyrus MAH 15274," *Mitteilungen Des Deutschen Archäologischen Instituts Abteilung Kairo* 15 (1957): 172–185.

103 Joris F. Borghouts, *Ancient Egyptian Magical Texts* (Leiden: Brill, 1978), 123.

prescribed enemas, suppositories, and purgatives to remove an illness. Alternatively, digestive disorders could be cured through cleansing the body with cool waters (Chester Beatty 6, 6.13): *k.t pẖr.t n sḳb ḥꜣ.tỉ sḳb pḥ.yt sꜥnḫ mt.w jrr.t m trỉ n šmw*, "Another remedy for cooling the heart, cooling the anus, and enlivening the *mt.w*-vessels. One made during Shemu." The need to *sḳbb*, 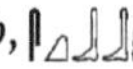 "cool," the body could serve the dual purposes of relieving an individual and purifying them as an act of conceptual ritual cleansing.[104]

Venomous bites and stings also reoccur frequently in the Chester Beatty papyri. The proximity between Deir el-Medina and the cultivated and deserted spaces of Western Thebes would have made it a prime location for scorpion stings and snake bites, as evidenced by at least seven examples of scorpion stings occurring in texts documenting workmen absences,[105] with two additional citations of undefined bites/stings.[106] Indeed, the presence of the *ḫrp-Srq.t* may even be required because of the frequent concerns over the venomous bites and stings of scorpions and snakes. Treatments for these afflictions in the Chester Beatty Papyri frequently focus on spoken spells recited to either draw out the venom or protect a workman from future bites/stings. For example, P. Chester Beatty 5, 3.1–3.2: *ky r n(.ỉ) ḏꜥry.t r mḥ m r⸗s tm dỉ.t pzḥ⸗s* "another spell against a scorpion in order to seize him by his mouth and not allow him to bite." Whereas many treatments in the Chester Beatty papyri focus on reacting to illnesses through preparing medicines, these focus on spoken incantations meant to appease or combat dangerous animals. The inclusion of both examples suggest that these private medical texts included the kinds of treatments that were the purview of both the *zwn.w* and *ḫrp-Srq.t*.

Among the medical texts from Deir el-Medina are amuletic texts and treatments for protections against divine forces. These may have similarly served to treat individuals with illnesses that showed signs of infection. For example, in P. DEM 36,[107] the foreman *ꜣny-nḫt*[108] is protected from a fever of three days. The text was written as a royal decree from Osiris to Geb, asking that he sail to the fields of Yaru and bring with him the male and female *nsy/nsy.t* demons,

104 Cooling serves to counteract venom/poison, and thus decontaminate the body as is demonstrated in O. Cairo JE 69771: *r sḳbb tꜣ mtw.t nšn.tỉ*, "in order to cool the venom/poison that was raging."

105 O. Ashmolean Museum 0174; O. Cairo CG 25517, verso 13; O. Cairo CG 25519, verso6–7; O. Cairo CG 25521, verso 2–3; O. BM 5634, verso 7.

106 O. Cairo CG 25517, verso 19; O. Varille 26, recto 15. This latter text is broken and could have included "of a scorpion."

107 Serge Sauneron, "Le Rhume d'Anynakhte (Pap. Deir El-Medineh 36)," *Kemi* 20 (1970): 7–18.

108 Davies, *Who's Who at Deir El-Medina*, 75.

opponents (*ḏʿ.yw*[109]), and dead. Once these disease agents are taken away, the symptoms of burning (*srf*[110] and *rmn.t*[111]) would also be removed quickly. The amuletic text was written in conjunction with drawings of two divine barks, two wadjet eyes, and two khepri beetles. Then the papyrus was folded[112] and placed on a cord with seven knots, which was meant to be worn as a necklace (as indicated in line 6). The knots would have both sealed and blocked out divine beings from entering the seven orifices of the head,[113] and its placement at the neck in combination with ritual folding and knotting would have simultaneously served to enclose and thus protect the individual. It was written in a fast, cursive hand,[114] rather than the more intentional hands used for medical texts in the Chester Beatty Papyri. Within this context, one can see that the amulet was written as a response to a specific illness of *ꜣny-nḫt*, and even though it appeared to be short-term (three days), the illness was serious enough to warrant the hasty production of a customized amulet calling for divine intervention to remove the demons or dead that are contaminating *ꜣny-nḫt* immediately. This amuletic text of *ꜣny-nḫt* was clearly designed to treat one individual, likely at the onset of an illness as a form of treatment owing to its hasty execution. Its ultimate disposal in the grand pit further suggests that it retained no value after this one-time use.

Some medical texts also address the need to bandage wounds and may have been used to treat injuries using simple ingredients similar to those distributed to the workforce in O. Gardiner 246. P. Chester Beatty 6, verso 1.7–2.2 mentions *pẖr.t n.t dr nkn m ʿ.t nb.t*, "a treatment for an injury in any limb." The treatment combines multiple plants, fat, fine oil (*tp.ỉt*), and honey, bandaging the wound for four days.[115] The author of the text includes at the end of

---

109 TLA lemma 181880; Wb 5, 517.10–12.

110 TLA lemma 139380; Wb 4, 195.11–13; MedWb 781f.

111 For the correction *rmn.t* from *r-ḫn.t*, see Joachim Friedrich Quack, "Beiträge Zu Einigen Religiösen Und Magischen Texte," in *Ramesside Studies in Honour of K.A. Kitchen*, ed. Mark Collier and Steven Snape (Bolton: Rutherford Press, 2011), 415. For the association of *rmn.t* with burning, see Iorwerth Eiddon Stephen Edwards, *Oracular Amuletic Decrees of the Late New Kingdom*, vol. 1. Text (London: Trustees of the British Museum, 1960), 20, nt. 16.

112 It was folded eight times lengthwise, five times widthwise, and two additional folds from both the right and the left. Bernard Bruyère, *Rapport sur les fouilles de Deir el Médineh (1948 à 1951)*, Fouilles de l'Institut français d'archéologie orientale 26 (Cairo: Institut français d'archéologie orientale, 1953), 72.

113 Willeke Wendrich, "Entangled, Connected or Protected? The Power of Knots and Knotting in Ancient Egypt," in *Through a Glass Darkly: Magic, Dreams and Prophecy in Ancient Egypt*, ed. Kasia Maria Szpakowska (Swansea: Classical Press of Wales, 2006), 243–269.

114 Sauneron, "Le Rhume d'Anynakhte (Pap. Deir El-Medineh 36)," 7–8.

115 The plants included are *ỉbzꜣ*, *šꜣšꜣ*, and *ḥbt*.

the treatment, *nfr nfr*, "good, good," a phrase sometimes used to indicate that a treatment was particularly effective. P. Chester Beatty 6, 6.1–6.2 includes a similar treatment for bandaging a wound, calling for fat, cumin, incense, myrrh, and honey. Both examples contain several similar ingredients to those distributed among the workforce—namely oil, honey, incense, and fat—making it possible that these kinds of salves were used by workman when bandaging each other's injuries.

Some of the documented treatments likely did help in ways known to biomedicine by preventing infection, improving digestion, and reducing pain. The use of honey, for example, in bandaging wounds would have aided healing through its antibacterial properties, maintaining a moist environment, and acting as a protective barrier to infection.[116] Enemas are commonly used today at home and in hospitals, and in some cases are composed of similar active ingredients to those described in the Chester Beatty papyri. For example, P. Chester Beatty 6, 6.12–6.13 is a prescription for an enema made of milk and honey. This could have operated similarly to the milk and molasses enemas used by many nurses to relieve constipation.[117] Recent studies have also identified how several known plants used in Egyptian medical texts had anti-inflammatory, antimicrobial, and analgesic properties.[118] These include ingredients found among the medical texts at Deir el-Medina such as myrrh.[119] The extra note *nfr nfr*, "good, good" to indicate when a treatment was particularly effective

---

116 Manisha Deb Mandal and Shyamapada Mandal, "Honey: Its Medicinal Property and Antibacterial Activity," *Asian Pacific Journal of Tropical Biomedicine* 1, no. 2 (April 2011): 154–160, https://doi.org/10.1016/S2221-1691(11)60016-6.

117 Sarah E. Hansen et al., "Safety and Efficacy of Milk and Molasses Enemas Compared With Sodium Phosphate Enemas for the Treatment of Constipation in a Pediatric Emergency Department," *Pediatric Emergency Care* 27, no. 12 (December 2011): 1118, https://doi.org/10.1097/PEC.0b013e31823b0088; Gary M. Vilke et al., "Safety and Efficacy of Milk and Molasses Enemas in the Emergency Department," *The Journal of Emergency Medicine* 48, no. 6 (June 2015): 667–670, https://doi.org/10.1016/j.jemermed.2015.01.035; Kimberley Walaker et al., "Milk and Molasses Enemas: Clearing Things Up," *Journal of Emergency Nursing* 40, no. 6 (November 2014): 546–551, https://doi.org/10.1016/j.jen.2013.08.012; Jackline Wangui-Verry et al., "CE: Original Research: Are Milk and Molasses Enemas Safe for Hospitalized Adults? A Retrospective Electronic Health Record Review," *The American Journal of Nursing* 119, no. 9 (September 2019): 24–28, https://doi.org/10.1097/01.NAJ.0000580148.43193.76.

118 Victor Kuete et al., "Antibacterial Activity and Cytotoxicity of Selected Egyptian Medicinal Plants," *Planta Medica* 78, no. 2 (January 2012): 193–199, https://doi.org/10.1055/s-0031-1280319; Mostafa Abbas Shalaby and Ashraf Abd-Elkhalik Hammouda, "Analgesic, Anti-Inflammatory and Anti-Hyperlipidemic Activities of Commiphora Molmol Extract (Myrrh)," *Journal of Intercultural Ethnopharmacology* 3, no. 2 (2014): 56–62.

119 Used in three treatments in P Chester Beatty 6 (lines 2.2, 5.11, and 6.1).

also shows that within the village, people were aware and tracking which treatments had more effective outcomes than others. The people of Deir el-Medina were, therefore, capable of evaluating and improving their medical treatments, using ones that they knew were effective and ones that modern research has suggested would have benefited their health.

Even in cases where the medical treatment acted only as a placebo, medical care at Deir el-Medina could still reduce stress due to the placebo effect's impact on symptoms associated with the stress response. Placebo treatments consistently result in increased pain relief, stimulated immune responses, and adjusted serotonin and dopamine levels.[120] These placebos can even be significantly effective when the recipient realizes they are receiving a placebo.[121] The kind of ritual involved in medicine further affects its efficacy; in one study, personal care and attention during treatments with a placebo pill generated 18 % more pain relief than the pill alone, and 34 % more relief than no treatment.[122] Even treatments traditionally deemed magical—which often involve personal attention and care—can offer significant health benefits of their own.

4 Healthcare Access in the Human Remains: Three Case Studies

Most texts documenting Egyptian medical treatments—including those referenced in this chapter—acted as reference volumes for individuals to turn to in the event someone is ill. They, therefore, represent the concerns related to illness in the community but do not usually attest to individual illness experiences. Medical texts were also more frequently recorded when one needed to remember a list of ingredients; more common issues like injuries do not appear in most medical papyri and are not attested at Deir el-Medina. Case studies from the human remains can fill this gap, offering a window into illness experiences at the site and insights into medicine often missing from the medical papyri and ostraca. The following three case studies represent examples where healthcare access would have impacted health outcomes in the village. Like

120 Damien G. Finniss et al., "Biological, Clinical, and Ethical Advances of Placebo Effects," *The Lancet* 375, no. 9715 (February 2010): 686–695, https://doi.org/10.1016/S0140-6736(09)61706-2.

121 Ted J. Kaptchuk et al., "Placebos without Deception: A Randomized Controlled Trial in Irritable Bowel Syndrome," *PLoS ONE* 5, no. 12 (December 2010): e15591, https://doi.org/10.1371/journal.pone.0015591.

122 Ted J. Kaptchuk et al., "Components of Placebo Effect: Randomised Controlled Trial in Patients with Irritable Bowel Syndrome," *BMJ* 336, no. 7651 (May 2008): 999–1003, https://doi.org/10.1136/bmj.39524.439618.25.

the case-studies in Chapter 5, these three osteological examples come from the Ramesside-era commingled remains in TT 290 and TT 298.

One well-healed fracture shows the potential for how a *zwn.w* for the workmen, well-trained in treating injuries related to the workforce, may have improved overall health outcomes. One ulna (DEM 290.14.124) of an adult who was possibly male[123] has a transverse fracture in the distal third of the bone. The callus from this lower arm fracture is smooth with no evidence of infection (i.e., no pitting or periosteal reactions around the callus). The cause of this fracture can only remain speculative. Its location is typical of so-called parry fractures which can result from either violence or an accident where the forearm is used in protection (e.g., from being hit or from falling).[124] The bone is straight with no angulation on either side of the callus (Figure 23), and there appears to have been minimal rotational deformity during healing. The ulna is thus fully healed and well-aligned. This bone alone does not tell us how fractures were treated at Deir el-Medina, and indeed, the example from Chapter 5 of a poorly aligned fracture of a woman's femur even contradicts this example. However, the broader awareness for how to align fractures in earlier medical texts (i.e., P. Edwin Smith) indicates that it is possible the village *zwn.w* would have known how to set a bone in order to improve healing. This may also explain health patterns at other state-building sites. At Giza, for example, workers and elites had similar rates of well-aligned fractures—90% and 89% respectively.[125] Although the workers had higher rates of fractures overall and higher cases of multiple fractures,[126] they also likely benefitted from state-supported medical care with a *zwn.w* who was consequently well-versed in how to align and treat fractures.

123 Age is based on fusion; however, a more specific adult age estimate is not possible. Sex estimation for ulnae is based on methods outlined in: L.S. Cowal and R.F. Pastor, 'Dimensional variation in the proximal ulna: Evaluation of a metric method for sex assessment', *American Journal of Physical Anthropology*, 135/4 (2008), 469–478.

124 One distinguishing criterion for parry fractures is isolated fractures in the ulna and not in the radius. Because this was identified among commingled human remains, it could not be compared to its paired radius. For further discussion on identifying and interpreting parry fractures, see Margaret A. Judd, "The Parry Problem," *Journal of Archaeological Science* 35, no. 6 (June 2008): 1658–1666, https://doi.org/10.1016/j.jas.2007.11.005.

125 Fawzia Hussien et al., "Similarity of Fracture Treatment of Workers and High Officials of the Pyramid Builders," in *Pharmacy and Medicine in Ancient Egypt: Proceedings of the Conferences Held in Cairo (2007) and Manchester (2008)*, ed. Jenefer Cockitt and A. Rosalie David, Bar International Series 2141 (Oxford: Archaeopress, 2010), 85–89.

126 El-Din Sarry and Azza Mohamed, "Bone Fractures in Ancient Egyptians From Giza, Old Kingdom," *Egyptian Medical Journal* 2, no. 2 (2003): 1–13.

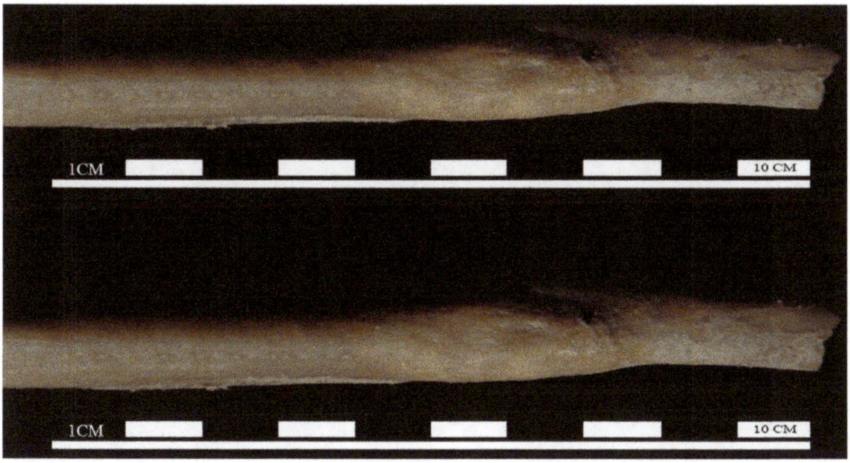

FIGURE 23 Ulna DEM 290.14.124 with a transverse fracture in the distal third of the bone.

Fighting infection was likely a common issue in the village based both on the data from human remains and medical texts from the site. One pair of adult articulated tibiae and fibulae (DEM 290.14.208–290.14.211) show extensive, bilateral periosteal reactions that may have even involved the marrow (i.e., osteomyelitis), as there are irregular areas of radiolucency within the medullary cavity and cloacae on the shaft of one tibia (Figure 24). While periosteal reactions such as these can be the result of direct injury, the bilateral distribution of the lesions across all four bones suggests that it is more likely to be the consequence of systemic infection. This bilateral inflammation of the periosteum would have initially resulted in the formation of woven bone on the shaft. Over several months, this woven bone was replaced by compact bone. This individual survived the infection long enough to show evidence of extensive healing. Like the example above, we cannot know whether this person received medical care, but they certainly could have benefitted from the kinds of treatments detailed in the medical texts for extensive infections, including spoken recitations and pharmacological ingredients with known antiseptic properties that were combined and applied either as ointments, drinks, enemas, or suppositories.

One final example shows direct evidence of medical intervention. DEM 298.20.232 is a partially complete mandible (Figure 8) with a possible dental filling.[127] The second molar has a large carious lesion measuring 4 mm wide by

127 There may also be a second filling identified by Bruyère based on his report describing human remains found in TT 337: "une momie de vieillard préparée au natron, dont les

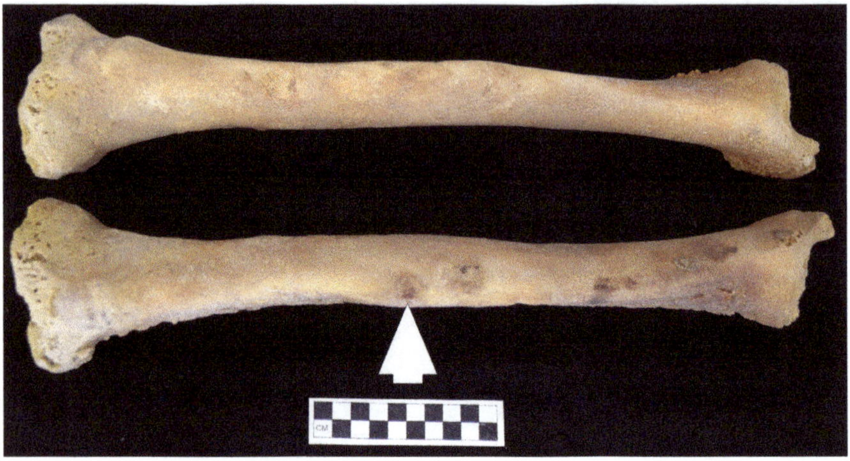

FIGURE 24 Extensive periosteal reactions on tibiae (DEM 290.14.208, DEM 290.14.210) from an adult including possible cloacae present on the anterior shaft of the right tibia (white arrow)

at least 4 mm deep that can be seen both at the occlusal surface and along a post-mortem break in the crown (Figure 25). This carious lesion is filled with a mass of fibrous material which has a light brown color. It fills most of the cavity and lips over the occlusal surface appearing attached to it. This suggests that the cavity was intentionally packed. While no mentions of tooth fillings appear in the published medical texts from Deir el-Medina, two texts from the contemporaneous P. Ebers describe such a treatment.[128] While the substance of this filling remains unknown, it appears homogenous. Such a treatment falls well within the purview of the *zwn.w* or the kinds of treatments described in private medical texts like the Chester Beatty papyri.

These examples illustrate some ways the villagers could benefit from professional and private medical care. Regular access to medical professionals and even common ingredients from the state would have allowed them to receive more consistent care. The presence of private medical texts would also have given the most literate members of the community unusually high degrees of

dents cariées portent, semble-t-il, des traces d'obturation" [a mummy of an old man prepared with natron, whose carious teeth seem to bear traces of filling]. Bernard Bruyère, *Rapport sur les fouilles de Deir el Médineh (1924–1925)*, Fouilles de l'Institut français d'archéologie orientale 3 (Cairo: Institut français d'archéologie orientale, 1926), 76–80.

128 Anne E. Austin, "Dental Health and Dentistry in Ancient Egypt: Possible Evidence for Dental Filling and Extraction at Deir El-Medina," *International Journal of Paleopathology* 38 (2022): 95–106, https://doi.org/10.1016/j.ijpp.2022.06.005.

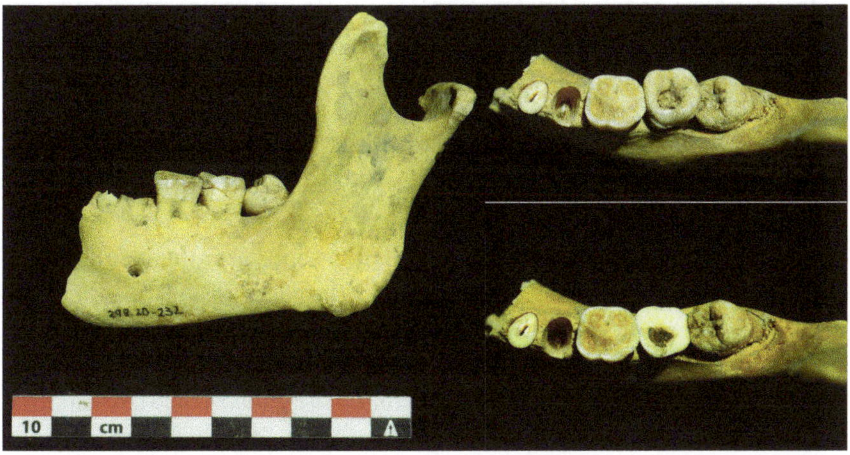

FIGURE 25 DEM 298.20.232 is a partially complete mandible (left) with a possible dental filling (upper right) and demineralized dentine visible below the filling (bottom right)

medical knowledge, thus allowing them to advocate for or even treat themselves and other members of the community when state-funded care was insufficient. State-supported healthcare and the community's high degree of medical literacy would have been particularly beneficial for illnesses and injuries common to the Deir el-Medina community because there was a consistent person to turn to when sick (e.g., *zwn.w*) who had access to extensive medical texts with treatments known to be effective. Those illnesses and injuries most common to the community would have included injuries like the ulnar fracture described above as well as infections, evidenced by the paired tibiae and fibulae with extensive periosteal reactions. Through both direct and indirect means, medical access at Deir el-Medina likely improved health outcomes by decreasing stress response, reducing pain, protecting against infection, and stimulating immune responses.

5 Healthcare Access and Health Outcomes at Deir el-Medina

Evidence from the medical texts, the kinds of healthcare professionals at the site, and the case studies from human remains demonstrate how healthcare access benefitted families at Deir el-Medina. Reflecting on the six health patterns from Chapter 4, healthcare access can also explain the rates of degenerative joint disease (DJD), periosteal reactions, and trauma at Deir el-Medina.

In some cases, medical treatments at Deir el-Medina do not reflect concerns around health indicators, explaining why stress indicators like DJD tended to be higher than non-working and elite cemeteries. None of the medical texts mention joint treatments or joint pain. This may be due to the nature of the texts as memory aids; however, the impact of joint degeneration may have also been simply seen as a natural part of aging and therefore did not require seeking healthcare.[129]

Conversely, treatments for infectious diseases appear in the medical texts, but higher rates of periosteal reactions and cranial porosities may indicate malaria and other infectious diseases still impacted health outcomes at Deir el-Medina. Examples of periosteal reactions with extensive healing, such as in the case study above, also suggest that the *Osteological Paradox* could bias interpretations of periosteal reactions since healed and unhealed lesions were reported together. Individuals who had healthcare support may have been more likely to survive a serious infection long enough to develop periosteal reactions and/or recover from them. Consequently, the irregular distribution of periosteal reactions and cranial porosities may alternatively reflect survival and healing.

Similarly, the high degree of healing in traumatic injuries at Deir el-Medina, including the case study of a well-aligned ulna, could also be a consequence of healthcare access. While social support (Chapter 5) could have benefitted healing by ensuring caretaking and provisioning after injuries, access to a healthcare professional who could set fractures and bandage wounds with honey would also have impacted survival rates.

Finally, the villagers had access to a combination of support from both private, family medical care, including those with high degrees of medical literacy, and a state-supported network of care. This may help to explain cases where the people of Deir el-Medina had even better health outcomes than elites elsewhere in Egypt, who may have had enough wealth and knowledge to access healthcare, but without the benefit of state support.

This system could function well during periods of relative stability but is vulnerable to changes in state funding or leadership. At the end of the New Kingdom, state support collapsed leaving the villagers without consistent rations.

---

129 This is true more broadly in published Egyptian medical texts from the New Kingdom. However, Papyrus Brooklyn 47.218.75+86, possibly from Elephantine and dating to the 26th Dynasty, evidences treatments for back pain. See Juliane Unger, "Ancient Egyptian Prescriptions for the Back and Abdomen and Their Mesopotamian and Mediterranean Counterparts," in *Systems of Classification in Premodern Medical Cultures: Sickness, Health, and Local Epistemologies*, ed. Ulrike Steinert (New York: Routledge, 2020), 123–126.

What happens when that second tier of support is no longer available? The next chapter evaluates just such a shift, examining how the economic uncertainty of the late 20th and early 21st Dynasty impacted health patterns at Deir el-Medina.

CHAPTER 7

Maintaining Economic Stability

While having a socially cohesive and supportive community at Deir el-Medina is one way to improve individual health outcomes, its success is also partially dependent on the community's success. Once a community—or even a state—starts to falter and there are insufficient resources to share, social support and healthcare access are far less likely to be available. Therefore, economic stability is one key *Social Determinant of Health* that can have trickle-down consequences and operate synergistically with social support and healthcare access.

Deir el-Medina's unique social circumstances ensured far more economic stability than the average Egyptian town. As evidenced in the last chapter, the village had the unusual benefit of both state and private support simultaneously. This chapter explores the various ways the villagers benefited from these social circumstances to ensure their economic stability even during the ultimate collapse of royal authority at the end of the New Kingdom.

I begin the chapter by reviewing the connections between economic stability and health outcomes. The chapter continues by identifying how the Egyptian state created economic stability at Deir el-Medina. Because of the unique skills of the Deir el-Medina workforce, the king provided them with a rich array of resources to ensure they could work daily on the royal tombs—a kind of *royal pact*. This gave them the housing and food security they needed to hone their craft, and their position as craftsmen for the king meant they could also seek out private avenues to enhance their economic status. The royal pact also impacted the working conditions at Deir el-Medina, bringing benefits to economic stability above and beyond comparable private workforces. As the state collapsed, and these resources became unstable, the workforce's social cohesion and valuable skills allowed them to adapt quickly. The chapter ends with the osteobiographies of two individuals whose experiences expand on how economic stability operated in the 18th Dynasty. Since texts focus on the Ramesside evidence for economic stability, the human remains also expand what we can say about daily life in Deir el-Medina's earliest period of occupation.

 | DOI:10.1163/9789004700871_008

1 Economic Stability and its Connection to Improved Health Outcomes

In modern contexts, the study of economic stability encompasses not just the stability of an individual's access to wealth, but relatedly, necessities such as food and housing. Short-term and long-term food insecurity can lead to major health problems as people grapple with reduced food intake; food of less quality, variety, or desirability; and ultimately malnutrition. These negative health outcomes can be particularly acute for children and teens who exhibit poorer overall health and more mental health issues.[1] Childhood impacts can be long-lasting given the connections between malnutrition and decreased immune response, making those experiencing food insecurity also more prone to infections.[2] Similarly, housing security has impacts on health that extend beyond the obvious benefits of consistent access to shelter. People with housing security also experience a greater sense of control, autonomy, and well-being, and they develop a stronger investment in their neighborhood and neighbors when their housing does not change.[3] For both food and housing security, health is not only connected to accessing these necessities, but also the mental and social benefits of getting them consistently.

While for many, economic stability is directly correlated with employment, those who are employed also face different health costs and benefits of their working environments.[4] Occupations may require different physical risks, expose people to more or fewer illnesses, and bring with them different degrees of mental stress. Therefore, the connection between economic stability and health is also dependent on the nature of the health risks associated with a given job.[5]

---

1 Michael P. Burke et al., "Severity of Household Food Insecurity Is Positively Associated with Mental Disorders among Children and Adolescents in the United States," *The Journal of Nutrition* 146, no. 10 (October 1, 2016): 2019–2026, https://doi.org/10.3945/jn.116.232298; Craig Gundersen and Brent Kreider, "Bounding the Effects of Food Insecurity on Children's Health Outcomes," *Journal of Health Economics* 28, no. 5 (September 2009): 971–983, https://doi.org/10.1016/j.jhealeco.2009.06.012.

2 Ulrich E. Schaible and Stefan H.E. Kaufmann, "Malnutrition and Infection: Complex Mechanisms and Global Impacts," *PLoS Medicine* 4, no. 5 (May 2007), https://doi.org/10.1371/journal.pmed.0040115.

3 Steve Rolfe et al., "Housing as a Social Determinant of Health and Wellbeing: Developing an Empirically-Informed Realist Theoretical Framework," *BMC Public Health* 20, no. 1 (July 20, 2020): 1138, https://doi.org/10.1186/s12889-020-09224-0.

4 Daniel S. Friedland and Richard H. Price, "Underemployment: Consequences for the Health and Well-Being of Workers," *American Journal of Community Psychology* 32, no. 1 (2003): 33–45, https://doi.org/10.1023/A:1025638705649.

5 Lisa F. Berkman, Ichiro Kawachi, and M. Maria Glymour, eds., *Social Epidemiology*, 2nd ed. (Oxford: Oxford University Press, 2014).

Relatedly, whether employers offer contingencies for an individual's illness or their family members' illness can also have a direct impact on communal health. For example, workers with paid sick leave are more likely to take time off than those without this benefit, and this holds true when considering not only leave for their own illnesses but also to take care of sick family members.[6] Relatedly, researchers have suggested population health can be dramatically improved through paid parental leave by comparing health statistics between the United States, which has no such federal policies, and other countries with paid parental leave built into their infrastructure (e.g., Sweden).[7] They found indirect evidence to support their findings including lower infant mortality rates, fewer delivery complications, and higher birthweight. These factors influence not only childhood health outcomes, but can also impact later adult health experiences because of the variety of ways childhood health later impacts adult health.[8]

These correlations in modern contexts point to two broader trends in the ways economic stability impacts health. First, when economic stability carries with it consistent access to necessities including food and shelter, it improves health not only by avoiding deprivation, but also through the mental and social benefits of expected, consistent access. While many people can accomplish this through steady employment, the second trend focuses on the nature of working environments. If work requires heightened risk or if it prevents someone from taking the time they or their family need to caretake, community health outcomes worsen.

2 Placing Economic Stability into the Past

Because economic stability as a concept carries with it some notion of an economy, it is important to consider how applicable this *Social Determinant*

6 Lisa Clemans-Cope et al., "Access to and Use of Paid Sick Leave among Low-Income Families with Children," *Pediatrics* 122, no. 2 (2008): e480–486, https://doi.org/10.1542/peds.2007-3294; LeaAnne DeRigne, Patricia Stoddard-Dare, and Linda Quinn, "Workers Without Paid Sick Leave Less Likely To Take Time Off For Illness Or Injury Compared To Those With Paid Sick Leave," *Health Affairs* 35, no. 3 (2016): 520–527; LeaAnne DeRigne et al., "Working U.S. Adults without Paid Sick Leave Report More Worries about Finances," *Journal of Social Service Research* 45, no. 4 (2019): 570–581.

7 Adam Burtle and Stephen Bezruchka, "Population Health and Paid Parental Leave: What the United States Can Learn from Two Decades of Research," *Healthcare* 4, no. 2 (2016): 30, https://doi.org/10.3390/healthcare4020030.

8 Julia Gamble and Gilian R. Bentley, "Developmental Origins of Health and Disease (DOHaD): Perspectives from Bioarchaeology," in *Palaeopathology and Evolutionary Medicine: An Integrated Approach*, ed. Kimberly A. Plomp et al. (Oxford: Oxford University Press, 2022), 17–41.

of Health is in the past. Describing or even defining an ancient economy is a fraught and debated task, especially given the potential errors when one assumes a modern economic model can be used to describe ancient economic practices.[9] In Pharaonic Egypt—where no set currency existed—this has been especially debated.[10] The economy of Deir el-Medina has also been widely published addressing issues of value, pricing, and private economic activity—topics that require entire books rather than a mere chapter.[11] However, the issues brought up by economic stability as a *Social Determinant of Health* avoid the need to define how the economy operated more broadly because it instead focuses on the two broader trends in economic stability as a *Social Determinant of Heath*:

1. How, when, and why does a community get consistent access to necessities like food and shelter?
2. What are the impacts of working conditions on health in a community and how were these accommodated?

I use these two questions to investigate economic stability at Deir el-Medina and how variations like private versus state-supported tomb construction, the collapsing state economy, and diachronic changes impacted how economic stability operated in the village.

3 Accessing Necessities through the Royal Pact

As royal artisans, the workmen at Deir el-Medina and their families were provided with the housing, food, and services necessary to allow the workforce to flourish. One stela, Cairo CGC 34504, dedicated by Ramesses II summarizes both the esteem afforded to skilled workmen and the rich variety of ways the king supplied his artisans:[12]

---

9 In reference to Deir el-Medina, see the short summary on these issues in Sofia Häggman, *Directing Deir El-Medina: The External Administration of the Necropolis*, Uppsala Studies in Egyptology 4 (Uppsala: Uppsala University, 2002), 76–78.

10 Ben J.J. Haring, "Economy," ed. Elizabeth Frood, Willeke Wendrich, and Jacco Dieleman, *UCLA Encyclopedia of Egyptology* 1, no. 1 (February 4, 2009), https://escholarship.org/uc/item/2t01s4qj.

11 Cooney, *The Cost of Death: The Social and Economic Value of Ancient Egyptian Funerary Art in the Rameside Period*; Janssen, *Commodity Prices from the Ramessid Period*; Jac J. Janssen, *Donkeys at Deir El-Medîna*, Egyptologische Uitgaven 19 (Leiden: Nederlands Instituut voor het Nabije Oosten, 2005).

12 Kenneth A. Kitchen, *Ramesside Inscriptions. Translated & Annotated.*, vol. 2 (Oxford: Wiley-Blackwell, 1996), 194. This stela contains several unusual signs that required it to

> I shall deal with your needs in every respect, so that you shall work for me devotedly ... I know that your labours are energetic and efficient, and that only on a full stomach are people glad to work on it ... I have filled the stores for you with everything; with bread, meat, cakes, to sustain you; sandals, clothing, unguent enough to anoint your heads every 10 days and your clothing (issued) annually, that you may persevere daily. None of you (need) pass the night moaning about poverty. I have assigned many people to supply you against need ... I have done all of this so that you may be united in working for me.

This text was written for royal sculptors, but its description connects to the variety of benefits afforded to the workmen at Deir el-Medina and suggests a *royal pact* made between a king and his artisans.[13] Like the royal sculptors, the workmen at Deir el-Medina and their families also received *ḥtrỉ*, a variety of goods most often provided by the *smd.t* including fish, water, vegetables, wood, and pottery.[14] The *smd.t* delivered these goods to Deir el-Medina regularly. Less often, the workforce received more luxury goods, including linen, beer, wine, oils, and meats. The frequent distribution of *ḥtrỉ* ensured not only regular access to food but also a varied diet.

The workmen also received pay in the form of grain rations regularly given to the crew, and these rations allowed them to trade for other necessities.[15] A normal workman would have received 4 *ẖꜣr* of emmer and 1 ½ *ẖꜣr* of barley each month—far more than what they would need to feed their family, especially given the variety of other foods given to the workforce.[16] This surplus would have even been higher for senior members of the workforce (i.e., the scribes and foremen) as well as the *zwn.w* and *ẖrp-Srq.t* who were given supplementary rations. The surplus grain rations could then be exchanged for other necessities. Many ostraca attest to these transactions with extra *ẖꜣr* of grain traded for

---

be republished in Ahmed Hamada, "A Stela from Manshîyet Eṣ-Ṣadr," *Annales Du Service Des Antiquités de l'Égypte* 38 (1938): 217–230. Owing to this, I present it in translation.

13 Valbelle, *Les ouvriers de la Tombe*, 148.

14 Davies, *Life Within the Five Walls*, 266–267; Häggman, *Directing Deir El-Medina*, 83–84; Valbelle, *Les ouvriers de la Tombe*, 148.

15 Grain rations were distributed both as an initial payment and smaller and more irregular subsequent amounts serving as arrears or advances. For detailed discussion on the nature of these payments, see Mandeville, *Wage Accounting in Deir El-Medina*, 2014.

16 Miller estimates that just 1 *ẖꜣr* of wheat and ¼ *ẖꜣr* of barley would have been sufficient to feed four adults 2,000 calories per day. Robert L. Miller, "Counting Calories in Egyptian Ration Texts," *Journal of the Economic and Social History of the Orient* 34, no. 3 (1991): 257–269, https://doi.org/10.1163/156852091X00021.

things like vegetables, fat, thread, basketry, and sandals.[17] These various regular rations and distributions to the workforce demonstrate that when the state was delivering goods, food security was incredibly high for a family of a workman.

Similarly, housing was also secure for the workmen as the state provided both the village houses and temporary huts near the royal wadis to members of the crew.[18] The "stato civile" texts—records from the late 20th Dynasty listing household membership—offer a kind of census for the village, telling us the composition of households of the workmen.[19] The households are listed as the house of a workman, identified by his name and parentage. After this, the text lists the household members and their relation to the workman. Across the records, we see repeated examples of workmen's households consisting of their wives, sons, and daughters. Many records also attest to close female relatives—sisters and mothers—as members of the household. Notably absent are brothers and fathers who presumably would have lived in a household of their own if they were also part of the workforce.

These benefits for workmen and their families from the *royal pact* demonstrate how both food and housing stability was contingent on being a member of the crew. However, this was a competitive task since most workmen had multiple sons, leading to more men in the village than available positions on the crew. As the size of the workforce at Deir el-Medina grew or shrunk based on the decisions of individual kings and the lengths of their reigns,[20] workmen had to invest in ensuring their sons' skills met expectations for those working on the royal tomb or risk losing these coveted positions to other workmen's sons or even artisans from outside the village.

Because of this uncertainty, fathers in the village used multiple strategies to ensure their sons' employment. One way was through the early apprenticeship of boys in the community as demonstrated by the variety of terms used to describe boys and young men who were not yet appointed as full workmen,

---

17 Jaroslav Černý, "Prices and Wages in Egypt during the Ramesside Period," *Cahiers d'histoire Mondial* 1, no. 4 (1954): 903–921.

18 Davies, *Life Within the Five Walls*, 151.

19 Demarée and Valbelle, *Les registres de recensement du village de Dier el-Médineh*; Robert J. Demarée, Andreas Dorn, and Stéphane Polis, "Les Listes de Maisonnées de Deir El-Médina («Stato Civile»). Nouveaux Fragments de l'Ifao et Localisation de l'archive d'une Ligne de Scribes," *Bulletin de l'Institut Français d'Archéologie Orientale*, no. 120 (2020): 171–220.

20 Dominique Valbelle, *Les ouvriers de la Tombe*, Biobliothèque d'Étude 96 (Cairo: Institut français d'archéologie orientale du Caire, 1985); Benedict G. Davies, *Life Within the Five Walls: A Handbook to Deir El-Medina* (Wallasey: Abercromby Press, 2018), 379–381.

including *ms-ḫr* ("child of the tomb"), *ꜥḏd* ("boy"), and *mnḥ* ("stripling").[21] These titles show successive growth in responsibilities and pay, with individuals being promoted from positions as boys to striplings and ultimately to workmen if a position was available. When their skills were in doubt, fathers might even use bribes to the scribe and foremen to ensure their sons were recommended for promotion to the vizier's office.[22] Families with sons who were not on the workforce could still secure employment elsewhere. Some may have joined the support staff (*smd.t*),[23] allowing them to stay in daily proximity to their families. Alternatively, the high degrees of literacy within the village meant that some sons were able to get positions outside of Deir el-Medina acting as scribes and administrators. For example, two of the sons of *Nfr-ḥtp* (i) were able to secure such positions, serving in one case as an army scribe and the other as a chief transport officer.[24] Whether by skill, opportunity, or bribery, these various strategies demonstrate the value of the housing and food secured by one of these positions.

Conversely, there was potential economic risk when retiring, given the number of benefits lost when a workman was no longer part of the crew. As discussed in Chapter 5, workmen managed this transition by replacing themselves with their apprenticed and appointed son. In recompense for the position, sons would then give some portion of their salary to their retired father, since these men were no longer regularly paid. McDowell presents several examples that suggest a transition period between elderly workmen who were retiring and the hiring of their children.[25] For example, soon after *Wsḫ-nmt.t*[26] joins the workforce, his father disappears from the rosters. During this period, *Wsḫ-nmt.t* gives half of his salary to his father for ten months.[27] McDowell suggests this and other examples mean that when a workman was transitioning out of the workforce or needed prolonged support completing their

21 Černý, *A community of workmen at Thebes in the Ramesside period*, pp. 113–117. Janssen, *Village varia*, pp. 19–21.

22 A.G. McDowell, *Village Life in Ancient Egypt: Laundry Lists and Love Songs*, (Oxford University Press, 1999), 230.

23 This was most noticeable in the reign of Ramesses V when the workforce, after being briefly doubled in size, reverted back to its original size with the fired workmen taking positions on the *smd.t* as described in O. Berlin O. 12654. For further discussion, see Davies, *Life Within the Five Walls*, 383.

24 Davies, *Who's Who at Deir El-Medina*, 31.

25 A.G. McDowell, 'Legal aspects of care of the elderly in Egypt to the end of the New Kingdom', in M. Stol, S.P. Vleeming (eds.), *The care of the elderly in the ancient Near East* (Brill, 1998), p. 211.

26 Davies, *Who's who at Deir el-Medina*, p. 258.

27 O. Glasgow D.1925.71.

work, they would ration half their salary to make up for the loss in productivity. In this case, village expectations dictated that new workmen take care of their aging fathers because the state offered no support for them once they left the workforce. Village expectations likely predicted a reciprocation of wages between sons and fathers that would have helped them navigate potential periods of economic instability as they were hired and retired from the crew.

4 The Royal Pact and its impact on Working Conditions

Ramesses II's stela above reveals the royal motivation behind state support for royal artisans—they were provided with their "needs in every respect" so that as a united workforce, they could construct the royal tombs "devotedly," "energetically," and "efficiently." This *royal pact* carried with it a promise and expectation—the workforce's many benefits are guaranteed so long as their work meets these royal standards.

Since the vizier's office was responsible for paying rations and appointing members of the crew, their visits were likely a pivotal moment for economic stability as they could include major decisions for the entire community; it was the vizier who informed the crew about when it was to be expanded or reduced, and visits could also come with news of bonuses for the crew's productivity based on their progress.[28] For example, in O. Cairo CG 25504, workmen were given loaves, oxen, beer, fish, fine cloth, and much more as rewards by the vizier for their work completing the king's tomb.[29] Alternatively, in O. OIM 16991, the scribe specifically mentions the tomb's progress as proof that the vizier should pay the workmen their regular rations, presumably because their pay had been delayed.[30] Economic stability was thus deeply interconnected with the vizier given his role as Overseer of Royal Works and the vizier's visits were critical moments to ensure that economic stability continued. This oversight also offered a means for the vizier's office to ensure the workforce maintained the productivity expected of them in the *royal pact*.

---

28 Häggman, *Directing Deir El-Medina*, 123.

29 Wolfgang Helck, *Die datierten und datierbaren Ostraka, Papyri und Graffiti von Deir el-Medineh*, Ägyptologische Abhandlungen 63 (Wiesbaden: Harrassowitz Verlag, 2002), 87–88; Kitchen, *Ramesside Inscriptions. Translated & Annotated.*, 1996.

30 Edward F. Wente, "A Letter of Complaint to the Vizier To," *Journal of Near Eastern Studies* 20, no. 4 (1961): 252–257.

These expectations for the crew's productivity meant that workmen also had to endure potential injury and occupational stress through the very nature of their working conditions. As already seen in Chapter 4, higher rates of osteoarthritis at Deir el-Medina—particularly in the knees and ankles of males—may have been a consequence of the workmen's regular hikes to and from the royal tomb in combination with the heavy workloads required to cut and remove stone from the rock-cut tombs. While these arduous tasks primarily fell to the ordinary workmen, the draftsmen were sometimes required to help with removing stone.[31] Additionally, the tombs were poorly ventilated, especially during excavation when there would be constant debris in the air. In the earliest days of a tomb's construction, the space would have been densely packed with other workers excavating stones to form the tomb's central corridor. Workmen risked falling debris as they excavated and removed heavy loads of limestone. The crew's working conditions could easily lead to injury or sickness that may result in a worker's short-term, prolonged, or permanent absence from the crew.

The scribe of the workforce recorded the daily absences of workmen, keeping a record of the reasons and dates that workmen were not at the tomb, which provides a wealth of texts documenting illnesses and injuries in the workforce as well as the administrative response to these related absences. Over 150 of these absence texts have been uncovered for the Ramesside period.[32] Of these, 69 absence texts have a complete regnal date and describe daily absences for one or more workmen. These texts consist of 2,043 total absences recorded over a 127-year period beginning in year 40 of Ramses II and ending in year 14 of Ramses IX. The recording of absences varied greatly over Deir el-Medina's occupation (Figure 26), reflecting the broader change in accounting during the Ramesside period, where absences were recorded more frequently and in more detail in the 19th Dynasty—an average 128 absences per year[33]—than the 20th Dynasty where the total number of absences in any given year drops to just 25. Consequently, though it is not possible to compare total absences over time, a closer look at the types of absences gives insight into the frequency and nature of illnesses and injuries at Deir el-Medina.

These texts often listed the reason for absence with illness (*mr*)[34] being one of the most common reasons, accounting for 29% of absences

31 Davies, *Life Within the Five Walls*, pp. 296–297.

32 For a more detailed discussion of this corpus, see Anne E. Austin, "Accounting for Sick Days: A Scalar Approach to Health and Disease at Deir El-Medina," *Journal of Near Eastern Studies* 74, no. 1 (2015): 75–85.

33 For years with one or more absence recorded.

34 There is debate whether Gardiner U23 should be transliterated as *mr* or *mḥr*. For con-

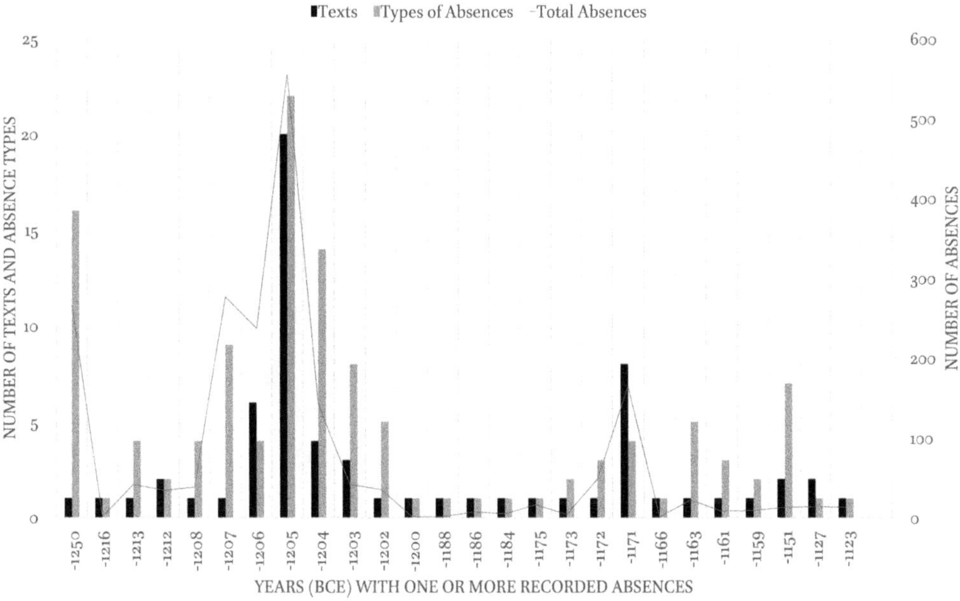

FIGURE 26 Distribution of Absence from Work Texts by estimated date. Dates are based on regnal year and reign when available.

(Figure 27).[35] This value is likely an underestimate as well, as in some cases, the reason listed for a likely sick workman was the generic *wsf*;[36] this term alone accounts for 40 % of all absences from work. Additionally, some scribes recorded the location of the workman when he was sick, such as "in the village," which can be reconstructed in some cases as due to illness, but is otherwise ambiguous.

In the rare cases where absences due to illness include more information, the scribe described illnesses of specific body parts, perhaps because these were work-related injuries. Thirteen absences list specific parts of the body, includ-

sistency with the *Thesaurus Linguae Aegyptiae*, I have chosen to transliterate as *mr*. See Simon D. Schweitzer, "Zum Lautwert Einiger Hieroglyphen," *Zeitschrift Für Ägyptische Sprache Und Altertumskunde* 138, no. 2 (2011): 132–149, https://doi.org/10.1524/zaes.2011.0011; Joachim Friedrich Quack, "Nochmals Zum Lautwert von Gardiner Sign-List U 23," *Lingua Aegyptia* 30 (2022): 271–289, https://doi.org/10.37011/lingaeg.30.09.

35 For a more detailed discussion of these texts, see Janssen, 'Absence from Work by the Necropolis Workmen of Thebes'.

36 This term has been discussed more fully by Janssen, where he connects the word etymologically to the phrase "to be slack, to neglect." Janssen, "Absence from Work by the Necropolis Workmen of Thebes," 145; Janssen, *Village Varia*, 1997, 93–95.

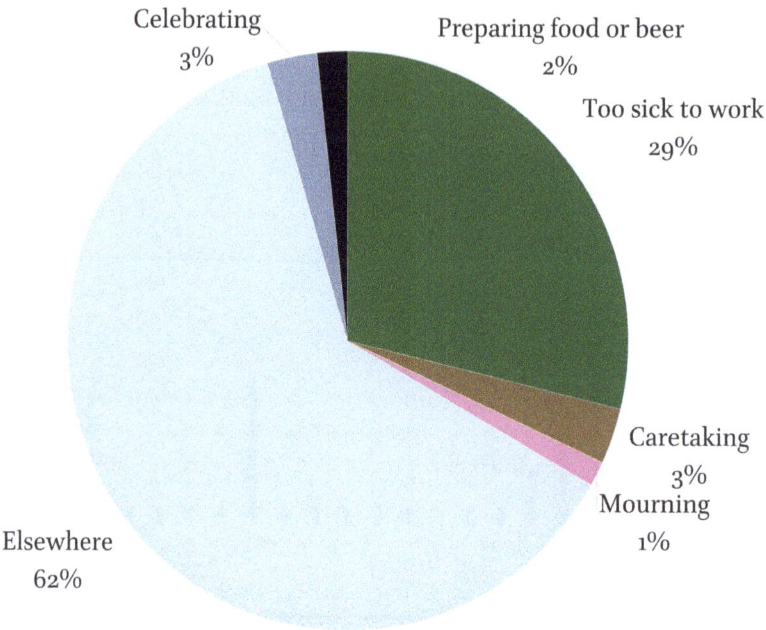

FIGURE 27 Distribution of absences where specific reasons were recorded (n = 1,937 absences)

ing the legs, hands, eyes, and ears.[37] Additionally, there are seven examples of scorpion stings[38] and two additional bites/stings mentioned.[39] If these were due to injuries, it is difficult to know their severity. Many texts are too fragmentary to determine whether there were additional days off. In other cases, an individual who was sick for only one or two days could have been placed on a longer leave and not be part of subsequent daily accounting. Some workers disappear from records for the workforce entirely after these absences, but these disappearances may be more of an attestation to the fragmentary nature of archaeological data rather than long-term injury.[40]

37 These are found in O. BM 5634, O. Cairo CG 25532, O. Cairo CG 25533, O. Cairo CG 25787, O. Gardiner 0037, and O. BTdK 614.

38 O. Ashmolean Museum 0174; O. Cairo CG 25517, verso 13; O. Cairo CG 25519, verso 6–7; O. Cairo CG 25521, verso 2–3; O. BM 5634, verso 7.

39 O. Cairo CG 25517, verso 19; O. Varille 26, recto 15. This latter text is broken and could have included "of a scorpion."

40 *Rt* (i), for example, is absent due to an illness in his leg in regnal year 4 of Siptah (O. Gardiner 0037). This workman disappears from the textual record for decades, not reappearing again until year 13 of Ramesses III. Davies tentatively suggests this is the same individual, and the lack of documentation for him during this time is due to the dearth

Infectious diseases likely accounted for many of these absences. Indeed, the seasonal distribution of sickness-related absences suggests infectious disease was a key cause of absence.[41] When comparing the ratio of days workmen were absent due to illness against total absences, there are growing numbers of sickness-related absences beginning in November and peaking in March–May (Figure 28).[42] This distribution could be due to a wide variety of ecological factors impacted by the annual inundation in July, leading to an agricultural cycle that made March through May a particularly dangerous period. Sicknesses were not only higher during this time, but historic accounts suggest infectious diseases tended to be more plentiful in April and May, causing similar seasonal mortality patterns in Upper Egypt more broadly.[43] It is also at this same time—the end of the growing season and beginning of harvest—that grain from the previous season would have been at their most exhausted point,[44] potentially adding nutritional stress to the variety of reasons why workmen may have been more likely to get sick. One direct example of an infectious disease spreading through the crew is the growing number of workmen's absences on O. BM 5634 from 3 *šm.w* 5 to 1 *ꜣḫ.t* 13, which peaks when five workmen were absent, four of whom were sick and the sixth (*Pꜣ-ḥr.y-pḏ.t* [iii]) was caretaking most likely as the *zwn.w*.[45] Soon afterward, *Pꜣ-ḥr.y-pḏ.t* (iii) too is sick perhaps because he was infected after caretaking his colleague. The close working conditions within the tomb, poor tomb ventilation, and the constant interactions between the *zwn.w* and sick colleagues all could lead to more ready spread of infectious diseases within the crew.

---

of administrative documents in the early years of Ramesses III. However, Davies is also unclear whether this is alternatively another workman of the same name. B. Davies, *Who's who at Deir el-Medina*, pp. 245–246.

41 Austin, "Accounting for Sick Days."

42 Austin.

43 Walter Scheidel accounts for the seasonality of illness through documenting Roman mummy tags, Greek funerary inscriptions, and Coptic epitaths from Egypt, comparing variation across Alexandria, the Fayum, and Upper Egypt. He also compares these data sets to more recent European accounts documenting the seasonality of disease. See, Walter Scheidel, *Death on the Nile: Disease and the Demography of Roman Egypt* (Leiden: Brill, 2001).

44 It is also possible that we see this evidenced in grain ration delays from Deir el-Medina. See Jean-Christophe Antoine, "The Delay of the Grain Ration and Its Social Consequences at Deir El-Medina in the Twentieth Dynasty: A Statistical Analysis," *The Journal of Egyptian Archaeology* 95, no. 1 (2009): 223–234. For a rebuttal of these data, see Mandeville, *Wage Accounting in Deir El-Medina*, 2014.

45 For a transcription of this text, see Jaroslav Černý and Alan H. Gardiner, *Hieratic Ostraca* (Oxford: University Press, 1957), 22–23, pl. LXXXIII and LXXXIV.

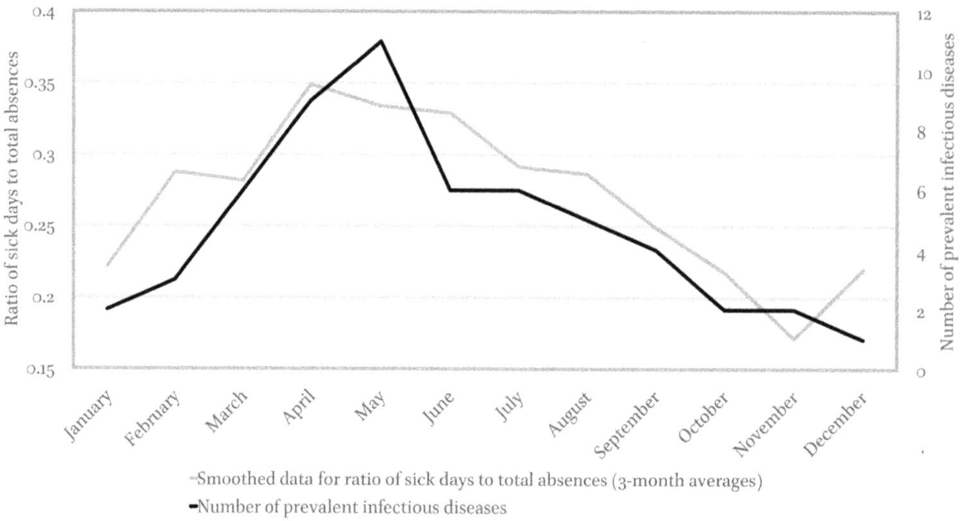

FIGURE 28 Seasonal distribution of absences due to illness in comparison to prevalent infectious diseases

These absences were still paid, however, ensuring economic stability even during long, sustained absences. In O. Cairo CG 25519 and 25521, *Pꜣ-ỉm.y-r-ỉḥ.w* (i) was marked as sick over a span of 47 days. He is accounted for in subsequent lists of workmen and absence records[46] indicating he was kept on the workforce despite this extended absence. Possibly just two months later, this same workman is documented as being absent due to an injured, burned hand.[47] Despite being absent for most if not all of the 1st month of *pr.t*, *Pꜣ-ỉm.y-r-ỉḥ.w* (i) is listed as receiving the same rations as his colleagues during this time.[48] More broadly, ration distributions across the Ramesside period do not appear to be calculated based on workmen's absences.[49] Permissible extended absences for these workmen not only allowed them to heal from their injuries and illnesses, but also ensured that they could return to continue their work once they recovered. This meant that the same workman could start and finish decorating a scene despite injury or illness.

46 E.g., O. Gardiner 0057, O. Cairo JE 72461, O. Cairo JE 72468.

47 See O. Cairo CG 25787. This has been tentatively dated to year 1 of Siptah. See W. Helck, *Die datierten und datierbaren Ostraka, Papyri und Graffiti von Deir el-Medineh*, (Otto Harrassowitz Verlag, 2002), p. 167.

48 O. DeM 00611 records rations paid during the third month of *šmw* for the first month of *pr.t* where *Pꜣ-ỉm.y-r-ỉḥ.w* (i) receives a normal workman's rations. The unusually long delay between issuance and work may be due to scribal error. This may mean this ostracon does not overlap with the extended illness.

49 Mandeville, *Wage Accounting in Deir El-Medina*, 2014, 97.

Even though workers were permitted sick leave, it is clear that these absences did not always allow for long-term leave, were not always taken, and sometimes required the workmen to make up for their impact on tomb construction. In O. OIM 16973, a workman faces legal accusations (*sḫꜣ-r*) for being away from work for five months.[50] In this case, the extended absence seems to exceed what was permissible. In O. Cairo CG 25785, the workman *Mry-Sḫm.t* (ii) was sick, attempted to go to the worksite but could not, and then returned to the village, recuperating for 10 days before returning to work.[51] His movement to and from the valley suggests he may have felt compelled to work through his illness, but being unable to, remained away from work until he recovered. As *Mry-Sḫm.t* (ii) was likely a draftsman,[52] he may have been in a more difficult position than most workmen during absences. Draftsmen were some of the least replaceable members of the workforce, and consequently their absences could have had an even larger impact than other workmen. In P. Ashmolean Museum 1958.112, *Ḥr-Mnw*,[53] a draftsman, asks his father for help because his brother is sick.[54] In this example, the absence from the left side of the crew has left them with a measurable deficit in their progress. To remedy this, *Ḥr-Mnw* possibly offers to share his own rations with a replacement.[55] Both of these examples reinforce the message from Ramesses II's stela to his artisans: workmen's absences were supported by the state so long as the crew maintained adequate progress on the tomb's construction.

These examples demonstrate that the *royal pact* meant that the workmen at Deir el-Medina were allowed to recover from illnesses and injuries so long as they maintained their productivity on the royal tomb. This state support at Deir el-Medina offered them measurable economic stability in comparison to the men who worked on private tombs of even the most successful non-royal elite.[56] Non-royal tomb construction had temporary work contracts and intermittent work, making it difficult for men to have economic stability. As Eyre notes, "the careful recording of daily quotes may be related to the temporary employment of various bodies of men on large scale works, whereas the crew-

50 Janssen, 'Absence from Work by the Necropolis Workmen of Thebes'.

51 Austin, "Accounting for Sick Days," 85.

52 Austin.

53 Davies, *Who's who at Deir el-Medina*, p. 168.

54 C.J. Eyre, 'A Draughtsman's Letter from Thebes', *SAK*, 11 (1984), 195–207.

55 Eyre notes that the final sentence is ambiguous since the suffix pronoun of rations is cramped and consequently unclear. This leads to a reading of either "his rations" or "my rations," though Eyre has translated it as "my."

56 Anne E. Austin, "Injuries, Illness, and Care While Constructing the Royal Tomb," in *Tomb Construction in New Kingdom Egypt*, ed. Fredrik Hagen, Daniel Soliman, and Rune Olsen (Cambridge: Cambridge University Press, Forthcoming).

men of Deir el-Medina were a permanent, salaried workforce."[57] Additionally, even if the same men could be reliably used in private tombs, their work may have been intermittent. In the tomb of the High Priest of Amun Mery (TT 95), Laboury argues that: "the same kinds of work were performed in the same parts of the tomb after several months and sometimes after several years, a fact that strongly suggests that the work was not continuous."[58]

Without a *royal pact*, illnesses or injuries would have had a much larger impact on the livelihood of non-royal tomb workers when compared to the royal crew. Even short-term injuries could have severely impacted a workman since he would not be guaranteed a position once he was able to work again. Additionally, he might not have benefitted from receiving rations during recovery from such an injury if compensation was based on his daily progress. Finally, while documentation at Deir el-Medina demonstrates they were provided care from medical practitioners, we have no mentions of medical practitioners, medical rations, or other forms of caretaking among ostraca from non-royal tomb construction.[59] Although these workers were exposed to similar working conditions and responsibilities as the crew at Deir el-Medina, they carried a much greater economic burden that would have directly impacted their health during tomb construction.

5 Maintaining Economic Stability outside of the State

The economic stability at Deir el-Medina discussed so far, especially in comparison to private tomb workers, is possible because of state support. During the 20th Dynasty, however, this state support becomes more erratic. Ration deliveries fall short and become less consistent, Libyans imperiled the villagers enough that they cannot safely leave the village, and royal control over Upper and Lower Egypt began to fracture. By the end of the 20th Dynasty, these impacts are great enough that some members of the Deir el-Medina community relocated to the nearby temple, Medinet Habu.[60] As the state collapsed

57 Eyre, C.J., 'Work and Organisation of Work in the New Kingdom', in M.A. Powell (ed.), *Labor in the ancient Near East*, (American Oriental Society, 1987), p. 185.

58 Laboury, 'Tracking Ancient Egyptian Artists, a Problem of Methodology. The Case of the Painters of Private Tombs in the Theban Necropolis during the Eighteenth Dynasty', p. 202.

59 Austin, "Injuries, Illness, and Care While Constructing the Royal Tomb"; William Christopher Hayes, *Ostraka and Name Stones from the Tomb of Sen-Mūt (No. 71) at Thebes* (New York: Metropolitan Museum of Art, 1942).

60 It is likely that the village was gradually abandoned rather than completely abandoned during this period, as discussed in Ben J.J. Haring, "Late Twentieth Dynasty Ostraca and

around them, so too did the *royal pact*. During these times when state support faltered, the people of Deir el-Medina showed remarkable solidarity and entrepreneurship to maintain their economic stability in an increasingly unstable world.

5.1 *Ensuring Rations in a Crumbling Economy*

In the final 80 years of the 20th Dynasty, the Egyptian state's crumbling finances lead to periods of shortfalls in rations for the workmen at Deir el-Medina. This made both the time between receiving rations longer[61] and the rations received often less than what they were owed. Rations were sometimes delayed, with supplementary deliveries necessary because they were in arrears.[62] Delays and shortages were not only in grain, but also goods from the *smd.t* such as fish[63] and wood.[64]

These issues with ration deliveries were exacerbated in the final years of the New Kingdom, but they were already visible decades earlier during the reign of Ramesses III. In O. Turin N 57072 a senior member of the workforce recorded the delivery of rations, regularly noting the unpaid balance. This document covers deliveries from regnal year 28 to 30 of Ramesses III, giving us an unusually long perspective on ration deliveries. While frequently the balance due was less than 1 *ḫꜣr*, there were also months where the author received considerably less, most notably in II *pr.t* of year 28 when the author received only 1 ½ *ḫꜣr* out of his total allotted 5 ½. By the end of year 29 and into year 30, the ration deliveries are consistently short with the author receiving only 59% of his allotted 5 ½ *ḫꜣr* between III *pr.t* of year 29 and III *šm.w* of year 30. These values reflect the loss of rations for a senior member of the workforce,[65] making the amount paid to regular workmen likely less—potentially as little as 1 *ḫꜣr*. When describ-

the End of the Necropolis Workmen's Settlement at Deir El-Medina," in *Deir El-Medina through the Kaleidoscope. Proceedings of the International Workshop Turin 8th–10th October 2018*, ed. Susanne Töpfer, Paolo Del Vesco, and Federico Poole (Modena: Formazione e ricerca, 2022), 44–62.

61 By the end of the 20th Dynasty, a large majority of rations were delivered in the final five days of the month rather than the more periodic distributions from the earlier Ramesside period. See Mandeville, *Wage Accounting in Deir El-Medina*, 2014, 73.

62 Antoine, "The Delay of the Grain Ration and Its Social Consequences at Deir El-Medina in the Twentieth Dynasty." Mandeville, however, argues that the delays were likely not as extensive as Antoine suggests. See Mandeville, *Wage Accounting in Deir El-Medina*, 2014.

63 Jean-Christophe Antoine, "Fluctuations of Fish Deliveries at Deir El-Medina in the Twentieth Dynasty. A Statistical Analysis," *Studien Zur Altägyptischen Kultur* 35 (2006): 25–41.

64 Jac J. Janssen, "The Year of the Strikes," *Bulletin de La Société d'Égyptologie de Genève* 16 (1992): 41–49.

65 Calculations assume a total of 5 ½ *ḫꜣr* and not the 4 *ḫꜣr* accorded to regular workmen.

ing these periods, the workmen frequently cite their hunger and thirst.[66] The rations listed in the worst months of O. Turin N 57072 were indeed insufficient to provide adequate beer and bread for the workforce and their families if the workmen relied on provisions from the state alone.[67]

While these texts claim that the workmen were without food, in some cases it is apparent that this was an exaggeration meant to call out the state for breaking the *royal pact*. In. P. Turin Cat. 1880, the scribe *ʾImn-nḫt* (v) wrote that:[68]

> |r2.2 *i͗.ir͗i͗=n pḥ nꜣ* |r2.3 *r-ḥꜥ.t ḥkr r-ḥꜥ.t i͗b mn ḥbsw mn sgnn mn rmw mn* |r2.4 *smw hꜣb n pr-ꜥꜣ pꜣy=n nb nfr ḥr r-r=sn mtw=tn hꜣb n ṯꜣty pꜣy=n* |R2.5 *ḥry-tp*
>
> |r2.2 Our arrival is because of |r2.3 hunger and because of thirst; there is no clothing, there is no oil, there are no |r2.4 fish, there are no vegetables. Send to Pharaoh, our good lord, about it, and send to the vizier, our |r2.5 superior.

Yet, other texts from the village suggest *ʾImn-nḫt* (v) exaggerated when he said there were no fish or vegetables; the workmen received 4,100 deben worth of fish just four days earlier (O. DeM 394) and a delivery of vegetables four days before that (O. Ifao 1405).[69] The issue was consequently not that the workmen were deprived, but that they were not receiving the amounts they were due from the state. *ʾImn-nḫt* (v) cited their thirst and hunger to frame the insufficient grain rations as part of a broken *royal pact*. He wrote about the very provisions promised by Ramesses II in his stela above and appealed directly to the king and vizier: those responsible for maintaining the *royal pact*. While P. Turin Cat. 1880 relates to a different pharaoh and period than Ramesses II's Cairo CGC 34504, the contract between the workforce and administration appeared to be the same: the crew worked so long as they had a full stomach and were supplied against need.

---

66 Hunger (*ḥkr*) is cited three times in the Turin Strike Papyrus and thirst is also mentioned once. Hunger is also mentioned in other related texts later during the 20th Dynasty, including P. Turin 1884 and the 20th Dynasty journal of the necropolis.

67 For example, in II *pr.t* of year 28, a regular workman likely received less than the 1 ½ *ḫꜣr* given to the author of this text. Miller estimates that 1 *ḫꜣr* of wheat and ¼ *ḫꜣr* of barley would have been sufficient to feed four adults 2,000 calories per day thus feeding a workman, his wife, and only two other family members which could include the workman's mother, sister(s), and children. For estimates of caloric value from grain rations, see Miller, "Counting Calories in Egyptian Ration Texts."

68 Transliteration based on Gardiner, *Ramesside Administrative Documents*, 54–55.

69 Helck, *Die datierten und datierbaren Ostraka, Papyri und Graffiti von Deir el-Medineh*, 307–308.

Consequently, the workmen at Deir el-Medina responded to these shortages by going on organized strike. Repeatedly, they left their worksite and village, passing the (5) walls (*sš tꜣ ỉnb.wt 5 n pꜣ ḫr*), a phrase that was used when the crew refused to work until they received some form of rations.[70] In year 29 of Ramesses III, they do so multiple times over the span of seven months.[71] In each case, they appeal to some of the highest authorities, including the vizier, and successfully received at least partial rations during or soon after their strike.

The workmen continued to use these strikes during later periods of the 20th Dynasty as well, often doing so as a collective, which led to their success at getting food even in the final years of state control. In one of the strikes, the villagers were even told to bring their families to the mortuary temple of Seti I, uniting the non-working members of the community. While repeated strikes suggest the workmen were still dealing with insufficient rations and the risk of hunger, these strikes also show the influence the men had on the state. In one case, the vizier wrote to them that the granaries were empty, but he would give them the grain he could find.[72] The crew was subsequently paid half their rations. While it is reasonable to question whether the state granaries were indeed as empty as the vizier claimed, the fact that so senior an official wrote to appease the crew and send them a portion of their rations shows the efficacy of their protest.

Their strikes also occurred during important political shifts for both the king and vizier, suggesting that the workmen took advantage of these political transitions to leverage their social power. The first strike recorded in the Turin Strike Papyrus took place at the moment To was promoted to vizier. Later strikes happened amid death and burial of Ramesses III (Figure 29), clearly a time when pressure was on the workforce to complete their work. Just weeks after recording one strike in O. DeM 38, the scribe recorded that Ramesses III had died (using another sherd, O. DeM 39, from the same broken vessel[73]). Between the king's death and his burial, the crew goes on strike again (O. Berlin 12631),

70 William F. Edgerton, "The Strikes in Ramses III's Twenty-Ninth Year," *Journal of Near Eastern Studies* 10, no. 3 (1951): 137–145; Paul J. Frandsen, "Editing Reality: The Turin Strike Papyrus," in *Studies in Egyptology Presented to Miriam Lichtheim*, ed. S. Israelit-Groll (Jerusalem: Magnes Press, 1990), 166–199.

71 Edgerton, "The Strikes in Ramses III's Twenty-Ninth Year"; Frandsen, "Editing Reality: The Turin Strike Papyrus."

72 Frandsen, "Editing Reality: The Turin Strike Papyrus," 188–189.

73 On their join from the same vessel, see Jaroslav Černý, *Catalogue des ostraca hiératiques non littéraires de Deir el-Médineh*, vol. I (Nos 1 à 113), Documents de fouilles 3 (Cairo: l'Institut français d'archéologie orientale, 1935), 10.

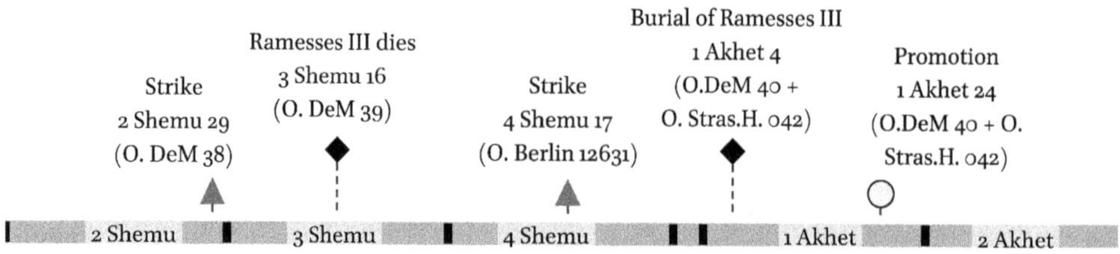

FIGURE 29 Timeline of strikes during the transition between the reigns of Ramesses III and IV

receiving their rations that same day. Ramesses IV handsomely rewarded the crew soon after Ramesses III's successful burial with a promotion of the next generation (*ḏꜣm*) of workmen. The crew strikes at least two more times in the very early years of Ramesses IV—once in year 2 (O. DeM 44) and another possibly in year 3 (O. Cairo CG 25533) when the workmen again seek sufficient rations. Simultaneously, it is in these early years of Ramesses IV that we see the greatest change in the size of the workforce documented at Deir el-Medina: the entire workforce grows to 120 workmen. While this does not last beyond Ramesses IV's reign, the continuous strikes in the uneasy transition between Ramesses III and Ramesses IV suggest they were at least temporarily effective at leveraging both rations and more positions on the crew.

Over 30 years later, the crew had another series of strikes in the reigns of Ramesses IX, X, and XI, demonstrating that these strikes are part of a broader strategy to ensure economic stability at Deir el-Medina throughout the Ramesside period and possibly as early as the 18th Dynasty.[74] The strikes consistently get results for the workforce—in most cases within days of the initial action of passing the five walls. This could even take greater measures to secure grain for the workforce; by the reign of Ramesses X, the administration supported sending the *smd.t* south in search of grain for the workforce.[75] These results ensure economic stability for the crew from the state even at times when the granaries are empty. Simultaneously, at least during the reign of Ramesses IV, they also appear to enable the crew to secure permanent positions for the next generation of the workforce.

74 Hans-Werner Fischer-Elfert, "A Strike in the Reign of Merenptah? Plus the Endowment of Three Cult Statue(Tte)s on Behalf of the Same King at Deir El-Medina (Pap. Berlin P. 23300 and P. 23301)," in *Forschung in Der Papyrussammlung: Eine Festgabe Für Das Neue Museum*, ed. Verena M. Lepper, Ägyptische Und Orientalische Papyri Und Handschriften Des Ägyptischen Museums Und Papyrussammlung Berlin 1 (Berlin: Akademie Verlag, 2012), 47–73.

75 Antoine, "The Delay of the Grain Ration and Its Social Consequences at Deir El-Medina in the Twentieth Dynasty," 233.

5.2 *Deir el-Medina in the Private Economy*

When state support became erratic, the villagers at Deir el-Medina ensured their economic stability through private economic opportunities, often available to them because of their status as royal artisans. In some cases, the members of the workforce at Deir el-Medina were compensated for the decoration of tomb chapels for upper elite tombs, and this may have been part of a private sector "informal workshop" led by the scribes and/or foremen of the crew.[76] More often, they were commissioned to make tomb equipment such as coffins or furniture as either draftsmen focused on the decoration of the object or carpenters.[77] These skillsets, therefore, prioritized the skills necessary for a private economy, including writing, drafting, painting, and woodworking. In theory, these private commissions could also afford workmen more economic power than their monthly grain rations, potentially doubling or tripling the total value of their earnings when funerary goods were in high demand.[78]

In some cases, the goods exchanged could help to mitigate the effects of insufficient grain rations during both the tumultuous years ending Ramesses III's reign and the final decades of the 20th Dynasty. For example, one text (O. Gardiner 171) dated to the midst of strikes during the reign of Ramesses IV indicates that *ꜣImn-pꜣ-Ḥꜥpy* completed 61 deben worth of carpentry work for a priest and scribe *ꜣImn-ḥtp*—a sizeable project that could be used to buy sufficient grain, vegetables, and fish during delays.[79] Even in examples like this, however, "craftsmen were never independent beings, but instead relied on their state training, official access to raw materials, on their co-workers in the official Deir el-Medina crew, as well as on craftsmen and patrons beyond the borders of the village to facilitate private sector earnings."[80] Indeed, many of the private commissions involved multiple crew members working collaboratively to

76 The few examples suggest the Deir el-Medina artisans were almost exclusively hired to decorate tombs with only one document O. Cairo CG 25243, evidencing the crew excavating a non-royal tomb. For further discussion, see Kathlyn M. Cooney, "Profit or Exploitation? The Production of Private Ramesside Tombs Within the West Theban Funerary Economy," *Journal of Egyptian History* 1, no. 1 (2008): 79–115, https://doi.org/10.1163/187416608784118776.

77 Cooney, *The Cost of Death: The Social and Economic Value of Ancient Egyptian Funerary Art in the Rameside Period.*

78 Cooney, 128.

79 Kitchen dates this ostracon to possibly year 2 of Ramesses IV in Kitchen, *Ramesside Inscriptions*, 1989, VII:223–224.

80 Kathlyn M. Cooney, "An Informal Workshop: Textual Evidence for Private Funerary Art Production in the Ramesside Period," in *Living and Writing in Deir El-Medine: Socio-Historical Embodiment of Deir El-Medine Texts*, ed. Andreas Dorn and Tobias Hofmann, Aegyptiaca Helvetica 19 (Basel: Schwabe AG, 2006), 55.

carve, assemble, and decorate coffins as evidenced by workshop records.[81] This large commission would have likely been distributed among multiple workmen offering additional income in the midst of poor grain supply to several families within the village.

There were additional economic opportunities outside of tomb preparation for both working and non-working members of the village. This included lending privately or possibly state-owned[82] donkeys to members of the *smd.t* in exchange for commodities.[83] Numerous texts attest to the use of donkeys as a way of extending income at Deir el-Medina, including legal disputes when workmen were not adequately compensated. Fortunately, several of these texts are securely dated. O. DeM 244 is a contract where the water-carrier *ỉmn-ḫʿ* hired a donkey from the workman *Nḫw-m-Mw.t* for a total of 5 ¼ *ḫꜣr* worth of goods—likely paid over the time of the donkey's use—around 83 days.[84] This text is dated to Ramesses III year 28, month 2 of *pr.t*, day 15. This same month, the workmen received their lowest grain ration payment from the state, according to O. Turin N 57072. The author only received 1 ½ *ḫꜣr* of grain, 27% of his normal allotted wage. While the text does not reveal the exact goods exchanged for the donkey hire, the workman's ability to hire out his donkey made it possible for him to make up some of the difference in wages not paid on time by the state. These loans were also most frequently made to water carriers—directly benefitting the villagers by making it more manageable to get water to the village and the royal wadis.

When economic stability from the state faltered, senior officials within the village used extra means to ensure food was available to the workforce. Wealthier members of the community could own fields and livestock that they cultivated and could have even used to supplement grain ration shortages for other members of the workforce. Throughout the Ramesside period, there is evidence that the chiefs owned both agricultural land and oxen to be used for plowing.[85] It is possible that other members of the crew also owned and cul-

81 Cooney, *The Cost of Death: The Social and Economic Value of Ancient Egyptian Funerary Art in the Rameside Period*, 46–50. Note that one such example, O. DeM 223, contains a payment by *ỉmn-Pꜣ-Ḥʿpy* to a carpenter *ʿꜣ-pꜣ-ṯꜣw* for his work on a set of 2–3 coffins. It is difficult, however, to know if this is the same *ỉmn-Pꜣ-Ḥʿpy* as the one mentioned in O. Gardiner 171.

82 Davies, *Life Within the Five Walls*, 85.

83 Janssen, *Donkeys at Deir El-Medîna*.

84 Janssen, 10.

85 Jean-Christophe Antoine, "Landholding and Agriculture in Late Ramesside Theban Documents," *Zeitschrift Für Ägyptische Sprache Und Altertumskunde* 142, no. 2 (2015): 104–119; Andrea G. McDowell, "Agricultural Activity by the Workmen of Deir El-Medina," *The Journal of Egyptian Archaeology* 78 (1992): 195–206, https://doi.org/10.2307/3822072.

tivated crops, but doing so would have required either non-working members of the community to farm or the wealth necessary to use forced labor from privately owned enslaved people and/or servants (*ḥm.w* and *bꜣk.w*).[86] This agricultural activity becomes increasingly visible by the reign of Ramesses XI when the workforce is no longer able to work on the royal tomb and the scribe of the necropolis instead focuses his efforts on cultivating both his own agricultural lands and ones belonging to the state and/or temples.[87] He does so in order to cultivate cereals, vegetables, and fruits that could supplement the grain ration shortages that became pervasive by the end of the village's occupation.[88]

6 Osteobiographies: Economic Stability during the 18th Dynasty

I began this chapter by looking at two questions to understand economic stability at Deir el-Medina. Ramesside-era texts answered the first question of how, when, and why the villagers got consistent access to necessities like food and shelter through the *royal pact*. Both the state's promise to provide for the workforce and the community's solidary response to state failures to maintain the *royal pact* ensured that food was always available, even in times of great instability at the end of the Ramesside period. The second question asked how working conditions and state responses to illness and injury impacted overall health in the community. Already, this was in part evidenced in Chapter 4, where the study of human remains revealed key differences in health outcomes between men and women in the village that could be explained by the arduous labor necessary to cut and decorate the royal tomb. In response to injuries and illnesses at work, Ramesside administrative texts demonstrated that the workmen were afforded paid leave, and these leaves gave them more economic stability in times of illness than private workforces. For both questions, texts have offered a wealth of detail about the way economic stability operated within the village, but exclusively during the Ramesside period.

---

86 McDowell, "Agricultural Activity by the Workmen of Deir El-Medina," 201. For discussion on the terms *bꜣk.w* and *ḥm.w*, see Endesfelder, "Sklaven (Hmw) in Der Nekropole von Deir El Medine"; Antonio Loprieno, "Slavery and Servitude," *UCLA Encyclopedia of Egyptology* 1, no. 1 (2012), https://escholarship.org/uc/item/8mx2073f.

87 As seen in the Late Ramesside Letters. For further discussion, see Antoine, "Landholding and Agriculture in Late Ramesside Theban Documents"; McDowell, "Agricultural Activity by the Workmen of Deir El-Medina."

88 Antoine, "Landholding and Agriculture in Late Ramesside Theban Documents."

Excluded from the discussion of economic stability so far is the 18th Dynasty. During this time, when administration for the village was handled orally, leaving no written record,[89] did economic stability operate the same way? Though the 18th Dynasty human remains from Deir el-Medina are only represented by a handful of individuals, these complete skeletons from known burial contexts provide an opportunity to understand economic stability during the 18th Dynasty through the use of osteobiographies[90]—life histories told through the study of both skeletons and burial contexts—to answer each of this chapter's main questions around economic stability. As these two osteobiographies reveal, economic stability during the 18th Dynasty may have operated similarly to the Ramesside period because the relative wealth of the community buffered them from stress, even in its most tenuous periods, though this also came at a greater physical cost because of more intense working conditions.

6.1 Stꜣw: *The Story of a Workman's Life during the Amarna Period*

The village at Deir el-Medina experienced some of its most extreme instability during the Amarna interlude—a period when the move of the capital to Akhetaten meant that the village was either partially abandoned or alternatively remained in use without full royal support.[91] Anyone staying or returning to Deir el-Medina had to contend with an extensive fire and an overall reorganization of the workforce. Any residents who moved to Amarna would have lived with the difficulties of a newly established capital. Given these differences, what do human remains from the Amarna period at Deir el-Medina reflect about working conditions and state responses to illness and injury during this time?

One workman, *Stꜣw*, who most likely came of age during the reign of Amenhotep III and subsequently stayed on the workforce through the Amarna period, is a testament to the working conditions during this time. His life story demonstrates the many and varied impacts these working conditions had on *Stꜣw* from his diet to his grave goods.

Stꜣw most likely died during or immediately after the Amarna period based on his tomb (P. 1352),[92] an ushabti that bears both his name and references

89 Haring, "From Oral Practice to Written Record in Ramesside Deir El-Medina."

90 At their simplest, osteobiographies are life narratives of single individuals. For an overview of osteobiographies, see Hosek and Robb, "Osteobiography."

91 Müller, "Deir El-Medina in the Dark—the Amarna Period in the History of the Village."

92 Bernard Bruyère, *Rapport sur les Fouilles de Deir el Médineh 1933–1934: I*, Fouilles de l'Institut français d'archéologie orientale (Le Caire: L'Institut Français d'Archéologie Orientale, 1937), 99.

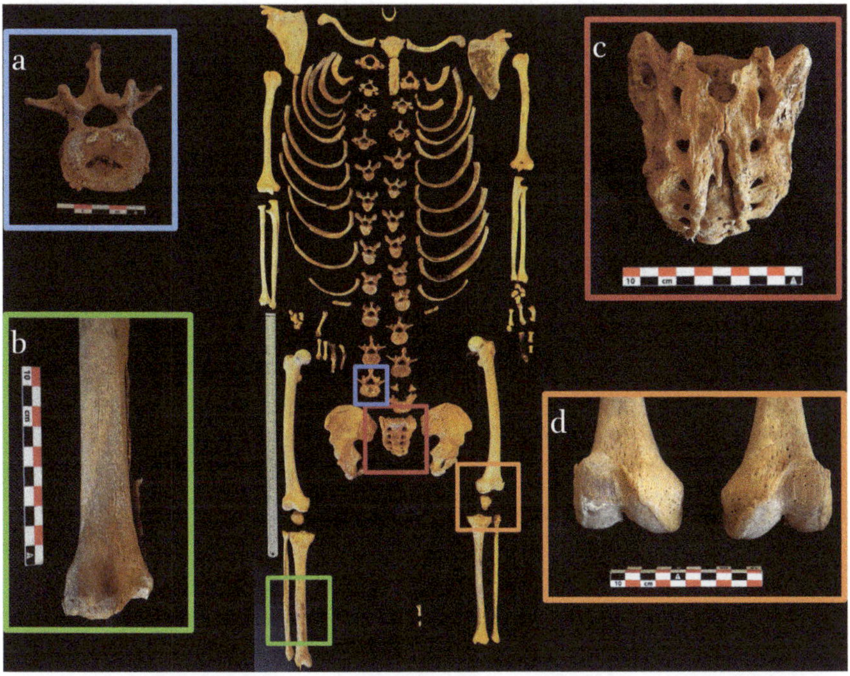

FIGURE 30 The articulated post-cranial skeleton of Stꜣw (DEM 217.23.001) exhibiting multiple paleopathological lesions including: (a) osteophytosis and a Schmorl's node on the T11 vertebra, (b) healed periosteal reactions on the tibia, (c) cleft neural arches on the sacrum, and (d) eburnation on both femora

to the Aten,[93] and his coffin decoration.[94] By that point, *Stꜣw* had lived a relatively long life—he was at least 50-years-old when he died and likely a decade or more older.[95] He was also found wearing a ring with the cartouche of Thutmosis IV[96]—a king who had personal meaning for *Stꜣw* given that Thutmosis IV

93 Bruyère, 95–109.

94 Gersande Eschenbrenner Diemer, Lisa Sartini, and Margaret Serpico, "Rediscovering Black Coffins from Deir El-Medina: A Comprehensive Approach," *Bulletin de l'Institut Français d'archéologie Orientale*, no. 121 (2021): 255–305, https://doi.org/10.4000/bifao.8189.

95 Age at death for *Stꜣw* was determined by observation of both the os coxae and skull. The composite score for the auricular surface was 15 (mean age 66.71, S.D. 11.88) using the Buckberry-Chamberlain method. The pubic symphysis scored 10 using the Todd System and 6 using Suchey-Brooks. These are the highest possible scores for the pubic symphysis for both methods. Cranial sutures also suggest an age over 50 based on a composite vault score of 19 and lateral-anterior score of 14. Additionally, there was extensive ossification of the laryngeal cartilage extending from the inferior to the superior horns as well as medially to the inferior thyroid notch, further suggesting an older adult age.

96 *Stꜣw* was found wearing a ring with the cartouche of Thutmosis IV on his left hand. See Bruyère, *Rapport sur les Fouilles de Deir el Médineh 1933–1934: I*, 103.

was most likely ruling when *Stȝw* was born.[97] This timeline indicates that *Stȝw* joined the workforce during the reign of Amenhotep III, and that he would have been on the workforce for decades by the time he died during or shortly after the Amarna period. His body, therefore, illustrates the working conditions at play during this volatile period for the village.

Stȝw was born with congenital defects in his spine that would not have been visible nor pathological but could be an indicator of issues in his mother's health during pregnancy. There are cleft neural arches along most segments of his sacrum (Figure 30.c) which likely led to spondylolysis of his 5th lumbar vertebra.[98] These genetic abnormalities are the result of a disruption of ossification of the two sides of the neural arch.[99] This leaves a gap in bone formation along the sacral spine and, in this case, an absent spinous process and incomplete laminae for the L5. In more extreme cases, such disruptions result in spina bifida which can have major consequences including paralysis or even death. Spina bifida has been linked to maternal nutritional deficiencies,[100] and consequently *Stȝw*'s cleft neural arches could be a sign of nutritional deficiency in his mother.

After birth, *Stȝw*'s health and life trajectory exemplify the broader patterns seen at Deir el-Medina. *Stȝw* shows no evidence of stress from childhood—enamel hypoplasias and cranial porosities are both absent. His adolescence similarly shows no obvious signs of stress—his stature (159 cm),[101] while below average for males at Deir el-Medina, is still within 2 S.D. of the average suggesting that he did not experience extreme deprivation.

He was at some point given an official role on the workforce, but his titles alone do not offer many indications of his specific activities. *Stȝw* has the nondescript title *sḏm-ʿš* (servant) that is connected to both the Valley of the Kings and the Valley of the Queens.[102] During the 18th Dynasty, the administration of

97 If *Stȝw* died somewhere between the reign of Akhenaten and Tutankhamun, then likely would not have been born any earlier than Tuthmosis IV's starting reign in 1396 BCE. It is possible he was alternatively born under the following reign of Amenhotep III, but only if he had lived to only 50 and died in the later range of possible dates.

98 Spondylolysis is a kind of vertebral stress fracture that has been linked to both repetitive stress and morphological weaknesses such as the cleft neural arches described here.

99 Ethne Barnes, *Atlas of Developmental Field Anomalies of the Human Skeleton: A Paleopathology Perspective* (Hoboken: Wiley-Blackwell, 2012), 72.

100 Barnes, 76.

101 Based on maximum femoral length and stature estimation formula from Raxter et al., "Stature Estimation in Ancient Egyptians."

102 Daniel M. Soliman, "Of Marks and Men: The Functional and Historical Context of the Workmen's Marks of the Royal Theban Necropolis" (Ph.D. Dissertation, Leiden, Leiden University, 2016), 35–36.

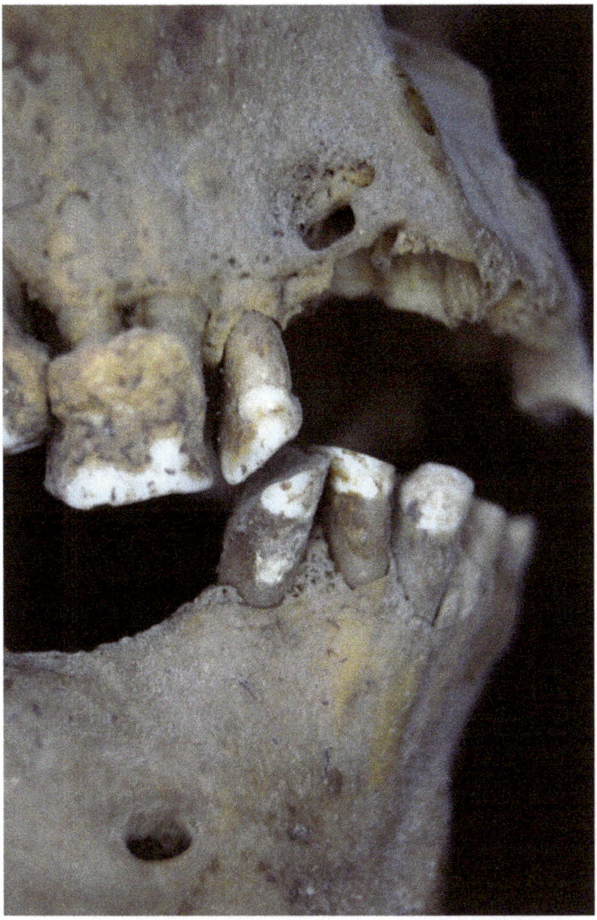

FIGURE 31 Stꜣw had an unusual wear on the right side of the mouth with a sharp inferior-posterior to superior-anterior angle of the second premolars. Additionally, an abscess is visible on the maxilla, antemortem tooth loss in the mandible, and large, calculus deposits on the maxillary, first molar.

the village may have involved less formal hierarchies than during the Ramesside periods with less obvious scribal practice, making it harder to differentiate workmen's responsibilities.[103]

Starting in young adulthood, likely in conjunction with his appointment to the workforce, *Stꜣw* began to have physical signs of occupational stress. He lost

103 Soliman, "Of Marks and Men."

both his first and second mandibular molars bilaterally early enough in life that, without a chewing surface, his remaining maxillary molars had minimal wear. Conversely, his third molars—all four of which remain in his mouth—were in occlusion. He prioritized chewing on the left side as large, coalesced dentine patches were present on the left side, though the right only has blunted cusps.

His early tooth loss may have been caused or exacerbated by using his teeth as tools as part of his work, as evidenced by an extremely unusual and asymmetrical tooth wear pattern. *Stꜣw*'s right, second premolars have a sharp inferior-posterior to superior-anterior angle (Figure 31), though no such wear is visible on the left side. This resulted in overall higher degrees of wear on the remaining teeth on the right side in all but the third molar. If *Stꜣw* was a draftsman, one possibility to explain his tooth wear could be consistent wetting and chewing of brushes, which can cause asymmetrical wear patterns that most often favor the right side.[104] Other activities where *Stꜣw* would have used his teeth as a "third hand" could have also led to such wear, though most responsibilities for the workforce (i.e., carpentry, quarrying, gypsum production, chiseling) would likely not have required such use.

Given this unusual wear pattern and the degree of antemortem tooth loss in his molars, it is possible *Stꜣw*'s diet was focused on softer foods that were easier to eat without extensive chewing. Unlike most individuals at Deir el-Medina where calculus is usually absent, *Stꜣw* has extensive calculus buildup on his remaining molars. He also has apical abscesses near both the left and right maxillary, first premolars with the left premolar almost completely destroyed from a carious lesion. Calculus, carious lesions, and abscesses all suggest that *Stꜣw*'s diet included softer and more sugary foods that ultimately impacted his overall dental health throughout his adult life.

Stꜣw likely spent decades on the workforce given his older age, and this is clearly evidenced by stress on his joints—particularly at his knees.[105] *Stꜣw*'s left and right femora and patellae exhibited so much osteoarthritis that they all show evidence of eburnation (Figure 30.d)—a polished appearance that develops after a joint breaks down to where bone is rubbing against bone. This

104 Theya Molleson, "A Method for the Study of Activity Related Skeletal Morphologies," *Bioarchaeology of the Near East* 1 (2007): 10.

105 I was first able to study the labeled skull of *Stꜣw* in 2012 (DEM 217.12.056 for the mandible and 217.12.057 for the skull) as it had been set aside and separated from the body. In the 2023 field season, we found the post-cranial skeleton (DEM 217.23.001) in the burial chamber of TT 217—this body not only matched Bruyère's description in terms of preservation and body positioning but also the atlas articulated with the occipital condyles.

joint degeneration resulted in lipping on the anterior and posterior of both femora and patellae, but eburnation was particularly visible on the lateral sides of the patellofemoral joints—the point of articulation when the knee is flexed. The right distal femur also has a stress fracture visible on the inferior aspect of the lateral condyle. This high degree of joint degeneration is among the most extreme I have observed at Deir el-Medina.

The stress on his knees is noticeably higher than the rest of his joints, where mild osteoarthritis was frequently observed in the form of small patches of pitting and lipping, but none were larger than 1 square centimeter. No other joint shows evidence of eburnation. Indeed, at such an old age, it is not surprising to see evidence of arthritic change more broadly, but the eburnation in his knees suggests it is not just age, but also repetitive strain that led to such extreme wear and tear. The only other area of the body showing more extreme joint degeneration is the lower lumbar vertebrae, where both osteophytic lipping and a Schmorl's node are present (Figure 30.a). *Stȝw* also exhibited small patches of periosteal reactions on both tibiae, though these were fully healed by the time he died (Figure 30.b).

Stȝw was buried in his coffin with a long staff made from a plain, straight, knotty stick that was wrapped in cloth and placed at his left side,[106] signifying his working conditions left him physically impaired in his old age. While staffs were frequently used in Egypt as a sign of authority and rank,[107] they also were depicted to assist with walking for the elderly and disabled. Here, the one placed with *Stȝw* likely assisted him in his aging years as he contended with increasingly deteriorating joints in his knees and lower back, especially given its plain and functional form. Indeed, another staff was also found in his tomb that Bruyère describes as being a ceremonial one made of acacia with a papyrus pommel and leather sheath attaching it in two parts.[108] Though undecorated, this seems more similar to other contemporary 18th Dynasty staffs meant for high officials such as those placed in the tomb of Kha.[109]

106 Bruyère, *Rapport sur les Fouilles de Deir el Médineh 1933–1934: I*, 104.

107 Henry G. Fischer, "Notes on Sticks and Staves in Ancient Egypt," *Metropolitan Museum Journal* 13 (1978): 5–32; Ali Hassan, *Stöcke und Stäbe im pharaonischen Ägypten bis zum Ende des Neuen Reiches*, Münchner ägyptologische Studien 33 (München: Deutscher Kunstverlag, 1976).

108 Bruyère, *Rapport sur les Fouilles de Deir el Médineh 1933–1934: I*, 101.

109 Barbara Russo, *Kha (TT 8) and His Colleagues: The Gifts in His Funerary Equipment and Related Artefacts from Western Thebes*, GHP Egyptology 18 (London: Golden House Publications, 2012), 19–20, 48.

Stꜣw's tomb was partially usurped during the Ramesside period, making it difficult to assess its architecture.[110] However, grave goods meant for *Stꜣw* and his family were still left intact. By the time he died, *Stꜣw* and his family had acquired enough wealth to be described by Egyptologists as a member of an upper-middle class—someone with considerable wealth in comparison to the average Egyptian, but who was not buried with the kinds of goods of the most elite.[111] Instead, based on his associated grave goods, *Stꜣw* was equivalent in wealth to a "midrange official."[112] Despite the fact that his tomb was likely partially plundered in antiquity,[113] he was still found with a well-decorated coffin, ushabti, and a variety of other burial goods suggesting that those who buried him could afford to furnish a well-equipped burial, though without the more expensive materials of the most elite.

Stꜣw's life history and burial exemplify how economic stability operated in a similar way during the 18th Dynasty as it did during the Ramesside period, but also how it impacted more than just *Stꜣw*'s health. His working conditions left visible marks on his body through both his deteriorating joints and asymmetrical teeth. These signs of stress only started to appear in his skeleton after adolescence and most likely in conjunction with joining the workforce. Because his working conditions left him with tooth loss and asymmetrical wear, *Stꜣw* also had to change his diet for most of his adult life. Because his joints in his knees and lower back had deteriorated substantially by his old age, *Stꜣw* was physically impaired, walking by aid of a staff. Yet in his death, it is clear that these working conditions also went hand-in-hand with relative wealth that may have in part protected him from the economic instability many faced during the Amarna period.

6.2 Nbw/Nb(.t)-tꜣ.wy *and Becoming a Woman in the 18th Dynasty*

The second osteobiography for this chapter focuses on how, when, and why the villagers got consistent access to necessities through one of the 18th Dynasty

110 Bruyère, *Rapport sur les Fouilles de Deir el Médineh 1933–1934: I*, 96.

111 Claudia Näser, "Zur Interpretation Funerärer Praktiken Im Neuen Reich: Der Ostfriedhof von Deir El-Medine," in *Begegnungen Antike Kulturen Im Niltal: Festgabe Für Erika Endesfelder, Karl-Heinz Priese, Walter Friedrich Reineke Und Steffen Wenig*, ed. Caris-Beatrice Arnst, Ingelore Hafemann, and Angelika Lohwasser (Leipzig, Germany: Wodtke and Stegbauer, 2001), 373–398.

112 Stuart Tyson Smith, "Intact Tombs of the Seventeenth and Eighteenth Dynasties from Thebes and the New Kingdom Burial System," *Mitteilungen Des Deutschen Archäologischen Instituts Kairo* 48 (1992): 218.

113 Bruyère, *Rapport sur les Fouilles de Deir el Médineh 1934–1935: II*, 97.

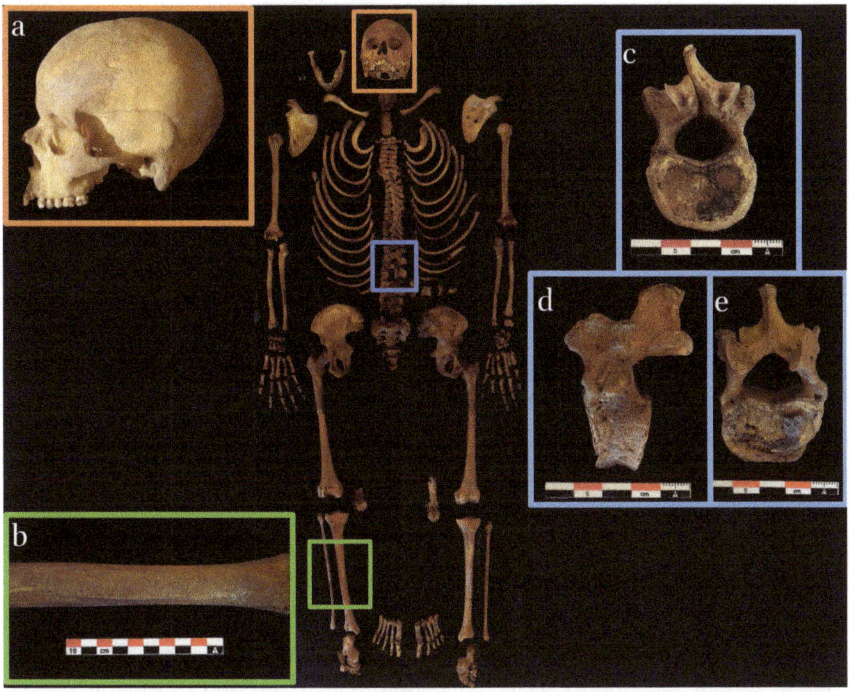

FIGURE 32 The skeleton of DEM 217.13.008 from P. 1371. (a) The lateral view of the skull shows enlarged mastoid processes possibly due to carrying loads on the skull. (b) Active periosteal lesions on the tibiae cover almost half the diaphyses. (c) The T11 has a cleft neural arch and (d, e) there was a compression fracture of the T12.

burials from the Eastern Cemetery. In P. 1371 a woman was buried alone[114]—her name is partially washed out from the coffin she was buried in with traces perhaps indicating *Nbw/Nb(.t)-tꜣ.wy*.[115] We do not know exactly when this woman lived and died, but her burial was found in the midst of other 18th Dynasty tombs, placed near the boundary of the tombs of the adults and adolescents, and her coffin was a type common during the Reign of Tuthmosis III and ear-

114 Sex estimation for this individual is based on morphological traits in the pelvis as described in Jane E. Buikstra and Douglas Ubelaker, *Standards for Data Collection from Human Skeletal Remains: Proceedings of a Seminar at the Field Museum of Natural History*, Arkansas Archeological Survey Research Series 44 (Fayetteville: Arkansas Archeological Survey, 1994).

115 Bruyère, *Rapport sur les Fouilles de Deir el Médineh 1934–1935: II*, 41; Näser, "Zur Interpretation Funerärer Praktiken Im Neuen Reich," 385. Unlike its surrounding text, this name is partially washed out. This may suggest that the coffin was first intended for another recipient, and then reused because of the untimely death of its current occupant.

lier.[116] As the sole person buried in P. 1371, *Nbw/Nb(.t)-tꜣ.wy* offers a means to see how health, burial goods, and access to necessities correlated in the 18th Dynasty.

There is no evidence of stress from enamel hypoplasias during her early childhood nor cranial porosities, but she died far earlier in her life than *Stꜣw*; she was only around 17 years old when she died.[117] By this young age, she had already accumulated multiple lesions in her skeleton evidencing her own battles with illness and injury.

Like her childhood, *Nbw/Nb(.t)-tꜣ.wy*'s adolescent years leading up to her death did not appear to be continually impacted by physiological stress. Her stature was at least 156 cm and she could have been taller given that her long bones were only partially fused.[118] This was slightly above the average at Deir el-Medina for females (154 cm) and suggests that the events leading to her death were not part of a much longer illness that was severe enough to stunt her growth. Like many other women from Deir el-Medina, it is hard to reconstruct what she was doing during these early years of her life since we have identified no written records mentioning her. Her skeleton does offer some clues, however, to her activities. She has some osteophytic lipping on her occipital condyles and both mastoids processes are unusually large for a female who died as a teenager (Figure 32.a). This could have been due to weight-bearing on the head,[119] a practice more broadly seen among women in Egypt such as in depictions of Middle Kingdom offering bearers (e.g., Metropolitan Museum of Art 20.3.7).

---

116 Dodson, "The Late Eighteenth Dynasty Necropolis at Deir El-Medina and the Earliest 'Yellow' Coffin of the New Kingdom," 97.

117 This is based on rates of epiphyseal fusion in Scheuer and Black, *The Juvenile Skeleton*. Whereas her humeral head was unfused, the medial and lateral epicondyles were fused. Similarly, the distal femoral epiphysis was unfused, while the femoral head and greater trochanter were both fused. The iliac crest is partially fused. Sex estimation was based on both metric and non-metric morphological observations of the os coxae. For the accuracy of sex estimation of the pelvis in late adolescents, see Jose Sanchez and Robert Hoppa, "Is Adulthood Required? Examining the Accuracy of Pelvic Sex Estimation Throughout Pubertal Growth," *Bioarchaeology International* 7, no. 2 (2023): 173–188, https://doi.org/10.5744/bi.2022.0005.

118 This is based on the Raxter formulae for maximum femoral length. Additionally, Bruyère, upon partially unwrapping the skeleton, indicated she was 159 cm. See Bruyère, *Rapport sur les Fouilles de Deir el Médineh 1934–1935: II*, 161.

119 Similarly, human remains from TT 34 have more developed mastoid processes and osteoarthritis on the occipital condyles, both suggesting weight-bearing on the head. See Jesús Herrerín and Mª Margarita Carmenate, "Sexual Dimorphism in Crania Belonging to the 1st Century AD from the Tomb of Mentuemhat (TT 34), Luxor, Egypt," *Anthropological Science* 130, no. 2 (2022): 135–145, https://doi.org/10.1537/ase.220128.

At some point, she experienced and survived a traumatic event that led to a compression fracture in her lower back. Her 12th thoracic vertebra was broken along the midline of its body to the right pedicle, leading to a compression fracture (Figure 32.d, e). Just above this, the 11th thoracic vertebra has a cleft neural arch (Figure 32.c), and the sacrum is also cleft, though it is ambiguous if these were congenital defects like *Stꜣw* or if they were fractures caused by the same event that led to the compression fracture in the 12th thoracic vertebra.[120] Regardless, the compression fracture could have had a short-term disabling impact as she negotiated recovery. After this traumatic event, osteophytes developed along the anterior edge of the fracture, indicating this woman survived long enough for lipping to form. Additionally, there are extensive periosteal reactions on both tibiae covering a large amount of the periosteum, though less than half of the total bone surface (Figure 32.b). While it is not clear whether these are or are not related to her fractured back, they have a fresh, woven appearance suggesting that her body was actively healing up until her time of death.

When she died, she was buried alone in P. 1371, and the decision to bury her in this specific location may also betray that her loved ones pictured her as dying in that transitional period between adolescence and adulthood. The tombs to the north and east of (and consequently above) hers belonged to adults, while to the south and west were the tombs of adolescents and infants. Her death as a late teenager positioned her in this liminal space between adolescence and adulthood.

Like many other tombs in the Eastern Cemetery, she was buried in a simple, rectangular pit measuring large enough (1 m. 65 wide, 2 m. 05 long, and 85 cm in height) to accommodate her coffin and several grave goods. When she was buried, she was given both food provisions and expensive jewelry, demonstrating that the dedication to economic stability not only extended for this life, but also the next. Among her grave goods were a rich variety of basketry and pottery filled with provisions for the afterlife: fruits (e.g., grapes, dates, doum), dried meat, grain, bread, and beer.[121] She was also buried with objects of considerable value including two pairs of golden earrings. There were likely even more grave goods present when she was first buried because sometime thereafter (long enough for her body to decompose), looters entered her tomb removing most of her jewelry, only leaving behind her golden earrings.[122] They then rewrapped

120 Cleft neural arches can increase the likelihood of getting spinal fractures more broadly. Barnes, *Atlas of Developmental Field Anomalies of the Human Skeleton*, 74.

121 Bruyère, *Rapport sur les Fouilles de Deir el Médineh 1934–1935: II*, 158–161.

122 It is unclear whether these were left behind for a reason, or simply missed if the looters avoided unwrapping her head. Bruyère, 158–161.

her body and placed the shrouds for the outside of her coffin back in their place, perhaps indicating this act of looting happened still during the occupation of the site, when such burial practices were known.[123] The fact that her grave was only robbed well after burial also suggests that the broader community had enough economic means to bury her with wealth in both commodities and food.

Her remaining grave goods were not only intended to provide for her in the afterlife but were also directly connected with childbirth by either providing for her own rebirth in the afterlife or because her death was connected with childbirth. Her grave goods included toiletry items found frequently in other 18th Dynasty graves, including needles, kohl, and a bronze mirror without handle that was placed between her wrappings. Mirrors and kohl were found in other women's burials at Deir el-Medina and in depictions of women at the site, not only indicating gender, but also marking them as sexually mature adults rather than children.[124] In some scenes, the act of giving a mirror and kohl was part of the offerings given to women after birth.[125] Notably, these scenes also often include perfumed fat that represented the end of the post-birth rituals and the reintroduction of a woman back into society as a purified, new mother.[126] Bruyère described finding a possible cone of fat placed on this woman's forehead.[127] At Amarna, researchers offered similar questions about whether the placement of a cone of fat in an adult woman's grave was part of "fertility-related problem-solving."[128]

As a post-pubescent late teen, *Nbw/Nb(.t)-tꜣ.wy*'s age-at-death could be related to childbirth, though there is currently no way to confirm whether or not she had given birth. If she had, this may also explain the compression fracture in her back since childbirth has been connected to cases of compression fractures in the lower spine of young, adult women.[129] When calcium is prioritized

123 Näser, "Zur Interpretation Funerärer Praktiken Im Neuen Reich."

124 Joanne Backhouse, *"Scènes de Gynécées" Figured Ostraca from New Kingdom Egypt: Iconography and Intent*, Archaeopress Egyptology 26 (Oxford: Archaeopress, 2020), 79–87.

125 Arnette, "Purification Du Post-Partum et Rites Des Relevailles Dans l'Égypte Ancienne," 31.

126 Arnette, "Purification Du Post-Partum et Rites Des Relevailles Dans l'Égypte Ancienne."

127 Bruyère described, "un amas de substance blanche qui à l'analyse donne les réactions des graisses animales altérées, posé sur le front même de la morte," Bruyère, *Rapport sur les Fouilles de Deir el Médineh 1934–1935: II*, 161.

128 Anna Stevens et al., "From Representation to Reality: Ancient Egyptian Wax Head Cones from Amarna," *Antiquity* 93, no. 372 (December 2019): 1529, https://doi.org/10.15184/aqy.2019.175.

129 Shailesh Hadgaonkar et al., "Post Pregnancy Severe Spinal Osteoporosis with Multiple Vertebral Fractures and Kyphoscoliosis in a Multigravida: A Rare Case with Management," *Asian Spine Journal* 9, no. 4 (2015): 625–628, https://doi.org/10.4184/asj.2015.9.4.625;

for the fetus/infant during pregnancy and lactation, there can be vitamin deficiencies that, when severe enough, cause osteoporosis and eventually fractures. For many women, this resolves after weaning, but if someone like *Nbw/Nb(.t)-tꜣ.wy* faced similar vitamin deficiencies, she may not have survived long enough for her body to recover, as evidenced by periosteal reactions on her tibiae that were still active up until her death.

Even after looting, one important grave good remained in situ at the side of *Nbw/Nb(.t)-tꜣ.wy*: a small stone sarcophagus containing within it a stone, female mummiform figurine replete with the provisions that one would need in the afterlife, including a blue-beaded necklace, food (i.e., grapes, grain, and dates), and a set of three clay balls filled with seeds.[130] Bruyère suggested this acted as a kind of ushabti both representing this woman's visage for eternity and serving on her behalf in the afterlife.[131] However, its placement by the side of her coffin, mimicking the placement of side-by-side burials in neighboring tombs, may have alternatively been meant as a substitution for another person, perhaps a mother, sister, or child buried or moved elsewhere, providing her body with companionship in a lone tomb.

When considering how, when, and why the people of Deir el-Medina were able to maintain economic stability, this young woman's burial suggests that during the 18th Dynasty, the community was able to and prioritized providing economic stability to both its living and deceased members. *Nbw/Nb(.t)-tꜣ.wy*'s burial goods suggest that she and/or her family had considerable wealth, enough to equip her with high-value grave goods in the afterlife, some of which were lost to looters in antiquity. However, her burial was solitary, and the grave goods included in her tomb give us an idea of the kinds of provisions necessary for a lone, young woman who died prematurely and whose health history betrays a broken back even before her death. The value of her grave goods can be considered as more than just a marker of her socioeconomic status. The inclusion of foods from seed to fruit shows the need to provision in the afterlife, and the placement of objects associated with childbirth either suggests she may have died during childbirth or that her family wanted to provide for her own successful rebirth inside the tomb. The inclusion of an unusual stone

---

C.S. Kovacs and S.H. Ralston, "Presentation and Management of Osteoporosis Presenting in Association with Pregnancy or Lactation," *Osteoporosis International* 26, no. 9 (2015): 2223–2241, https://doi.org/10.1007/s00198-015-3149-3.

130 The debated function of these clay balls likely varied based on context. Here, filling the clay balls with seeds and placing them in a burial context could have connected them with fertility and rebirth reminiscent of the so-called Osiris beds.

131 Bruyère, *Rapport sur les Fouilles de Deir el Médineh 1934–1935: II*, 130.

mummy at her side may even have provided her with companionship. These grave goods, therefore, not only allowed *Nbw/Nb(.t)-tꜣ.wy*'s to survive but also thrive in the afterlife.

7 Connecting Economic Stability to Health Outcomes at Deir el-Medina

Evidence from the medical texts, the kinds of healthcare professionals at the site, and the case studies from human remains demonstrates how equitable healthcare access benefitted families at Deir el-Medina. Reflecting on the patterns of stress indicators from Chapter 4, healthcare access can also explain some of the patterns seen at Deir el-Medina.

The combination of state and private efforts explains how and why rates of enamel hypoplasias remained remarkably low at Deir el-Medina even when compared to elite groups. Workmen and their families received state support even during illness or injury, making it possible to maintain economic stability when a workman was temporarily disabled. Simultaneously, when state economic stability faltered, the villagers supplemented their incomes, creating economic stability in the wake of workforce layoffs and state collapse. They used their social cohesion to emphasize the *royal pact* in strikes, effectively getting grain rations even when the vizier claimed the granaries were empty. This relative consistency meant that in the harshest times, when the granaries were almost or completely emptied because of seasonal cycles or bad inundations, the people of Deir el-Medina were comparatively buffered; many other groups did not have the institutional support or social cohesion to maintain the same degree of economic stability.

The impact of working conditions also connects economic stability to rates of DJD and trauma at Deir el-Medina. The *royal pact* demonstrates how important it was for the crew to make continuous, successful progress on the royal tombs. This puts into perspective why men had to work long enough to develop more joint degeneration than women in the village or elite groups. Paid sick leave, however, also explains the relatively high amount of healing observed at Deir el-Medina for traumatic injuries.

Economic stability also informs why wealth created health in ancient Egypt more broadly. The Egyptian agricultural cycle made food stability incredibly variable, both across seasons and years. The rations at Deir el-Medina, which were above and beyond what they needed to eat, allowed them to grow wealth that they could then capitalize on when the economy faltered. When grain rations were inconsistent, they also could take advantage of separate private enterprises like loaning their donkeys to secure additional grain.

This and previous chapters, however, also speak to the different forms of wealth visible at Deir el-Medina. While this chapter most explicitly discusses their economic capital, we also see how economic stability was possible because of social and knowledge capital; social capital allowed them to offer each other social support and strike together, while knowledge capital made it possible for them to secure private work outside of their royal duties. The next chapter, the conclusion, looks at how these three interwoven forms of capital explain how wealth made health in ancient Egypt.

CHAPTER 8

Conclusion

I began this book by describing a prevalent myth around the history of human health that people in the past, without germ theory, were unable to control their health and fight disease. The intervening chapters demonstrate that health outcomes in ancient Egypt were determined by more than medical practices alone. When we expand how people can control health outcomes to include social mechanisms, we also expand how people in the past could improve their health. This approach offers one example of how social mechanisms can reveal some of the hidden differences in health risk across individuals.

In many modern studies, *Social Determinants of Health*, such as social support, economic stability, and healthcare access, better explain heterogeneous health patterns than medicine alone. Research on health patterns in the past, however, rarely includes these social factors as systematic explanations for heterogeneous frailty—the often hidden differences in health risks and responses across individuals. Instead, environmental or chronological variables are more common in systematic studies. When social variables are included, they also often lack causal explanations. For example, when studies assume wealthier groups have better health outcomes, there are few explanations for *why*. Essentially, there is a lack of cohesive understanding in many contexts of how and why social factors influence health patterns in the past.

Deir el-Medina offers an ideal case study into the potential ways the *Social Determinants of Health* could have operated in the ancient world due to its rich variety of texts, small communal nature, and extensive existing scholarship. This village offers a unique lens given that its workforce had, on the one hand, high degrees of literacy and economic power and, on the other hand, hard labor that made them a combination of both a blue- and white-collar workforce.

Reconstructing health at Deir el-Medina requires combining evidence from texts and human remains, representing the broader occupation of the site beginning in the 18th Dynasty and extending to the gradual abandonment of the site by the beginning of the 21st Dynasty. The human remains from three tombs—TT 217, 290, and 298—represent the varied demography of the village, including men, women, children, and the elderly. They are a cross-section of the people of Deir el-Medina more broadly and, unlike texts from the village, more evenly represent the working and non-working members of the commu-

 | DOI:10.1163/9789004700871_009

nity. Although most of the human remains at Deir el-Medina were commingled from intermittent looting since antiquity, skeletal stress indicators make it possible to compare the villagers' experiences both within the village and with people from other Egyptian cemeteries.

Bioarchaeological research across these tombs reveals the life histories of their inhabitants, including the impact stressors had on the people of Deir el-Medina during childhood, adolescence, and adulthood. Six different skeletal stress indicators—enamel hypoplasias, cranial porosities, stature, trauma, degenerative joint disease (DJD), and periosteal reactions—each attest to a different life period and form of physiological stress in the skeleton. Data on these stress indicators from TT 217, 290, and 298 reveal broader health patterns visible at Deir el-Medina.

Some stress indicators like cranial porosities demonstrate that health outcomes were harder to control regardless of wealth—and a causal explanation for their patterns remains elusive. Other factors like period or site location do not explain the distribution of these stress indicators. Cranial porosities may have been particularly influenced by childhood exposures to malaria—a disease that even royalty could not elude. Similarly, tibial periosteal reactions do not neatly correlate with wealth in Egyptian populations and instead were more often dictated by sex or possibly site location, but they still showed no consistent patterning over time or space. For both cranial porosities and periosteal reactions, wealth did not predict whether a population had higher or lower rates of stress response. These conditions may have been impacted by stressors that wealth held little sway over such as exposure to infectious diseases.

Yet, the other skeletal stress indicators demonstrate that throughout their lives, people could use wealth to improve health. Enamel hypoplasias—indicators of early childhood stress—tended to be lower among elite populations than non-elite ones. Stature was also noticeably correlated with wealth during dynastic times when more elite populations had higher statures than their non-elite counterparts, indicating that wealth certainly affected adolescent health. As adults, those with harder labor had higher rates of DJD, even when compared to populations of elite groups where DJD could be a natural consequence of older populations. Trauma was more noticeable as well in working populations, perhaps as a byproduct of working conditions where traumatic injuries were more likely to occur. These results offer a more complete picture of the way health and wealth were correlated in ancient Egypt; during periods of physiological growth and development, people were much more likely to be able to use their wealth to protect their (or their loved ones) health. Simultaneously, as adults, wealth could protect individuals from enduring working conditions that led to DJD and traumatic injuries. Although a wide array of factors often invisible in the past (i.e., *hidden heterogeneity in frailty*) influence health outcomes, these results demonstrate that social factors were incredibly influential on structuring health outcomes in ancient Egypt.

Through this lens, we can see that the people of Deir el-Medina showed remarkable resilience to stressors in ways that were often consistent across tombs and periods, suggesting that throughout the site's history and across the community, the people of Deir el-Medina were able to buffer themselves from many major stressors that other communities could not. Consequently, their health outcomes tended to be better than other working populations—a result that, at first glance, is not surprising, given the many advantages the community had as a skilled, royal labor force. Although they still contended with the same problems as other working populations—especially DJD—they were more buffered in general, showing fewer injuries and fewer extreme manifestations of DJD (i.e., eburnation) than workers at Giza or Amarna.

More surprisingly, however, is the fact that even when compared to non-working elites, the people of Deir el-Medina were better at buffering stressors during childhood and adolescence. There were relatively few enamel hypoplasias at Deir el-Medina, and stature was remarkably uniform, suggesting that childhood, adolescent, and maternal health outcomes all tended to be better protected at Deir el-Medina than in most ancient Egyptian populations. This is even true when comparing Deir el-Medina to populations globally for stress indicators like enamel hypoplasias or variation in stature. These trends were consistent across tombs and suggest that it was not simply Deir el-Medina's wealthiest citizens but the whole community whose health benefitted. These results led me to two questions that structured the rest of this book:

1. How do ancient Egyptian attempts to control their health outcomes explain the relationship (or lack thereof) between health and wealth across skeletal stress indicators?
2. How is it that the people of Deir el-Medina were, in some cases, able to have better health outcomes than even wealthier, more elite populations with consistent results across the village community?

1 How Wealth made Health in Ancient Egypt

To answer these questions, I explored three *Social Determinants of Health* at Deir el-Medina to demonstrate tangible ways the social and cultural context of Deir el-Medina allowed the villagers to improve their health outcomes. Chapters dedicated to social support (Chapter 5), healthcare access (Chapter 6), and economic stability (Chapter 7) demonstrate that, in reality, wealth at Deir el-Medina consisted of more than simply what the people of Deir el-Medina could afford to own. Over the many generations of the site's occupation, the community built wealth through strengthening their social connections, knowledge, and economic access. These three forms of wealth enabled the villagers to buffer stress and respond to disease in ways that even surpassed non-working elite communities. While each of these forms of wealth tends to correlate to specific *Social Determinants of Health* (i.e., social wealth with social support, knowledge wealth with healthcare access, and economic wealth with economic stability), we can also see that they crosscut and interweave chapters. It is not just the sum of their social, knowledge, and economic wealth individually that benefited this community, but how these three forms of wealth worked together to allow the villagers at Deir el-Medina to thrive and control their health outcomes. Looking beyond Deir el-Medina, we can see how these three forms of wealth were healthmakers in ancient Egypt more broadly.

One way the people of Deir el-Medina made their health was through social support, the first *Social Determinant of Health* explored in more depth in this book. Texts referencing illnesses at Deir el-Medina consistently demonstrate that the villagers socially supported each other, offering to care for and provide necessities to the sick. They were aware of the benefits of social support and emphasized it in their teachings, social practices, and family interactions.

This social support translated to high degrees of social cohesion because of the village's close communal ties, unified purpose, and well-established families. The clear boundaries to the village and the importance of community membership meant that there was little ambiguity around who was and was not a member of the community. Intermarriage after many generations allowed the villagers to have widespread family networks. Social customs like gift-giving and wisdom texts demonstrate that the villagers emphasized the importance of supporting neighbors and family members through reciprocation.

The villagers built their social capital synergistically with their economic capital. The importance of reciprocation and close, family bonds was heightened for the residents of Deir el-Medina because of their intergenerational wealth. This gave them an edge compared to workers buried at Amarna or Giza, where laborers had minimal time to develop social ties and no opportunities to accumulate wealth. Because of a comparative lack of social capital, these individuals—even if they shared the same values—could not benefit from social support to the same extent as the villagers at Deir el-Medina.

The villagers also had communal and state support, providing them with the second *Social Determinant of Health* explored in this book, healthcare access. The state allowed time off and paid extra rations to a *zwn.w* and *ḫrp-Srq.t* on the crew. Most likely, only one workman took on each position at a time, and they could take time off to support and care for colleagues and their families. The wise woman also supported villagers when they wanted to understand the divine origins of illnesses, especially for women and children, though this role was not formalized through rations. Additionally, during illness, the state allowed workmen paid sick leave, making it easier for them to recover.

Medical texts from the village attest to high degrees of medical literacy at Deir el-Medina, and thus the degree of knowledge capital that families relied on to take care of each other outside of the healthcare available from the official *zwn.w* and *ḫrp-Srq.t*. These medical texts were accumulated to treat the various illnesses that concerned and affected the villagers. They attest to how, after multiple generations, medical texts grew and acted as a valuable resource to treat common, local illnesses. The high literacy rate and potential to inherit these documents along with state-supplied medical ingredients allowed the villagers two separate avenues for healthcare access.

It is difficult to assess how effective these treatments were, but they use ingredients that more broadly reduce inflammation, are antimicrobials, and are analgesics. Additionally, those reading and writing Egyptian medical texts used a process of prognosis and diagnosis. They would occasionally indicate when a treatment was particularly effective, demonstrating that they curated and assessed which treatments were more or less likely to get a positive outcome. Research on placebo medicine also suggests that even treatments traditionally deemed magical—which often involve personal attention and care—offer significant health benefits by buffering stress. Each of these lines of evidence suggests that healthcare access would have impacted health outcomes.

Consequently, healthcare access explains some of the relationships between health and wealth. In places where state support included medical care, non-elite groups could achieve similar health outcomes to their elite counterparts. For example, well-aligned fractures among the workers at Giza speak to the outcomes possible with an experienced and skilled state-appointed doctor. At Deir el-Medina, where residents received support from both the state and their own private medical records, the workforce achieved better health outcomes for some stress indicators because of this dual support.

The importance of both state and private support becomes even clearer when looking at the third *Social Determinant of Health* explored in this book, economic stability. This social determinant encompasses both the impacts of consistent access to necessities and working conditions on health outcomes.

At Deir el-Medina, the central role of the workforce to the king meant that they benefitted from a *royal pact* to ensure every need was met for the workmen and their families, providing them with unusually robust economic stability since they were provided regular access to a diverse diet and housing stability. It also was a mechanism for the workforce to demand rations from the king when the state failed to pay the workforce. This was especially important during periods of economic collapse and poor inundation when the state had to carefully prioritize who would and would not receive rations from their granaries.

The villager's economic success was equally entangled with their social cohesion. When the workmen were not paid their full rations, they used their social cohesion to strike. The success of the workmen's strikes was because of the involvement of the entire workforce and, in some cases, the entire village. The unified efforts paid off, allowing villagers to secure grain rations within a day of their demonstrations. Simultaneously, when they fell behind on the royal tomb, they relied on other members of the community to share the burden of catching up their work, ensuring the workforce met their part of the *royal pact*.

Additionally, the crew could rely on their own intergenerational wealth when the state failed. The workmen's allotted monthly grain rations were above and beyond what a family needed for nutrition, and this extra wealth could then be traded for goods that workmen and their wives passed on to future generations. Members of the workforce used their wealth to increase access to grain—for example, by loaning donkeys. Economic capital from the combined state support for the village and the villager's internal wealth meant that they could maintain food security both in times of state growth and collapse.

The *royal pact*, however, came at a cost. Working conditions required the workforce to labor long enough and consistently enough to develop more DJD than elites. The workmen likely encountered other health hazards due to the confined and physical labor necessary for cutting and decorating the royal tomb. In some cases, this required taking time off from work due to illness. Grain rations were still distributed despite prolonged absences, allowing the men at Deir el-Medina comparatively more economic stability than private workforces doing the same kind of labor and experiencing the same kinds of working conditions.

These working conditions impacted the health of the workforce even in the earliest periods of the site's occupation. Two osteobiographies from the 18th Dynasty exemplify the extreme joint degeneration and trauma that villagers had to face. Simultaneously, their burials—which included high-quality grave goods and provisions for the afterlife—indicate that even before the many generations of wealth growth in the village, the earliest residents would have had more wealth and thus more economic stability than other workforces.

2 Revealing *Hidden Heterogeneity in Frailty* in the Past beyond Ancient Egypt

These chapters demonstrate concrete explanations for why wealth, in its many forms, impacted health outcomes for the villagers of Deir el-Medina, revealing some of the *hidden heterogeneity in frailty* in ancient Egyptian populations. Communities like Deir el-Medina were able to protect children and adolescents from stress while also avoiding or ameliorating occupational stress for adults because of their economic, social, and knowledge capital. The combination of private and state support gave the residents of Deir el-Medina two different avenues for acquiring these three *Social Determinants of Health*, helping to explain how they could have better health outcomes than even elites in some cases.

These chapters also demonstrate how Deir el-Medina offers unusual and exceptional access to identifying the *Social Determinants of Health* in the past, and simultaneously, how critical social determinants are for explaining broader health outcomes. However, the very features that make Deir el-Medina an exceptional case study for researching health in the past should give us pause when considering how to translate this book beyond the site. As a village that is unusually well-documented, the kinds of sources available to study the *Social Determinants of Health* are rarely accessible in many other populations. Most bioarchaeologists and historians will not have access to personal letters attesting to caretaking or daily absence records revealing seasonal illnesses. In the absence of a strong written record, how might the *Social Determinants of Health*, as evidenced at Deir el-Medina, help to inform how to study and explain health patterns elsewhere?

To answer this question, let's return to other studies that have found unexpected health outcomes when comparing health patterns in the past. At face value, these suggest that *hidden heterogeneity in frailty* is a major issue for understanding why some people had better or worse health outcomes since these examples of health outcomes contradict conventional expectations. By considering the *Social Determinants of Health* systematically, however, it is possible to explain these health outcomes and reveal why these health differences existed. These three examples demonstrate how social support, economic stability, and healthcare access all likely influenced health outcomes in other studies on past health.

In the *Backbone of History*, a comparison of the relative health status of segregated Black and White cemeteries during the 19th century revealed health outcomes that were so startling and unexpected, "they border on the unbelievable."[1] Through the lens of the *Social Determinants of Health*, these results are actually not startling at all, and in fact, closely align with the experiences of the villagers at Deir el-Medina.

Specifically, the authors found that the free Black members of First African Baptist Church in Philadelphia had, by their measure, better health outcomes than all of the White groups they analyzed from the same period including those from the middle and upper classes. The researchers suggested that this discrepancy is less surprising than it first may seem because "In the absence of a reliable theory of disease causation, the rich and the well-educated did not know how to spend their wealth to improve health … Thus, socioeconomic status was probably a poor indicator of health in the nineteenth century."[2] In dismissing socioeconomic status, the authors suggest that without biomedicine, people in the past were too ignorant to use their wealth to control their health.

The authors go on to describe the Black community they studied, noting that one possible explanation for their improved health was high church membership. The church provided a "social and economic safety net for its members."[3] This included food provisioning, which was particularly effective given that many congregants were involved in catering. The authors suggest this could explain why childhood health indicators, including enamel hypoplasias, cranial porosities, and stature, were unusually robust for this group of Free Black Americans.

This example carries with it multiple clear parallels to Deir el-Medina. Both populations had high degrees of social support and in both cases, the nature of their work allowed them unusual degrees of economic stability, and more specifically, food stability. Both communities also could use their social wealth to improve health outcomes beyond wealthier, comparable groups. As a consequence, both communities also had surprisingly robust health during childhood specifically. The parallels between this example and Deir el-Medina demonstrate how important it is to consider not just economic wealth when evalu-

---

1 Rathbun and Steckel, "The Health of Slaves and Free Blacks in the East," 219.

2 Steckel and Rose, *The Backbone of History*, 219.

3 Rathbun and Steckel, "The Health of Slaves and Free Blacks in the East," 220.

ating how social context impacted health outcomes in the past, but also social support and social capital as key drivers of past health.

Researchers looking at health patterns in Europe also evaluated whether skeletal stress indicators attest to the presence of an urban penalty to health prior to germ theory. Previous research has suggested that many pre-modern populations suffered an urban penalty due to higher rates of infectious disease and poorer sanitation in areas with denser populations.[4] However, skeletal stress indicators, when compared over time in Europe, offered unexpected insights into the urban penalty. Data suggested that although urban penalties were sometimes present, in many periods and places there was no urban penalty or, surprisingly, an urban benefit.

In an attempt to explain the absence of an urban penalty, researchers suggested that isolated farming communities were more likely to suffer malnutrition because of inconsistent access to food.[5] The authors argue that during periods where market integration was poor, farming communities suffered because "food in regions producing a surplus could not easily be sold to the regions most severely hit by harvest failures."[6] Like in ancient Egypt, these communities were dependent on a successful agricultural cycle and vulnerable seasonally and in years of poor harvests. Whereas groups living in urban areas could benefit from trading for food in such times, thus maintaining economic stability, disconnected, rural communities were left in a particularly precarious position, and consequently suffered worse health outcomes. Though not explicitly stated, the researchers used economic stability, and in particular food stability, to explain why certain health outcomes like stature were better in urban contexts. Here, we see how research on food stability and stature at Deir el-Medina mirror the unexpected results on the urban penalty in Europe.

Separately, researchers also suggested that the urban penalty may have been offset by more medical literacy and access to a more varied diet that ultimately buffered childhood stress. They argued that "the types of food available in city markets and the possible access to health knowledge—even if on a very low level—in the settlement might have played a stronger role for promoting normal growth and development."[7] Here too, insights from Deir el-Medina carry

4 Christopher Dye, "Health and Urban Living," *Science* 319, no. 5864 (2008): 766–769, https://doi.org/10.1126/science.115019.

5 Joerg Baten et al., "Multidimensional Patterns of European Health, Work, and Violence over the Past Two Millen," in *The Backbone of Europe: Health, Diet, Work and Violence over Two Millennia*, ed. Richard H. Steckel et al., Cambridge Studies in Biological and Evolutionary Anthropology 80 (Cambridge: Cambridge University Press, 2018), 381–396.

6 Baten et al., 385.

7 Bereczki et al., "Growth Disruptions in Children," 189.

important parallels. The value of knowledge wealth and their impacts on diet might explain why children benefitted from living in urban environments for most of Europe's pre-medieval through modern periods.

In all three of these examples, researchers discussed possible explanations for unexpected health findings that ultimately concluded that social support, economic stability, and healthcare access (in the form of medical literacy) influenced health outcomes in the past. These conclusions, however, did not come from a systematic comparison of these variables across populations, but rather as deeper contextual research when results were unexpected. They demonstrate that bioarchaeologists and historians consider the *Social Determinants of Health* when explaining health patterns, but often as an afterthought rather than a unifying, systematic means for explaining past health outcomes. This book is only a case study of one ancient Egyptian village and the role *Social Determinants of Health* played in the residents' health outcomes. It demonstrates, however, the potential to use these social determinants more systematically in the past to explain how people maintained their health.

3 Healthmaking in Ancient Egypt

In the medical text P. Edwin Smith, when a patient's survival was uncertain, the *zwn.w* told patients it was an illness with which they would fight (*mr ꜥḥꜣ=ỉ ḥnꜥ*). This reveals the underlying cultural perception of treating illnesses as enemies in a battle, embedding this concept orthographically in the verb *ꜥḥꜣ*, "to fight" (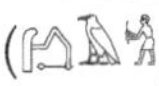).

Like the *zwn.w* in P. Edwin Smith, examples throughout this book demonstrate that the people of Deir el-Medina were not passive observers of their own or others' health; they too contended with illnesses. Their health was something they actively made by fighting for a stronger community, seeking medical knowledge, and ensuring economic success. This example shows us how health outcomes in the past were determined by more than medical practices alone and that past peoples were more than passengers on their health journeys. They were active healthmakers, who could use their social networks, knowledge, and resources to fight stressors. When we expand how we study health in the past to include the *Social Determinants of Health*, we also expand how people in the past made their health.

APPENDIX

The Osteological Datasets

Osteological data for this research comes from three assemblages of human remains stored in Theban tombs (TT) 217, 290, and 298 at Deir el-Medina. These data sets largely consist of commingled remains dating from the 18th to 21st Dynasty. Osteological methods employed in this study require modifications to suit working with commingled human remains when assessing demographic information like age and sex estimates. This appendix elucidates the methods, scoring criteria, and metadata recorded during fieldwork at Deir el-Medina to make data reuse easier and allow bioarchaeologists interested in this book more detailed information about the data collected at Deir el-Medina.

I recorded all data using OsteoSurvey—a series of digital osteological data collection forms used on Android-operated mobile devices via Open Data Kit (ODK) Collect.[1] I designed OsteoSurvey to follow existing bioarchaeological standards[2] while also streamlining data entry to improve the overall quantity and quality of data recorded. All data were recorded on tablets using ODK in the field, and then exported as comma-separated value files for analysis. I developed separate forms for each element as well as forms to record mummified human remains, the skull, and dentition. I then combined data across different years to develop Excel spreadsheets with all data entries for a given form recorded between 2013–2022. Each spreadsheet includes a metadata tab that describes the data-entry columns and controlled vocabularies used in OsteoSurvey. The processed data files are publicly available online at the Digital Archaeological Record (tDAR) database (https://core.tdar.org) under the tDAR ID number 394652 and title, "Deir el-Medina Human Remains."

As these remains are commingled, I assign numbers to any discrete element, skull, or individual. This number consists of the Theban Tomb number (e.g., 217), a two-digit year, and a three-digit sequential identification number (e.g., 217.13.005 was the fifth data entry from the 2013 field season in TT 217).

1 Anne E. Austin, "Mobilizing Archaeologists: Increasing the Quantity and Quality of Data Collected in the Field with Mobile Technology," *Advances in Archaeological Practice: A Journal of the Society for American Archaeology* 2, no. 1 (2014): 13–23.

2 Buikstra and Ubelaker, *Standards for Data Collection from Human Skeletal Remains*; J.L. Buckberry and A.T. Chamberlain, "Age Estimation from the Auricular Surface of the Ilium: A Revised Method," *American Journal of Physical Anthropology* 119, no. 3 (November 2002): 231–239, https://doi.org/10.1002/ajpa.10130; Steckel et al., *The Backbone of Europe*.

 | DOI:10.1163/9789004700871_010

These numbers are written on each element and are recorded during data collection. Numbers were not assigned to individual ribs, metacarpals, carpals, metatarsals, and tarsals aside from the calcaneus and talus.

Each data entry includes information on archaeological context. Because human remains were sometimes moved between tombs, particularly for TT 217, the location recorded may not be the original burial location. In the notes field, I indicated whether there was any additional information about the original tomb location in these cases. I also recorded a findspot for each data entry. The findspot for elements from TT 290 is a box or bag number since these human remains were previously packed and set aside in the tomb. For TT 298, I indicated a 1×1 meter grid location within the tomb.

Each element recorded includes an estimate of its completeness. For long bones, this is separately assessed for the proximal end, distal end, and shaft. Additionally, estimates for surface preservation are provided with a note field to indicate any additional explanations for issues with surface preservation (e.g., skin present).

Measurements for each long bone are based on those described in Buikstra and Ubelaker.[3] Additionally, some measurements were taken to align with comparable datasets. This includes additional measurements of the scapulae.[4] Instruments used for measurements vary based on those recommended in Buikstra and Ubelaker (i.e., osteometric board, sliding caliper, or scaling caliper).

Methods for aging are based on those outlined by Buikstra and Ubelaker.[5] Specifically, methods for aging adults include observations on cranial suture closure,[6] occlusal surface wear,[7] pubic symphyseal phasing,[8] and auricular sur-

3 Buikstra and Ubelaker, *Standards for Data Collection from Human Skeletal Remains.*

4 Gretchen R. Dabbs, "Sex Determination Using the Scapula in New Kingdom Skeletons from Tell El-Amarna," *HOMO—Journal of Comparative Human Biology* 61, no. 6 (December 2010): 413–420, https://doi.org/10.1016/j.jchb.2010.09.001.

5 Buikstra and Ubelaker, *Standards for Data Collection from Human Skeletal Remains.*

6 Richard S. Meindl and C. Owen Lovejoy, "Ectocranial Suture Closure: A Revised Method for the Determination of Skeletal Age at Death Based on the Lateral-Anterior Sutures," *American Journal of Physical Anthropology* 68, no. 1 (1985): 57–66.

7 B. Holly Smith, "Patterns of Molar Wear in Hunter–Gatherers and Agriculturalists," *American Journal of Physical Anthropology* 63, no. 1 (1984): 39–56; Phillip L. Walker, Gregory Dean, and Perry Shapiro, "Estimating Age from Tooth Wear in Archaeological Populations," in *Advances in Dental Anthropology*, ed. Marc A. Kelley and Clark Spencer Larsen (New York: Wiley-Liss, 1991), 169–178.

8 Sheilagh Brooks and Judy M. Suchey, "Skeletal Age Determination Based on the Os Pubis: A Comparison of the Acsádi-Nemeskéri and Suchey-Brooks Methods," *Human Evolution* 5, no. 3 (1990): 227–238; T. Wingate Todd, "Age Changes in the Pubic Bone. I: The Male White

face phasing.[9] Juvenile age estimates are determined based on dental development,[10] epiphyseal fusion rates,[11] and diaphyseal lengths.[12] Since crania and os coxae may have more than one adult age estimation, the final age estimate is assigned to a broader category (Under 20, 20–35 years old, 36–50 years old, over 50 years old).

Because of commingling, age estimates are also provided for each element, however, many elements cannot be given a more specific age category than differentiation between fully fused, partially fused, or unfused. As age estimates for epiphyseal union, dental development, and diaphyseal lengths are based on other populations, ages derived from these methods should be taken only as initial estimates. To accommodate this, the following categories are assigned to juveniles: Under 5, 5–11 years old, 12–20 years old, or Juvenile (unknown age).

Adult sex estimates for the os coxae and crania follow non-metric observations outlined by Buikstra and Ubelaker.[13] Additionally, when os coxae are incomplete or difficult to observe, I used metric sex estimates based on DSP2 functions.[14] For individual long bones, I used univariate and multivariate discriminant functions to estimate sex. These are based on previously established sectioning points and discriminant functions for other ancient Egyptian populations.[15] Previous research has demonstrated that metric sex estimation

Pubis.," *American Journal of Physical Anthropology*, no. 3 (1921): 285–334; T. Wingate Todd, "Age Changes in the Pubic Bone. III: The Pubis of the White Female," *American Journal of Physical Anthropology*, no. 4 (1921): 1–70.

9 C. Owen Lovejoy et al., "Chronological Metamorphosis of the Auricular Surface of the Ilium: A New Method for the Determination of Adult Skeletal Age at Death," *American Journal of Physical Anthropology* 68, no. 1 (1985): 15–28; Buckberry and Chamberlain, "Age Estimation from the Auricular Surface of the Ilium."

10 Sakher J. AlQahtani, Mark P. Hector, and Helen M. Liversidge, "Accuracy of Dental Age Estimation Charts: Schour and Massler, Ubelaker and the London Atlas," *American Journal of Physical Anthropology* 154, no. 1 (2014): 70–78, https://doi.org/10.1002/ajpa.22473.

11 Scheuer and Black, *The Juvenile Skeleton.*

12 Fazekas and Kósa, *Forensic Fetal Osteology*; Primeau et al., "A Method for Estimating Age of Medieval Sub-Adults from Infancy to Adulthood Based on Long Bone Length"; Ubelaker, "The Estimation of Age at Death from Immature Human Bone."

13 Buikstra and Ubelaker, *Standards for Data Collection from Human Skeletal Remains.*

14 Jaroslav Brůžek et al., "Validation and Reliability of the Sex Estimation of the Human Os Coxae Using Freely Available DSP2 Software for Bioarchaeology and Forensic Anthropology," *American Journal of Physical Anthropology* 164, no. 2 (2017): 440–449, https://doi.org/10.1002/ajpa.23282.

15 Raxter, "Metric Sex Estimation in an Ancient Egyptian Skeletal Sample"; Dabbs, "Sex Determination Using the Scapula in New Kingdom Skeletons from Tell El-Amarna"; Dabbs, "Estimating the Sex of Ancient Egyptian Skeletal Remains: Methods from Tell El-Amarna."

techniques derived from one ancient Egyptian population can be applied to another with similarly accurate results.[16] This appears to be consistent with Deir el-Medina since sample-specific univariate sectioning points derived from this sample are comparable to those previously published.[17] It should be noted, however, that accuracy varies across long bones and sex estimate functions. Because all long bones with sex estimates have multiple univariate or multivariate discriminant functions, sex estimates are attributed as definitely male or female only when all functions agree. When only one function is calculable, long bones are assigned as probably male or female. When the functions estimate both male and female or when any function estimates ambiguous, I designate the element as ambiguous. When there is not enough information to calculate any sex estimates, the element is recorded as indeterminate.

I observed each element macroscopically for the absence or presence of trauma.[18] When trauma was present, I recorded its degree of healing, location, size, and appearance. Additionally, I recorded the absence, presence, and severity of non-specific stress indicators, including cribrotic lesions (cribra orbitalia, cribra humeri, and cribra femora),[19] porotic hyperostosis, enamel hypoplasias, osteoarthritis, osteophytosis, and periosteal reactions. Scoring criteria for these are based on the *Global History of Health Project*[20] and additional descriptions of each are provided in Chapter 4. I additionally noted the absence or presence of indicators of infectious disease including lesions associated with scurvy or rickets, leprosy, and treponemal diseases.[21] However, given the commingled nature of the human remains, it was often impossible to evaluate if any of these diseases were present from lone skeletal lesions.

---

16 Emily Marlow, "Metric Sex Estimation of Ancient Egyptian Skeletal Remains Part 1: Testing of Published Methods," *Bioarchaeology of the Ancient Near East* 10 (2016): 1–25.

17 For example, the sample-specific sectioning point for femoral head diameter at Deir el-Medina is the same as that previously published in Raxter, "Metric Sex Estimation in an Ancient Egyptian Skeletal Sample"; Dabbs, "Estimating the Sex of Ancient Egyptian Skeletal Remains: Methods from Tell El-Amarna."

18 While some human remains from TT 290 were radiographed in 2015, we did not have permission to use x-ray equipment in subsequent years. Consequently, only macroscopic observations were possible for most human remains at Deir el-Medina.

19 Cribra femora and cribra humeri are scored based on absence or presence. Definitions for these conditions can be found in Nicole E. Smith-Guzmán, "The Skeletal Manifestation of Malaria: An Epidemiological Approach Using Documented Skeletal Collections," *American Journal of Physical Anthropology* 158, no. 4 (December 1, 2015): 624–635, https://doi.org/10.1002/ajpa.22819.

20 Steckel et al., *The Backbone of Europe*.

21 As described in Steckel et al.

I photographed human remains using DSLR cameras and photographs from the tablet during data recording. Photograph numbers are included in each data entry and photographs were separately logged with the photo number, element number, and a brief description of the photograph. Currently, photographs are not available in an online data repository. Researchers interested in photographs of specific elements can contact me for access to images.

Works Cited

Abdalla, Aly. "A Group of Osiris-Cloths of the Twenty-First Dynasty in the Cairo Museum." *The Journal of Egyptian Archaeology* 74, no. 1 (1988): 157–164.

Albrecht, Gary L., Katherine Delores Seelman, and Michael Bury. *Handbook of Disability Studies*. 1st ed. Thousand Oaks: Sage Publications, Inc, 2001.

Allen, James. *The Art of Medicine in Ancient Egypt*. New York: Metropolitan Museum of Art, 2005.

Allen, Lindsay H. "Nutritional Influences on Linear Growth: A General Review." *European Journal of Clinical Nutrition* 48 (1994): S75–89.

AlQahtani, Sakher J., Mark P. Hector, and Helen M. Liversidge. "Accuracy of Dental Age Estimation Charts: Schour and Massler, Ubelaker and the London Atlas." *American Journal of Physical Anthropology* 154, no. 1 (2014): 70–78. https://doi.org/10.1002/ajpa.22473.

Amick III, Benjamin C., Sol Levine, Alvin R. Tarlov, and Diana Chapman Walsh, eds. *Society and Health*. Oxford: Oxford University Press, 1995.

Andreu, Guillemette. *Les Artistes de Pharaon: Deir El-Médineh et La Vallée Des Rois*. Paris: Brepols Publishers, 2002.

Andrus, Miranda R., and Mary T. Roth. "Health Literacy: A Review." *Pharmacotherapy: The Journal of Human Pharmacology and Drug Therapy* 22, no. 3 (2002): 282–302. https://doi.org/10.1592/phco.22.5.282.33191.

Angel, J. Lawrence. "Porotic Hyperostosis, Anemias, Malarias, and Marshes in the Prehistoric Eastern Mediterranean." *Science* 153, no. 3737 (1966): 760–763.

Antoine, Jean-Christophe. "Fluctuations of Fish Deliveries at Deir El-Medina in the Twentieth Dynasty. A Statistical Analysis." *Studien Zur Altägyptischen Kultur* 35 (2006): 25–41.

Antoine, Jean-Christophe. "Landholding and Agriculture in Late Ramesside Theban Documents." *Zeitschrift Für Ägyptische Sprache Und Altertumskunde* 142, no. 2 (2015): 104–119.

Antoine, Jean-Christophe. "The Delay of the Grain Ration and Its Social Consequences at Deir El-Medina in the Twentieth Dynasty: A Statistical Analysis." *The Journal of Egyptian Archaeology* 95, no. 1 (2009): 223–234.

"APA Dictionary of Psychology." Accessed March 8, 2022. https://dictionary.apa.org/.

Armelagos, George J. "Disease in Ancient Nubia." *Science* 163, no. 3864 (1969): 255–259.

Armelagos, George J., and Peter J. Brown. "The Body as Evidence; the Body of Evidence." In *The Backbone of History*, 593–602. Cambridge: Cambridge University Press, 2002.

Armelagos, George J., James H. Mielke, Kipling H. Owen, Dennis P. Van Gerven, John R. Dewey, and Paul Emil Mahler. "Bone Growth and Development in Prehistoric

Populations from Sudanese Nubia." *Journal of Human Evolution* 1, no. 1 (1972): 89–119.

Arnette, Marie Lys. "Purification Du Post-Partum et Rites Des Relevailles Dans l'Égypte Ancienne." *Bulletin de l'Institut Français d'Archéologie Orientale*, no. 114 (2015): 19–72.

Assmann, Jan. *The Search for God in Ancient Egypt.* Ithaca: Cornell University Press, 2001.

Aufderheide, Arthur C. *The Scientific Study of Mummies*. Cambridge: Cambridge University Press, 2003.

Aufderheide, Arthur C., Conrado Rodríguez-Martín, and Odin Langsjoen. *The Cambridge Encyclopedia of Human Paleopathology*. Cambridge: Cambridge University Press, 1998.

Austin, Anne E. "Accounting for Sick Days: A Scalar Approach to Health and Disease at Deir El-Medina." *Journal of Near Eastern Studies* 74, no. 1 (2015): 75–85.

Austin, Anne E. "Dental Health and Dentistry in Ancient Egypt: Possible Evidence for Dental Filling and Extraction at Deir El-Medina." *International Journal of Paleopathology* 38 (2022): 95–106. https://doi.org/10.1016/j.ijpp.2022.06.005.

Austin, Anne E. "Injuries, Illness, and Care While Constructing the Royal Tomb." In *Tomb Construction in New Kingdom Egypt*, edited by Fredrik Hagen, Daniel Soliman, and Rune Olsen. Cambridge: Cambridge University Press, Forthcoming.

Austin, Anne E. "Living and Dying at Deir El-Medina: An Osteological Analysis of the TT 290 Assemblage." In *Outside the Box: Selected Papers from the Conference "Deir El-Medina and the Theban Necropolis in Contact,"* edited by Andreas Dorn and Stéphane Polis, 27–47. Liège: Presses Universitaires de Liège, 2018.

Austin, Anne E. "Mobilizing Archaeologists: Increasing the Quantity and Quality of Data Collected in the Field with Mobile Technology." *Advances in Archaeological Practice: A Journal of the Society for American Archaeology* 2, no. 1 (2014): 13–23.

Austin, Anne E. "The Cost of a Commute: A Multidisciplinary Approach to Osteoarthritis in New Kingdom Egypt." *International Journal of Osteoarchaeology* 27, no. 4 (July 2017): 537–550. https://doi.org/10.1002/oa.2575.

Austin, Anne E., and Marie-Lys Arnette. "Of Ink and Clay: Tattooed Mummified Human Remains and Female Figurines from Deir El-Medina." *The Journal of Egyptian Archaeology* 108, no. 1–2 (2022): 63–80. https://doi.org/10.1177/03075133221130089.

Austin, Anne E., and Cédric Gobeil. "Embodying the Divine: A Tattooed Female Mummy from Deir El-Medina." *Bulletin de l'Institut Français d'Archéologie Orientale*, no. 116 (2017): 23–46.

Backhouse, Joanne. *"Scènes de Gynécées" Figured Ostraca from New Kingdom Egypt: Iconography and Intent.* Archaeopress Egyptology 26. Oxford: Archaeopress, 2020.

Baines, John, and Christopher J. Eyre. "Four Notes on Literacy." *Göttinger Miszellen* 61 (1983): 65–96.

Barnes, Ethne. *Atlas of Developmental Field Anomalies of the Human Skeleton: A Paleopathology Perspective*. Hoboken: Wiley-Blackwell, 2012.

Baten, Joerg, and Richard H. Steckel. "The History of Violence in Europe." In *The Backbone of Europe: Health, Diet, Work and Violence over Two Millennia*, edited by Richard H. Steckel, Clark Spencer Larsen, Charlotte A. Roberts, and Joerg Baten, 300–324. Cambridge Studies in Biological and Evolutionary Anthropology 80. Cambridge: Cambridge University Press, 2018.

Baten, Joerg, Richard H. Steckel, Clark Spencer Larsen, and Charlotte A. Roberts. "Multidimensional Patterns of European Health, Work, and Violence over the Past Two Millen." In *The Backbone of Europe: Health, Diet, Work and Violence over Two Millennia*, edited by Richard H. Steckel, Clark Spencer Larsen, Charlotte A. Roberts, and Joerg Baten, 381–396. Cambridge Studies in Biological and Evolutionary Anthropology 80. Cambridge: Cambridge University Press, 2018.

Bereczki, Zsolt, Maria Teschler-Nicola, Antónia Marcsik, Nicholas J. Meinzer, and Joerg Baten. "Growth Disruptions in Children." In *The Backbone of Europe: Health, Diet, Work and Violence over Two Millennia*, edited by Richard H. Steckel, Clark Spencer Larsen, Charlotte A. Roberts, and Joerg Baten, 175–197. Cambridge Studies in Biological and Evolutionary Anthropology 80. Cambridge: Cambridge University Press, 2018.

Berkman, Lisa F., Ichiro Kawachi, and M. Maria Glymour, eds. *Social Epidemiology*. 2nd ed. Oxford: Oxford University Press, 2014.

Bertalanffy, Ludwig von. *General System Theory: Foundations, Development, Applications*. New York: George Braziller, 1969.

Bianucci, Raffaella, Michael E. Habicht, Stephen Buckley, Joann Fletcher, Roger Seiler, Lena M. Öhrström, Eleni Vassilika, Thomas Böni, and Frank J. Rühli. "Shedding New Light on the 18th Dynasty Mummies of the Royal Architect Kha and His Spouse Merit." *PLoS ONE* 10, no. 7 (July 22, 2015): e0131916. https://doi.org/10.1371/journal.pone.0131916.

Bianucci, Raffaella, Grazia Mattutino, Rudy Lallo, Philippe Charlier, Hélène Jouin-Spriet, Alberto Peluso, Thomas Higham, Carlo Torre, and Emma Rabino Massa. "Immunological Evidence of Plasmodium Falciparum Infection in an Egyptian Child Mummy from the Early Dynastic Period." *Journal of Archaeological Science* 35, no. 7 (July 2008): 1880–1885. https://doi.org/10.1016/j.jas.2007.11.019.

Bickel, Susanne, and Bernard Mathieu. "L'écrivain Amennakht et Son Enseignement." *Bulletin de l'Institut Français d'Archéologie Orientale*, no. 93 (1993): 31–51.

Bierbrier, Morris L. *The Late New Kingdom in Egypt* (*c. 1300–664* B.C.)*: A Genealogical and Chronological Investigation*. Liverpool Monographs in Archaeology and Oriental Studies. Warminster: Aris & Phillips Ltd., 1975.

Bierbrier, Morris L. *The Tomb-Builders of the Pharaohs*. London: British Museum Publications, 1982.

Borghouts, Joris F. *Ancient Egyptian Magical Texts*. Leiden: Brill, 1978.

Borghouts, Joris F. "Divine Intervention in Ancient Egypt and Its Manifestation (B3w)." In *Gleanings from Deir El-Medina*, edited by Robert J. Demarée and Jac J. Janssen, 1–70. Leiden: Nederlands Instituut voor het Nabije Oosten, 1982.

Borghouts, Joris F., K. Donker van Heel, Ben Haring, Robert J. Demarée, and Jaana Toivari-Viitala. "The Deir El-Medina Database." The Deir el-Medina Database, 2023. https://dmd.wepwawet.nl/.

Born, Gustav V.R. "The Wide-Ranging Family History of Max Born." *Notes and Records of the Royal Society of London* 56, no. 2 (2002): 219–262.

Bos, Kirsten I., Verena J. Schuenemann, G. Brian Golding, Hernán A. Burbano, Nicholas Waglechner, Brian K. Coombes, Joseph B. McPhee, Sharon N. DeWitte, Matthias Meyer, and Sarah Schmedes. "A Draft Genome of Yersinia Pestis from Victims of the Black Death." *Nature* 478, no. 7370 (2011): 506–510. https://doi.org/10.1038/nature105 49.

Boyd, Kenneth M. "Disease, Illness, Sickness, Health, Healing and Wholeness: Exploring Some Elusive Concepts." *Medical Humanities* 26 (June 1, 2000): 9–17. https://doi.org/ 10.1136/mh.26.1.9.

Brickley, Megan B. "Cribra Orbitalia and Porotic Hyperostosis: A Biological Approach to Diagnosis." *American Journal of Physical Anthropology* 167, no. 4 (2018): 896–902. https://doi.org/10.1002/ajpa.23701.

Brickley, Megan, and Rachel Ives. *The Bioarchaeology of Metabolic Bone Disease*. Amsterdam: Academic Press, 2008.

Brooks, Sheilagh, and Judy M. Suchey. "Skeletal Age Determination Based on the Os Pubis: A Comparison of the Acsádi-Nemeskéri and Suchey-Brooks Methods." *Human Evolution* 5, no. 3 (1990): 227–238.

Bruyère, Bernard. *Rapport sur les fouilles de Deir el Médineh (1923–1924)*. Fouilles de l'Institut français d'archéologie orientale 2. Cairo: Institut français d'archéologie orientale, 1925.

Bruyère, Bernard. *Rapport sur les fouilles de Deir el Médineh (1924–1925)*. Fouilles de l'Institut français d'archéologie orientale 3. Cairo: Institut français d'archéologie orientale, 1926.

Bruyère, Bernard. *Rapport sur les Fouilles de Deir el Médineh 1933–1934: I*. Fouilles de l'Institut français d'archéologie orientale. Le Caire: L'Institut Français d'Archéologie Orientale, 1937.

Bruyère, Bernard. *Rapport sur les Fouilles de Deir el Médineh 1934–1935: II*. Fouilles de l'Institut français d'archéologie orientale. Le Caire: L'Institut Français d'Archéologie Orientale, 1937.

Bruyère, Bernard. *Rapport sur les fouilles de Deir el Médineh (1948 à 1951)*,. Fouilles de l'Institut français d'archéologie orientale 26. Cairo: Institut français d'archéologie orientale, 1953.

Bruyère, Bernard, and Charles Kuentz. *Tombes thébaines: la nécropole de Deir el-Médineh; la tombe de Nakht-Min et la tombe d'Ari-Nefer*. Mémoires publiés par les membres de l'Institut français d'archéologie du Caire 54. Cairo: L'Institut français d'archéologie orientale, 1926.

Brůžek, Jaroslav, Frédéric Santos, Bruno Dutailly, Pascal Murail, and Eugenia Cunha. "Validation and Reliability of the Sex Estimation of the Human Os Coxae Using Freely Available DSP2 Software for Bioarchaeology and Forensic Anthropology." *American Journal of Physical Anthropology* 164, no. 2 (2017): 440–449. https://doi.org/10.1002/ajpa.23282.

Buckberry, J.L., and A.T. Chamberlain. "Age Estimation from the Auricular Surface of the Ilium: A Revised Method." *American Journal of Physical Anthropology* 119, no. 3 (November 2002): 231–239. https://doi.org/10.1002/ajpa.10130.

Buckingham, Jane. "Indian and British Concepts of Leprosy and of the Leprosy Sufferer." In *Leprosy in Colonial South India: Medicine and Confinement*, 7–35. London: Palgrave Macmillan, 2002. https://doi.org/10.1057/9781403932730_2.

Buikstra, Jane E., B.J. Baker, and D.C. Cook. "What Diseases Plagued Ancient Egyptians? A Century of Controversy Considered." In *Biological Anthropology and the Study of Ancient Egypt*, edited by W. Vivan Davies and Roxie Walker, 24–53. London: British Museum Press, 1993.

Buikstra, Jane E., and Douglas Ubelaker. *Standards for Data Collection from Human Skeletal Remains: Proceedings of a Seminar at the Field Museum of Natural History*. Arkansas Archeological Survey Research Series 44. Fayetteville: Arkansas Archeological Survey, 1994.

Burke, Michael P, Lauren H. Martini, Ebru Çayır, Heather L. Hartline-Grafton, and Randa L. Meade. "Severity of Household Food Insecurity Is Positively Associated with Mental Disorders among Children and Adolescents in the United States." *The Journal of Nutrition* 146, no. 10 (October 1, 2016): 2019–2026. https://doi.org/10.3945/jn.116.232298.

Burtle, Adam, and Stephen Bezruchka. "Population Health and Paid Parental Leave: What the United States Can Learn from Two Decades of Research." *Healthcare* 4, no. 2 (2016): 30. https://doi.org/10.3390/healthcare4020030.

Buzon, Michele R. 2004. "A Bioarchaeological Perspective on State Formation in the Nile Valley." Ph.D. Dissertation, University of California - Santa Barbara.

Buzon, Michele R. "Health of the Non-Elites at Tombos: Nutritional and Disease Stress in New Kingdom Nubia." *American Journal of Physical Anthropology* 130, no. 1 (2006): 26–37. https://doi.org/10.1002/ajpa.20303.

Buzon, Michele R. "Tombos during the Napatan Period (~750–660 BC): Exploring the Consequences of Sociopolitical Transitions in Ancient Nubia." *International Journal of Paleopathology* 7 (December 2014): 1–7. https://doi.org/10.1016/j.ijpp.2014.05.002.

Buzon, Michele R., and Margaret A. Judd. "Investigating Health at Kerma: Sacrificial versus Nonsacrificial Individuals." *American Journal of Physical Anthropology* 136, no. 1 (2008): 93–99. https://doi.org/10.1002/ajpa.20781.

Buzon, Michele R., and Rebecca Richman. "Traumatic Injuries and Imperialism: The Effects of Egyptian Colonial Strategies at Tombos in Upper Nubia." *American Journal of Physical Anthropology* 133, no. 2 (2007): 783–791. https://doi.org/10.1002/ajpa.20585.

Buzon, Michele R., and Antonio Simonetti. "Strontium Isotope (87Sr/86Sr) Variability in the Nile Valley: Identifying Residential Mobility during Ancient Egyptian and Nubian Sociopolitical Changes in the New Kingdom and Napatan Periods." *American Journal of Physical Anthropology* 151, no. 1 (2013): 1–9. https://doi.org/10.1002/ajpa.22235.

Buzon, Michele R., Stuart Tyson Smith, and Antonio Simonetti. "Entanglement and the Formation of the Ancient Nubian Napatan State." *American Anthropologist* 118, no. 2 (2016): 284–300. https://doi.org/10.1111/aman.12524.

Byrnes, Jennifer F., and Jennifer L. Muller, eds. *Bioarchaeology of Impairment and Disability: Theoretical, Ethnohistorical, and Methodological Perspectives*. Bioarchaeology and Social Theory. Cham: Springer, 2017.

Callahan, Daniel. "The WHO Definition of 'Health.'" *The Hastings Center Studies* 1, no. 3 (January 1, 1973): 77–87. https://doi.org/10.2307/3527467.

Cassel, John. "The Contribution of the Social Environment to Host Resistance." *American Journal of Epidemiology* 104, no. 2 (1976): 107–123.

Černý, Jaroslav. *A Community of Workmen at Thebes in the Ramesside Period*. Bibliothèque d'étude 50. Cairo: Institut français d'archéologie orientale, 1973.

Černý, Jaroslav. *Catalogue des ostraca hiératiques non littéraires de Deir el-Médineh*. Vol. I (Nos 1 à 113). Documents de fouilles 3. Cairo: l'Institut français d'archéologie orientale, 1935.

Černý, Jaroslav. "Prices and Wages in Egypt during the Ramesside Period." *Cahiers d'histoire Mondial* 1, no. 4 (1954): 903–921.

Černý, Jaroslav. "The Will of Naunakhte and the Related Documents." *The Journal of Egyptian Archaeology* 31 (1945): 29–53. https://doi.org/10.2307/3855381.

Černý, Jaroslav, and Alan H. Gardiner. *Hieratic Ostraca*. Oxford: University Press, 1957.

Chamberlain, Geoffrey. "Historical Perspectives on Health: Childbirth in Ancient Egypt." *The Journal of the Royal Society for the Promotion of Health* 124, no. 6 (November 1, 2004): 284–286. https://doi.org/10.1177/146642400412400618.

Chen, Eric M., Sulabha Masih, Kira Chow, George Matcuk, and Dakshesh Patel. "Periosteal Reaction: Review of Various Patterns Associated With Specific Pathology." *Contemporary Diagnostic Radiology* 35, no. 17 (2012): 1–5. https://doi.org/10.1097/01.CDR.0000418464.79923.5c.

Christakis, Nicholas A., and James H. Fowler. "The Collective Dynamics of Smoking in a Large Social Network." *New England Journal of Medicine* 358, no. 21 (2008): 2249–2258. https://doi.org/10.1056/NEJMsa0706154.

Clemans-Cope, Lisa, Cynthia D. Perry, Genevieve M. Kenney, Jennifer E. Pelletier, and Matthew S. Pantell. "Access to and Use of Paid Sick Leave among Low-Income Families with Children." *Pediatrics* 122, no. 2 (2008): e480–486. https://doi.org/10.1542/peds.2007-3294.

Cobb, Sidney. "Social Support as a Moderator of Life Stress." *Psychosomatic Medicine* 38, no. 5 (1976): 300–314. https://doi.org/10.1097/00006842-197609000-00003.

Cockburn, Aidan, Eve Cockburn, and Theodore A. Reyman, eds. *Mummies, Disease and Ancient Cultures*. 2nd ed. Cambridge: Cambridge University Press, 1998.

Cohen, Mark Nathan. *Health and the Rise of Civilization*. New Haven: Yale University Press, 1989.

Cohen, Mark Nathan. "The Osteological Paradox Reconsidered." *Current Anthropology* 35, no. 5 (December 1994): 629–637.

Cohen, Mark Nathan, and George J. Armelagos, eds. *Paleopathology at the Origins of Agriculture*. Proceedings of the Conference on Paleopathology and Socioeconomic Change at the Origins of Agriculture. New York: Academic Press, 1984.

Cohen, Sheldon, Ian Brissette, David P. Skoner, and William J. Doyle. "Social Integration and Health: The Case of the Common Cold." *Journal of Social Structure* 1, no. 3 (2000): 1–7.

Cole, Garrard, and Tony Waldron. "Cribra Orbitalia: Dissecting an Ill-Defined Phenomenon." *International Journal of Osteoarchaeology* 29, no. 4 (2019): 613–621. https://doi.org/10.1002/oa.2757.

Commission on Social Determinants of Health. *Closing the Gap in a Generation: Health Equity through Action on the Social Determinants of Health: Commission on Social Determinants of Health Final Report*. Geneva: World Health Organization, 2008.

Cook, Della Collins, and Mary Lucas Powell. "The Evolution of American Paleopathology." In *Bioarchaeology: The Contextual Analysis of Human Remains*, edited by Jane E. Buikstra and Lane A. Beck, 281–323. Amsterdam: Academic Press, 2006.

Cooney, Kathlyn M. "An Informal Workshop: Textual Evidence for Private Funerary Art Production in the Ramesside Period." In *Living and Writing in Deir El-Medine: Socio-Historical Embodiment of Deir El-Medine Texts*, edited by Andreas Dorn and Tobias Hofmann, 43–55. Aegyptiaca Helvetica 19. Basel: Schwabe AG, 2006.

Cooney, Kathlyn M. "Profit or Exploitation? The Production of Private Ramesside Tombs Within the West Theban Funerary Economy." *Journal of Egyptian History* 1, no. 1 (2008): 79–115. https://doi.org/10.1163/187416608784118776.

Cooney, Kathlyn M. *The Cost of Death: The Social and Economic Value of Ancient Egyptian Funerary Art in the Rameside Period*. Egyptologische Uitgaven 22. Leiden: Nederlands Instituut voor het Nabije Oosten, 2007.

Corwin, Anna I. "Lord, Hear Our Prayer: Prayer, Social Support, and Well-Being in a Catholic Convent." *Journal of Linguistic Anthropology* 24, no. 2 (2014): 174–192. https://doi.org/10.1111/jola.12047.

Cross, Morag. "Accessing the Inaccessible: Disability and Archaeology." In *Disability and Archaeology*, edited by Nyree Finlay, 7–30. New York: Routledge, 1999.

Dabbs, Gretchen R. "Bioarchaeology of the Non-Elite North Tombs Cemetery at Amarna: A Preliminary Assessment of the Non-Elite Individuals of the North Tombs Cemetery at Tell El-Amarna, Egypt." *Bioarchaeology International* 3, no. 3 (2019): 174–186. https://doi.org/10.5744/bi.2019.1012.

Dabbs, Gretchen R. "Estimating the Sex of Ancient Egyptian Skeletal Remains: Methods from Tell El-Amarna." *Bioarchaeology of the Near East* 14 (2020): 11–26.

Dabbs, Gretchen R. "Menarche at Amarna: Timing and the Further Implications." *American Journal of Biological Anthropology* n/a, no. n/a (2023). https://doi.org/10.1002/ajpa.24856.

Dabbs, Gretchen R. "Sex Determination Using the Scapula in New Kingdom Skeletons from Tell El-Amarna." *HOMO—Journal of Comparative Human Biology* 61, no. 6 (December 2010): 413–420. https://doi.org/10.1016/j.jchb.2010.09.001.

Dabbs, Gretchen R., and Melissa Zabecki. "Abandoned Memories. A Cemetery of Forgotten Souls." In *Remembering the Dead in the Ancient Near East*, edited by Benjamin W. Porter and Alexis T. Boutin, 217–250. Boulder: University Press of Colorado, 2014.

Dabbs, Gretchen R., and Melissa Zabecki. "Slot-Type Fractures of the Scapula at New Kingdom Tell El-Amarna, Egypt." *International Journal of Paleopathology* 11 (December 2015): 12–22. https://doi.org/10.1016/j.ijpp.2015.07.003.

Dar, Gali, Youssef Masharawi, Smadar Peleg, Nili Steinberg, Hila May, Bahaa Medlej, Natan Peled, and Israel Hershkovitz. "Schmorl's Nodes Distribution in the Human Spine and Its Possible Etiology." *European Spine Journal* 19, no. 4 (April 2010): 670–675. https://doi.org/10.1007/s00586-009-1238-8.

David, Arlette. *The Legal Register of Ramesside Private Law Instruments*. Göttinger Orientforschungen IV. Reihe Ägypten 38. Wiesbaden: Harrassowitz Verlag, 2010.

Davidson, Alan. *Social Determinants of Health: A Comparative Approach*. Oxford: Oxford University Press, 2019.

Davies, Benedict. *Who's Who at Deir El-Medina. A Prosopographic Study of the Royal Workmen's Community*. Egyptologische Uitgaven 13. Leiden: Nederlands Instituut voor het Nabije Oosten, 1999.

Davies, Benedict G. *Life Within the Five Walls: A Handbook to Deir El-Medina*. Robb de Peyster Tytus Memorial Series 5. Wallasey: Abercromby Press, 2018.

Davies, Norman de Garis. *Two Ramesside Tombs at Thebes*. New York: The Metropolitan Museum of Art, 1927.

Dawson, Warren Royal, and Peter Hugh Ker Gray. *Catalogue of Egyptian Antiquities in the British Museum: 1 Mummies and Human Remains*. Vol. 1. London: British Museum Press, 1968.

Deines, Hildegard von, and Wolfhart Westendorf. *Wörterbuch der medizinischen Texte*. Vol. VII, 2. Grundriss der Medizin der Alten Ägypter. Berlin: Akademie-Verlag, 1962.

"Deir El Medine Online," 2009. https://dem-online.gwi.uni-muenchen.de/.

Demarée, Robert J. "A House Is Not a Home—What Exactly Is a Hut?" In *Living and Writing in Deir El-Medine*, edited by Andreas Dorn and Tobias Hofmann, 57–66. Aegyptiaca Helvetica 19. Basel: Schwabe Verlag, 2006.

Demarée, Robert J., Andreas Dorn, and Stéphane Polis. "Les Listes de Maisonnées de Deir El-Médina («Stato Civile»). Nouveaux Fragments de l'Ifao et Localisation de l'archive d'une Ligne de Scribes." *Bulletin de l'Institut Français d'Archéologie Orientale*, no. 120 (2020): 171–220.

Demarée, Robert J., and Dominique Valbelle. *Les registres de recensement du village de Deir el-Médineh (le "Stato Civile")*. Leuven: Peeters, 2011.

DeRigne, LeaAnne, Patricia Stoddard Dare, Cyleste Collins, Linda M. Quinn, and Kimberly Fuller. "Working U.S. Adults without Paid Sick Leave Report More Worries about Finances." *Journal of Social Service Research* 45, no. 4 (2019): 570–581.

DeRigne, LeaAnne, Patricia Stoddard-Dare, and Linda Quinn. "Workers Without Paid Sick Leave Less Likely To Take Time Off For Illness Or Injury Compared To Those With Paid Sick Leave." *Health Affairs* 35, no. 3 (2016): 520–527.

DeWitte, Sharon N. "Differential Survival among Individuals with Active and Healed Periosteal New Bone Formation." *International Journal of Paleopathology* 7 (2014): 38–44. https://doi.org/10.1016/j.ijpp.2014.06.001.

DeWitte, Sharon N. "Health in Post-Black Death London (1350–1538): Age Patterns of Periosteal New Bone Formation in a Post-Epidemic Population." *American Journal of Physical Anthropology* 155, no. 2 (2014): 260–267. https://doi.org/10.1002/ajpa.22510.

DeWitte, Sharon N., and Christopher M. Stojanowski. "The Osteological Paradox 20 Years Later: Past Perspectives, Future Directions." *Journal of Archaeological Research* 23 (2015): 397–450. https://doi.org/10.1007/s10814-015-9084-1.

Dodson, Aidan. "The Late Eighteenth Dynasty Necropolis at Deir El-Medina and the Earliest 'Yellow' Coffin of the New Kingdom." In *Deir El-Medina in the Third Millenium AD: A Tribute to Jac. J. Janssen*, edited by Robert J. Demarée and Arno Egberts, 89–100. Egyptologische Uitgaven 14. Leiden: Nederlands Instituut voor het Nabije Oosten, 2000.

Donker van Heel, Koenraad. *Mrs. Naunakhte & Family: The Women of Ramesside Deir al-Medina*. Cairo: American University in Cairo Press, 2016.

Dorn, Andreas. *Arbeiterhütten im Tal der Könige: ein Beitrag zur altägyptischen Sozialgeschichte aufgrund von neuem Quellenmaterial aus der Mitte der 20. Dynastie (ca. 1150 v. Chr.)*. 3 vols. Aegyptiaca Helvetica 23. Basel: Schwabe Verlag, 2011.

Douthit, Nathan, S. Kiv, Tzvi Dwolatzky, and S. Biswas. "Exposing Some Important Barriers to Health Care Access in the Rural USA." *Public Health* 129, no. 6 (June 2015): 611–620. https://doi.org/10.1016/j.puhe.2015.04.001.

Dressler, W.W., A. Mata, A. Chavez, F.E. Viteri, and P. Gallagher. "Social Support and Arterial Pressure in a Central Mexican Community." *Psychosomatic Medicine* 48, no. 5 (June 1986): 338.

Dressler, William W. "Cross-Cultural Differences and Social Influences in Social Support and Cardiovascular Disease." In *Social Support and Cardiovascular Disease*, edited by Sally A. Shumaker and Susan M. Czajkowski, 167–192. The Springer Series in Behavioral Psychophysiology and Medicine. Boston, MA: Springer US, 1994. https://doi.org/10.1007/978-1-4899-2572-5_8.

Dressler, William W. "Cultural Consonance: Linking Culture, the Individual and Health." *Preventive Medicine* 55, no. 5 (November 2012): 390–393. https://doi.org/10.1016/j.ypmed.2011.12.022.

Dressler, William W., Mauro Campos Balieiro, and Jose Ernesto Dos Santos. "The Cultural Construction of Social Support in Brazil: Associations with Health Outcomes." *Culture, Medicine and Psychiatry* 21, no. 3 (September 1, 1997): 303–335. https://doi.org/10.1023/A:1005394416255.

Duhig, Corinne. "'They Are Eating People Here!' Skeletal Indicators of Stress in the Egyptian First Intermediate Period." Ph.D. Dissertation, University of Cambridge, 2000.

Dunand, Françoise, and Roger Lichtenberg. *Mummies And Death in Egypt*. Ithaca: Cornell University Press, 2006.

Duray, Stephen M. "Dental Indicators of Stress and Reduced Age at Death in Prehistoric Native Americans." *American Journal of Physical Anthropology* 99, no. 2 (1996): 275–286.

Dye, Christopher. "Health and Urban Living." *Science* 319, no. 5864 (2008): 766–769. https://doi.org/10.1126/science.115019.

Edgerton, William F. "The Strikes in Ramses III's Twenty-Ninth Year." *Journal of Near Eastern Studies* 10, no. 3 (1951): 137–145.

Edinborough, Marija, and Carolyn Rando. "Stressed Out: Reconsidering Stress in the Study of Archaeological Human Remains." *Journal of Archaeological Science* 121 (September 2020): 105197. https://doi.org/10.1016/j.jas.2020.105197.

Edwards, Iorwerth Eiddon Stephen. *Oracular Amuletic Decrees of the Late New Kingdom*. Vol. I. Text. London: Trustees of the British Museum, 1960.

El-Najjar, Mahmoud Y., Dennis J. Ryan, Christy G. Turner, and Betsy Lozoff. "The Etiology of Porotic Hyperostosis among the Prehistoric and Historic Anasazi Indians of Southwestern United States." *American Journal of Physical Anthropology* 44, no. 3 (1976): 477–487. https://doi.org/10.1002/ajpa.1330440311.

Endesfelder, Erika. "Sklaven (Hmw) in Der Nekropole von Deir El Medine." *Altorientalische Forschungen* 5, no. JG (1978): 17–24. https://doi.org/10.1524/aofo.1978.5.jg.17.

Engel, George L. "The Need for a New Medical Model: A Challenge for Biomedicine." *Science* 196, no. 4286 (April 8, 1977): 129–136. https://doi.org/10.1126/science.847460.

Engelmann, Heinz, and Jochen Hallof. "Der Sachmetpriester, Ein Früher Repräsentant Der Hygiene Und Des Seuchenschutzes." *Studien Zur Altägyptischen Kultur* 23 (1996): 103–146.

Eschenbrenner Diemer, Gersande, Lisa Sartini, and Margaret Serpico. "Rediscovering Black Coffins from Deir El-Medina: A Comprehensive Approach." *Bulletin de l'Institut Français d'archéologie Orientale*, no. 121 (2021): 255–305. https://doi.org/10.4000/bifao.8189.

Evans, Robert G., Morris L. Barer, and Theodore R. Marmor, eds. *Evans, Robert G., Barer, Morris L. and Marmor, Theodore R.. Why Are Some People Healthy and Others Not?: The Determinants of Health of Populations*. Social Institutions and Social Change. Boston: De Gruyer, 1994. https://doi.org/10.4324/9781315135755.

Eyre, Christopher J. "The Market Women of Pharaonic Egypt." In *Le Commerce En Égypte Ancienne*, edited by Nicolás Grimal and Bernadette Menu, 173–191. Bibliothèque d'étude 121. Cairo: Institut Français d'Archéologie Orientale, 1998.

Eyre, Christopher J. *The Use of Documents in Pharaonic Egypt*. Oxford Studies in Ancient Documents. Oxford: Oxford University Press, 2013.

Fazekas, István Gyula, and F. Kósa. *Forensic Fetal Osteology*. Akadémiai Kiadó, 1978.

Feucht, Erika. *Das Kind im Alten Ägypten: die Stellung des Kindes in Familie und Gesellschaft nach altägyptischen Texten und Darstellungen*. Frankfurt: Campus, 1995.

Finniss, Damien G., Ted J. Kaptchuk, Franklin Miller, and Fabrizio Benedetti. "Biological, Clinical, and Ethical Advances of Placebo Effects." *The Lancet* 375, no. 9715 (February 2010): 686–695. https://doi.org/10.1016/S0140-6736(09)61706-2.

Fischer, Henry G. "Notes on Sticks and Staves in Ancient Egypt." *Metropolitan Museum Journal* 13 (1978): 5–32.

Fischer-Elfert, Hans-Werner. "A Strike in the Reign of Merenptah? Plus the Endowment of Three Cult Statue(Tte)s on Behalf of the Same King at Deir El-Medina (Pap. Berlin P. 23300 and P. 23301)." In *Forschung in Der Papyrussammlung: Eine Festgabe Für Das Neue Museum*, edited by Verena M. Lepper, 47–73. Ägyptische Und Orientalische Papyri Und Handschriften Des Ägyptischen Museums Und Papyrussammlung Berlin 1. Berlin: Akademie Verlag, 2012.

Fischer-Elfert, Hans-Werner, ed. "Pap. Ebers Nr. 1–3—Reflexionen eines altägyptischen Heilers über seine Initiation?" In *Papyrus Ebers und die antike Heilkunde: Akten der Tagung vom 15.–16. 3. 2002 in der Albertina/UB der Universität Leipzig*, 133–148. Marburger altertumskundliche Abhandlungen 7. Wiesbaden: Harrassowitz Verlag, 2005.

Fox, Sherry C., and Kathryn Marklein. "Primary and Secondary Burials with Commingled Remains from Archaeological Contexts in Cyprus, Greece, and Turkey." In *Commingled and Disarticulated Human Remains*, edited by Anna J. Osterholtz,

Kathryn M. Baustian, and Debra L. Martin, 193–211. Springer New York, 2014. http://link.springer.com/chapter/10.1007/978-1-4614-7560-6_11.

Frandsen, Paul J. "Editing Reality: The Turin Strike Papyrus." In *Studies in Egyptology Presented to Miriam Lichtheim*, edited by S. Israelit-Groll, 166–199. Jerusalem: Magnes Press, 1990.

Frandsen, Paul J. "The Menstrual 'Taboo' in Ancient Egypt." *Journal of Near Eastern Studies* 66, no. 2 (2007): 81–106.

Frank, John W., and J. Fraser Mustard. "The Determinants of Health from a Historical Perspective." *Daedalus* 123, no. 4 (1994): 1–19.

Franks, Peter, Carolyn M. Clancy, and Marthe R. Gold. "Health Insurance and Mortality. Evidence from a National Cohort." *Journal of the American Medical Association* 270, no. 6 (1993): 737–741. https://doi.org/10.1001/jama.1993.03510060083037.

Friedland, Daniel S., and Richard H. Price. "Underemployment: Consequences for the Health and Well-Being of Workers." *American Journal of Community Psychology* 32, no. 1 (2003): 33–45. https://doi.org/10.1023/A:1025638705649.

Gabler, Kathrin. "Can I Stay or Must I Go? Relations between the Deir El-Medina Community and Their Service Personnel." In *Outside the Box: Selected Papers from the Conference "Deir El-Medina and the Theban Necropolis in Contact,"* edited by Andreas Dorn and Stéphane Polis, 157–189. Liège: Presses Universitaires de Liège, 2018.

Gabler, Kathrin. *Who's who around Deir el-Medina. Untersuchungen zur Organisation, Prosopographie und Entwicklung des Versorgungspersonals für die Arbeitersiedlung und das Tal der Könige*. Egyptologische Uitgaven 31. Leiden: Peeters Publishers, 2018.

Gamble, Julia, and Gilian R. Bentley. "Developmental Origins of Health and Disease (DOHaD): Perspectives from Bioarchaeology." In *Palaeopathology and Evolutionary Medicine: An Integrated Approach*, edited by Kimberly A. Plomp, Charlotte A. Roberts, Sarah Elton, and Gilian R. Bentley, 17–41. Oxford: Oxford University Press, 2022.

Gamble, Julia, and Gillian Bentley. Developmental origins of health and disease (DOHaD): perspectives from bioarchaeology (2022).

Gardiner, Alan H., ed. *Hieratic Papyri in the British Museum*. Vol. 1. Third Series Chester Beatty Gift. London: British Museum Press, 1935.

Gardiner, Alan H., ed. "Professional Magicians in Ancient Egypt." *Proceedings of the Society of Biblical Archaeology* 39 (1917): 31–44.

Gardiner, Alan H., ed. *Ramesside Administrative Documents*. Oxford: Oxford University Press, 1948.

Ghalioungui, Paul. *La Médecine Des Pharaons: Magie et science medicale dans l'Egypte ancienne*. Paris: Robert Laffont, 1983.

Gleason, Robyn Panther, and Shawn M. Kneipp. "Employment-Related Constraints: Determinants of Primary Health Care Access?" *Policy, Politics, & Nursing Practice* 5, no. 2 (May 2004): 73–83. https://doi.org/10.1177/1527154404263265.

Gobeil, Cédric. "The IFAO Excavations at Deir El-Medina." *Oxford University Press, Oxford Handbooks Online*, 2015. https://doi.org/10.1093/oxfordhb/9780199935413.013.32.

Goddard, Maria, and Peter Smith. "Equity of Access to Health Care Services: Theory and Evidence from the UK." *Social Science & Medicine* 53, no. 9 (2001): 1149–1162. https://doi.org/10.1016/S0277-9536(00)00415-9.

Gomez, Jose Alba. "Some Oils in Ancient Egypt: Debate between Moringa, Olive and Sesame Oils." In *Olive Oil and Wine Production in Eastern Mediterranean during Antiquity: International Symposium Proceedings, 17–19 November 2011, Urla–Turkey*, edited by Adnan Diler, Ahmet Kaan Şenol, and Ümit Aydınoğlu, 209–220. İzmir: Ege Üniversitesi Basımevi, 2015.

Goodman, Alan H., and George J. Armelagos. "Factors Affecting the Distribution of Enamel Hypoplasias within the Human Permanent Dentition." *American Journal of Physical Anthropology* 68, no. 4 (1985): 479–493. https://doi.org/10.1002/ajpa.1330680404.

Goodman, Alan H., and Jerome C. Rose. "Assessment of Systemic Physiological Perturbations from Dental Enamel Hypoplasias and Associated Histological Structures." *American Journal of Physical Anthropology* 33, no. S11 (1990): 59–110. https://doi.org/10.1002/ajpa.1330330506.

Goodman, Alan, and Debra Martin. "Reconstructing Health Profiles from Skeletal Remains." In *The Backbone of History: Health and Nutrition in the Western Hemisphere*, edited by Richard H. Steckel and Jerome C. Rose, 11–60. Cambridge: Cambridge University Press, 2002.

Goodman, Alan, Debra L. Martin, and George Armelagos. "Indicators of Stress from Bones and Teeth." In *Paleopathology at the Origins of Agriculture*, edited by George J. Armelagos and Mark Nathan Cohen, 13–49. New York: Academic Press, 1984.

Gowland, Rebecca L. "Entangled Lives: Implications of the Developmental Origins of Health and Disease Hypothesis for Bioarchaeology and the Life Course." *American Journal of Physical Anthropology* 158, no. 4 (2015): 530–540. https://doi.org/10.1002/ajpa.22820.

Gowland, Rebecca L., and A. Gaynor Western. "Morbidity in the Marshes: Using Spatial Epidemiology to Investigate Skeletal Evidence for Malaria in Anglo-Saxon England (AD 410–1050)." *American Journal of Physical Anthropology* 147, no. 2 (February 2012): 301–311. https://doi.org/10.1002/ajpa.21648.

Grandet, Pierre. *Catalogue des ostraca hieratiques non litteraires de Deir el-Medineh Tome IX*. Cairo: Institut français d'archéologie orientale, 2003.

Grapow, Hermann, Wolfhart Westendorf, and Hildegard von Deines. *Grundriss der Medizin der alten Ägypter*. Vol. 6. Berlin: Akademie-Verlag, 1959.

Guilmot, Max. "Une Lettre de Remontrances, l'Ostracon Berlin P. 10627." *Chronique d'Egypte* 40, no. 80 (1965): 235–248. https://doi.org/10.1484/J.CDE.2.308019.

Gundersen, Craig, and Brent Kreider. "Bounding the Effects of Food Insecurity on Children's Health Outcomes." *Journal of Health Economics* 28, no. 5 (September 2009): 971–983. https://doi.org/10.1016/j.jhealeco.2009.06.012.

Gunn, Battiscombe. "The Decree of Amonrasonthēr for Neskhons." *The Journal of Egyptian Archaeology* 41 (December 1955): 83–105.

Guy, Hervé, Claude Masset, and Charles-Albert Baud. "Infant Taphonomy." *International Journal of Osteoarchaeology* 7, no. 3 (1997): 221–229.

Hadgaonkar, Shailesh, Kunal Chandrakant Shah, Hrutvij Bhatt, Ashok Shyam, and Parag Sancheti. "Post Pregnancy Severe Spinal Osteoporosis with Multiple Vertebral Fractures and Kyphoscoliosis in a Multigravida: A Rare Case with Management." *Asian Spine Journal* 9, no. 4 (2015): 625–628. https://doi.org/10.4184/asj.2015.9.4.625.

Hagen, Fredrik. "'The Prohibitions': A New Kingdom Didactic Text." *The Journal of Egyptian Archaeology* 91 (2005): 125–164.

Häggman, Sofia. *Directing Deir El-Medina: The External Administration of the Necropolis*. Uppsala Studies in Egyptology 4. Uppsala: Uppsala University, 2002.

Halioua, Bruno, Bernard Ziskind, and M.B. DeBevoise. *Medicine in the Days of the Pharaohs*. Cambridge: Belknap Press of Harvard University Press, 2005.

Hamada, Ahmed. "A Stela from Manshîyet Eṣ-Ṣadr." *Annales Du Service Des Antiquités de l'Égypte* 38 (1938): 217–230.

Hansen, Sarah E., Jordan L. Whitehill, Collin S. Goto, Cheryl A. Quintero, Brenda E. Darling, and Jacqueline Davis. "Safety and Efficacy of Milk and Molasses Enemas Compared With Sodium Phosphate Enemas for the Treatment of Constipation in a Pediatric Emergency Department." *Pediatric Emergency Care* 27, no. 12 (December 2011): 1118. https://doi.org/10.1097/PEC.0b013e31823b0088.

Harari, Yuval Noah. *Homo Deus: A Brief History of Tomorrow*. New York: Harper Collins, 2017.

Haring, Ben J.J. "Economy." Edited by Elizabeth Frood, Willeke Wendrich, and Jacco Dieleman. *UCLA Encyclopedia of Egyptology* 1, no. 1 (February 4, 2009). https://escholarship.org/uc/item/2t01s4qj.

Haring, Ben J.J. "From Oral Practice to Written Record in Ramesside Deir El-Medina." *Journal of the Economic and Social History of the Orient* 46, no. 3 (2003): 249–272.

Haring, Ben J.J. "'In Life, Prosperity, Health!' Introductory Formulae in Letters from the Theban Necropolis." In *Texte–Theben–Tonfragmente: Festschrift Für Günter Burkard*, edited by Dieter Kessler, Regine Schulz, Martina Ullmann, Alexandra Verbovsek, and Stefan J. Wimmer, 180–191. Wiesbaden: Harrassowitz, 2009.

Haring, Ben J.J. "Late Twentieth Dynasty Ostraca and the End of the Necropolis Workmen's Settlement at Deir El-Medina." In *Deir El-Medina through the Kaleidoscope. Proceedings of the International Workshop Turin 8th–10th October 2018*, edited by Susanne Töpfer, Paolo Del Vesco, and Federico Poole, 44–62. Modena: Formazione e ricerca, 2022.

Harris, James E., and Kent R. Weeks. *X-Raying the Pharaohs*. New York: Charles Scribner's Sons, 1973.

Hassan, Ali. *Stöcke und Stäbe im pharaonischen Ägypten bis zum Ende des Neuen Reiches*. Münchner ägyptologische Studien 33. München: Deutscher Kunstverlag, 1976.

Hawass, Zahi A., ed. *The Treasures of the Pyramids*. Vercelli: White Star, 2003.

Hawass, Zahi, Yehia Z. Gad, Somaia Ismail, Rabab Khairat, Dina Fathalla, Naglaa Hasan, Amal Ahmed, et al. "Ancestry and Pathology in King Tutankhamun's Family." *Journal of the American Medical Association* 303, no. 7 (February 17, 2010): 638–647. https://doi.org/10.1001/jama.2010.121.

Hayes, William Christopher. *Ostraka and Name Stones from the Tomb of Sen-Mūt (No. 71) at Thebes*. New York: Metropolitan Museum of Art, 1942.

Helck, Wolfgang. *Die datierten und datierbaren Ostraka, Papyri und Graffiti von Deir el-Medineh*. Ägyptologische Abhandlungen 63. Wiesbaden: Harrassowitz Verlag, 2002.

Herrerín, Jesús, and Mª Margarita Carmenate. "Sexual Dimorphism in Crania Belonging to the 1st Century AD from the Tomb of Mentuemhat (TT 34), Luxor, Egypt." *Anthropological Science* 130, no. 2 (2022): 135–145. https://doi.org/10.1537/ase.220128.

Hertzman, C., J. Frank, and Robert G. Evans. "Heterogeneities in Health Status and the Determinants of Population Health." In *Why Are Some People Healthy and Others Not?*, edited by Robert G. Evans, Morris L. Barer, and Theodore R. Marmor, 67–92. Boston: De Gruyter, 1994.

Hill, Jacqueline, Marcia Nielsen, and Michael H. Fox. "Understanding the Social Factors That Contribute to Diabetes: A Means to Informing Health Care and Social Policies for the Chronically Ill." *The Permanente Journal* 17, no. 2 (2013): 67–72. https://doi.org/10.7812/TPP/12-099.

Hill, Kirsty B., B. Chadwick, R. Freeman, I. O'Sullivan, and J.J. Murray. "Adult Dental Health Survey 2009: Relationships between Dental Attendance, Patterns Oral Health Behaviour and the Current Barriers to Dental Care." *British Dental Journal* 214, no. 1 (2013): 25–32. https://doi.org/10.1038/sj.bdj.2012.1176.

Hinson, Benjamin Samuel Paul. "Coming of Age or an Age of Becoming? The Role of Childhood in Identity Formation at Deir El-Medina, New Kingdom Egypt." Ph.D. Dissertation, University of Cambridge, 2018. https://doi.org/10.17863/CAM.22076.

Holt-Lunstad, Julianne, Timothy B. Smith, and J. Bradley Layton. "Social Relationships and Mortality Risk: A Meta-Analytic Review." *PLOS Medicine* 7, no. 7 (2010): e1000316. https://doi.org/10.1371/journal.pmed.1000316.

Hooton, Earnest Albert. *The Indians of Pecos Pueblo: A Study of Their Skeletal Remains*. New Haven: Yale University Press, 1930.

Hosek, Lauren, and John Robb. "Osteobiography: A Platform for Bioarchaeological Research." *Bioarchaeology International* 3, no. 1 (2019): 1–15. https://doi.org/10.5744/bi.2019.1005.

House, James S., Debra Umberson, and K.R. Landis. "Structures and Processes of Social Support." *Annual Review of Sociology* 14, no. 1 (1988): 293–318. https://doi.org/10.1146/annurev.so.14.080188.001453.

Hudson, Stephanie E. "Ashmolean HO 774 and Ashmolean HO 804: New Light on Accounting Texts from Deir El-Medina." *Chronique d'Egypte* 89, no. 178 (July 2014): 236–247. https://doi.org/10.1484/J.CDE.5.103550.

Hue-Arcé, Christine. *La Violence Interpersonnelle En Égypte Au Nouvel Empire et à l'époque Gréco-Romaine*. Wallasey: Abercromby Press, 2020.

Hue-Arcé, Christine. "The Legal Treatment of Interpersonal Violence in Deir El-Medina." In *Outside the Box: Selected Papers from the Conference "Deir El-Medina and the Theban Necropolis in Contact" Liège, 27–29 2014*, edited by Andreas Dorn and Stéphane Polis, 265–279. Ægyptiaca Leodiensia. Liège, Belgium: Presses Universitaires de Liège, 2014.

Hussien, Fawzia, Rokia El Banna, W. Kandeel, and A. Sarry El-Din. "Similarity of Fracture Treatment of Workers and High Officials of the Pyramid Builders." In *Pharmacy and Medicine in Ancient Egypt: Proceedings of the Conferences Held in Cairo (2007) and Manchester (2008)*, edited by Jenefer Cockitt and A. Rosalie David, 85–89. Bar International Series 2141. Oxford: Archaeopress, 2010.

Hussien, Fawzia H., Rokia A. El Banna, and Azza M. Sarry El Din. "Non-Specific Stress Indicators in Ancient Egyptians from Giza and Bahriyah Oasis." *Journal of the Arab Society for Medical Research* 1 (2006): 13–27.

Hussien, Fawzia H., Soad Shabaan, Zahi Hawass, and Azza M. Sarry El Din. "Anthropological Differences between Workers and High Officials from the Old Kingdom at Giza." In *Egyptology at the Dawn of the Twenty-First Century*, edited by Zahi Hawass, 2:324–331. Cairo: American University in Cairo Press, 2003.

Ikram, Salima, and Aidan Dodson. *The Mummy in Ancient Egypt: Equipping the Dead for Eternity*. London: Thames & Hudson, 1998.

Institut français d'archéologie orientale au Caire. "Tombes de Deir el Medina," October 19, 2015. https://www.ifao.egnet.net/bases/archives/ttdem/.

Jacobi, Keith P., and Marie Elaine Danforth. "Analysis of Interobserver Scoring Patterns in Porotic Hyperostosis and Cribra Orbitalia." *International Journal of Osteoarchaeology* 12, no. 4 (2002): 248–258. https://doi.org/10.1002/oa.619.

Janssen, Jac J. "Absence from Work by the Necropolis Workmen of Thebes." *Studien Zur Altägyptischen Kultur* 8 (1980): 127–152.

Janssen, Jac J. *Commodity Prices from the Ramessid Period: An Economic Study of the Village of Necropolis Workmen at Thebes*. Leiden: Brill, 1975.

Janssen, Jac J. *Donkeys at Deir El-Medîna*. Egyptologische Uitgaven 19. Leiden: Nederlands Instituut voor het Nabije Oosten, 2005.

Janssen, Jac J. "Gift-Giving in Ancient Egypt as an Economic Feature." *The Journal of Egyptian Archaeology* 68 (1982): 253–258. https://doi.org/10.2307/3821641.

Janssen, Jac J. "Literacy and Letters at Deir El-Medîna." In *Village Voices: Proceedings of the Symposium "Texts from Deir El-Medîna and Their Interpretation", Leiden, May 31-June 1, 1991*, edited by Robert J. Demarée and A. Egberts, 81–94. CNWS Publications 13. Leiden: Centre of Non-Western Studies, Leiden University, 1992.

Janssen, Jac J. "The Year of the Strikes." *Bulletin de La Société d'Égyptologie de Genève* 16 (1992): 41–49.

Janssen, Jac J. *Village Varia: Ten Studies on the History and Administration of Deir El-Medina.* Egyptologische Uitgaven 11. Leiden: Nederlands Instituut voor het Nabije Oosten, 1997.

Janssen, Jac J. *Village Varia: Ten Studies on the History and Administration of Deir El-Medina.* Leiden: Nederlands Instituut voor het Nabije Oosten, 1997.

Jarcho, Saul. "Paleopathology." *Science* 147, no. 3662 (1965): 1160–1163.

Jauhiainen, Heidi. "'Do Not Celebrate Your Feast without Your Neighbours': A Study of References to Feasts and Festivals in Non-Literary Documents from Ramesside Period Deir El-Medina." Ph.D. Dissertation, University of Helsinki, 2009.

Jonckheere, Frans. *Les Médecins de l'Egypte Pharaonique: Essai de Prosopographie.* La Médecine Égyptienne 3. Bruxelles: Fondation égyptologique reine Élisabeth, 1958.

Judd, Margaret A. "Continuity of Interpersonal Violence between Nubian Communities." *American Journal of Physical Anthropology* 131, no. 3 (2006): 324–333.

Judd, Margaret A. "The Parry Problem." *Journal of Archaeological Science* 35, no. 6 (June 2008): 1658–1666. https://doi.org/10.1016/j.jas.2007.11.005.

Känel, Frédérique von. *Les prêtres-ouâb de Sekhmet et les conjurateurs de Serket.* Bibliothèque de l'École des hautes études. Sciences religieuses 87. Paris: Presses Universitaires de France, 1984.

Kaptchuk, Ted J., Elizabeth Friedlander, John M. Kelley, M. Norma Sanchez, Efi Kokkotou, Joyce P. Singer, Magda Kowalczykowski, Franklin G. Miller, Irving Kirsch, and Anthony J. Lembo. "Placebos without Deception: A Randomized Controlled Trial in Irritable Bowel Syndrome." *PLoS ONE* 5, no. 12 (December 2010): e15591. https://doi.org/10.1371/journal.pone.0015591.

Kaptchuk, Ted J., John M. Kelley, Lisa A. Conboy, Roger B. Davis, Catherine E. Kerr, Eric E. Jacobson, Irving Kirsch, et al. "Components of Placebo Effect: Randomised Controlled Trial in Patients with Irritable Bowel Syndrome." *BMJ* 336, no. 7651 (May 2008): 999–1003. https://doi.org/10.1136/bmj.39524.439618.25.

Karl, Doris. "Funktion Und Bedeutung Einer Weisen Frau Im Alten Ägypten." *Studien Zur Altägyptischen Kultur* 28 (2000): 131–160.

Kawachi, Ichiro, and Lisa F. Berkman. "Social Epidemiology." In *Social Capital, Social Cohesion, and Health*, edited by Lisa F. Berkman, Ichiro Kawachi, and M. Maria Glymour, 2nd ed., 174–190. Oxford University Press, 2014. https://oxfordmedicine.com/view/10.1093/med/9780195377903.001.0001/med-9780195377903-chapter-8.

Keita, S.O.Y., and A.J. Boyce. "Variation in Porotic Hyperostosis in the Royal Cemetery

Complex at Abydos, Upper Egypt: A Social Interpretation." *Antiquity* 80, no. 307 (March 2006): 64–73. https://doi.org/10.1017/S0003598X00093261.

Kemp, Barry, Anna Stevens, Gretchen R. Dabbs, Melissa Zabecki, and Jerome C. Rose. "Life, Death and beyond in Akhenaten's Egypt: Excavating the South Tombs Cemetery at Amarna." *Antiquity* 87, no. 335 (March 2013): 64–78. https://doi.org/10.1017/S0003598X00048626.

Kerley, Ellis R., and William M. Bass. "Paleopathology: Meeting Ground for Many Disciplines." *Science* 157, no. 3789 (1967): 638–644.

Kimmerle, Erin H., and José Pablo Baraybar, eds. *Skeletal Trauma*. Boca Raton: CRC Press, 2008.

King, Lester S. "What Is Disease?" *Philosophy of Science* 21, no. 3 (July 1954): 193–203.

Kitchen, Kenneth A. *Ramesside Inscriptions*. Vol. VI. Oxford: B.H. Blackwell, 1983.

Kitchen, Kenneth A. *Ramesside Inscriptions*. Vol. V. Oxford: B.H. Blackwell, 1983.

Kitchen, Kenneth A. *Ramesside Inscriptions*. Vol. VII. Oxford: B.H. Blackwell, 1989.

Kitchen, Kenneth A. *Ramesside Inscriptions. Translated & Annotated*. Vol. 2. Oxford: Wiley-Blackwell, 1996.

Kitchen, Kenneth A. *Ramesside Inscriptions. Translated & Annotated*. Vol. 6. Oxford: Wiley-Blackwell, 2012.

Klaus, Haagen D. "Frontiers in the Bioarchaeology of Stress and Disease: Cross-Disciplinary Perspectives from Pathophysiology, Human Biology, and Epidemiology." *American Journal of Physical Anthropology* 155, no. 2 (October 2014): 294–308. https://doi.org/10.1002/ajpa.22574.

Kleinman, Arthur. *Patients and Healers in the Context of Culture: An Exploration of the Borderland Between Anthropology, Medicine, and Psychiatry*. Berkeley: University of California Press, 1980.

Kleinman, Arthur, Leon Eisenberg, and Byron Good. "Culture, Illness, and Care: Clinical Lessons from Anthropologic and Cross-Cultural Research." *Annals of Internal Medicine* 88, no. 2 (February 1978): 251–258. https://doi.org/10.7326/0003-4819-88-2-251.

Koenig, Yvan. "Les Effrois de Keniherkhepeshef (Papyrus Deir El-Médineh 40)." *Revue d'Egyptologie Paris* 33 (1981): 29–37.

Kovacs, C.S., and S.H. Ralston. "Presentation and Management of Osteoporosis Presenting in Association with Pregnancy or Lactation." *Osteoporosis International* 26, no. 9 (2015): 2223–2241. https://doi.org/10.1007/s00198-015-3149-3.

Kremer, Célia, Stéphanie Racette, Charles-Antoine Dionne, and Anny Sauvageau. "Discrimination of Falls and Blows in Blunt Head Trauma: Systematic Study of the Hat Brim Line Rule in Relation to Skull Fractures." *Journal of Forensic Sciences* 53, no. 3 (2008): 716–719. https://doi.org/10.1111/j.1556-4029.2008.00725.x.

Kuete, Victor, Benjamin Wiench, Mohamed-Elamir F. Hegazy, Tarik A. Mohamed, Aimé G. Fankam, Abdelaaty A. Shahat, and Thomas Efferth. "Antibacterial Activity and

Cytotoxicity of Selected Egyptian Medicinal Plants." *Planta Medica* 78, no. 2 (January 2012): 193–199. https://doi.org/10.1055/s-0031-1280319.

Kumar, Ankita. "Health at Hierakonpolis, a Predynastic Settlement in Upper Egypt." Ph.D. Dissertation, University of Arkansas, 2009.

Lang, Philippa. *Medicine and Society in Ptolemaic Egypt*. Leiden: Brill, 2013.

Larcher, Cédric, Marie-Lys Arnette, Eweis Abdelrady Ateya, Anne Austin, Andreas Dorn, Kathrin Gabler, Rahel Glanzmann, et al. "Deir el-Médina (2022)." *Bulletin archéologique des Écoles françaises à l'étranger*, June 1, 2023. https://doi.org/10.4000/baefe.8324.

Lawrence, Julie, Christopher M. Stojanowski, Kathleen S. Paul, Andrew C. Seidel, and Debbie Guatelli-Steinberg. "Heterogeneous Frailty and the Expression of Linear Enamel Hypoplasia in a Genealogical Population." *American Journal of Physical Anthropology* 176, no. 4 (2021): 638–651.

Leake, Chauncey Depew. *The Old Egyptian Medical Papyri*. Lawrence: University of Kansas Press, 1952.

Lehner, Mark, and Zahi Hawass. *Giza and the Pyramids*. London: Thames Hudson, 2017.

Lesko, Barbara S. "Rank, Roles, and Rights." In *Pharaoh's Workers: The Villagers of Deir El Medina*, edited by Leonard Lesko, 15–40. Ithaca: Cornell University Press, 1994.

Lesko, Leonard H, and Barbara S. Lesko. *A Dictionary of Late Egyptian*. Vol. I–V. Berkeley: B.C. Scribe Publications, 1982.

Letellier, Bernadette. "La Destinée de Deux Enfants, Un Ostracon Ramesside Inédit." In *IFAO Livre Du Centenaire, 1880–1980*, edited by Jean Vercoutter, 127–133. Mémoires Publiés Par Les Membres de l'Institut Français d'archéologie Orientale Du Caire 104. Cairo: Institut français d'archéologie orientale, 1980.

Lichtheim, Miriam. *Ancient Egyptian Literature: The New Kingdom*. Berkeley: University of California Press, 1976.

Loprieno, Antonio. "Slavery and Servitude." *UCLA Encyclopedia of Egyptology* 1, no. 1 (2012). https://escholarship.org/uc/item/8mx2073f.

Lovejoy, C. Owen, Richard S. Meindl, Thomas R. Pryzbeck, and Robert P. Mensforth. "Chronological Metamorphosis of the Auricular Surface of the Ilium: A New Method for the Determination of Adult Skeletal Age at Death." *American Journal of Physical Anthropology* 68, no. 1 (1985): 15–28.

Lovell, Nancy C. "Analysis and Interpretation of Skeletal Trauma." In *Biological Anthropology of the Human Skeleton*, edited by Mary Anne Katzenberg and Shelley Rae Saunders, 2nd ed., 341–386. Hoboken: Wiley-Liss, 2008.

Lovell, Nancy C. "Trauma Analysis in Paleopathology." *American Journal of Physical Anthropology* 104, no. S25 (1997): 139–170.

Lovell, Nancy C., and Ira Whyte. "Patterns of Dental Enamel Defects at Ancient Mendes, Egypt." *American Journal of Physical Anthropology* 110, no. 1 (1999): 69–80.

Mandal, Manisha Deb, and Shyamapada Mandal. "Honey: Its Medicinal Property and Antibacterial Activity." *Asian Pacific Journal of Tropical Biomedicine* 1, no. 2 (April 2011): 154–160. https://doi.org/10.1016/S2221-1691(11)60016-6.

Manderson, Lenore, and Pascale Allotey. "Cultural Politics and Clinical Competence in Australian Health Services." *Anthropology & Medicine* 10, no. 1 (2003): 71–85. https://doi.org/10.1080/13648470301266.

Mandeville, Richard. "Wage Accounting in Deir El-Medina." PhD Dissertation, University of Liverpool, 2010.

Mandeville, Richard. *Wage Accounting in Deir El-Medina*. Wallasey: Abercromby Press, 2014.

Marlow, Emily. "Metric Sex Estimation of Ancient Egyptian Skeletal Remains Part I: Testing of Published Methods." *Bioarchaeology of the Ancient Near East* 10 (2016): 1–25.

Marmot, Michael, and Richard G. Wilkinson. *Social Determinants of Health*. 2nd ed. Oxford: Oxford University Press, 2006.

Marques, Carina, Vitor Matos, and Nicholas J. Meinzer. "Proliferative Periosteal Reactions." In *The Backbone of Europe*, edited by Clark Spencer Larsen, Charlotte A. Roberts, and Joerg Baten, 137–174, 2018.

Martin, Debra L., Ryan P. Harrod, and Ventura R. Pérez. *The Bioarchaeology of Violence*. Gainesville: University Press of Florida, 2013.

Martorell, R., L.K. Khan, and D.G. Schroeder. "Reversibility of Stunting: Epidemiological Findings in Children from Developing Countries." *European Journal of Clinical Nutrition* 48 Suppl 1 (February 1994): S45–57.

Martorell, Reynaldo. "Body Size, Adaptation and Function." *Human Organization* 48, no. 1 (Spring 1989): 15–20.

Massa, E. Rabino, Nicoletta Cerutti, and Martin Savoia. "Malaria in Ancient Egypt: Paleoimmunological Investigation on Predynastic Mummified Remains." *Chungará (Arica)* 32, no. 1 (January 2000). https://doi.org/10.4067/S0717-73562000000100003.

Massart, Adhémar. "The Egyptian Geneva Papyrus MAH 15274." *Mitteilungen Des Deutschen Archäologischen Instituts Abteilung Kairo* 15 (1957): 172–185.

Mathieu, Bernard. "Sur Quelques Ostraca Hiératiques Littéraires Récemment Publiés." *Bulletin de l'Institut Français d'Archéologie Orientale* 93 (1994): 335–348.

McDowell, Andrea G. "Agricultural Activity by the Workmen of Deir El-Medina." *The Journal of Egyptian Archaeology* 78 (1992): 195–206. https://doi.org/10.2307/3822072.

McDowell, Andrea G. *Jurisdiction in the Workmen's Community of Deir El-Medîna*. Egyptologische Uitgaven 5. Leiden: Nederlands Instituut voor het Nabije Oosten, 1990.

McDowell, Andrea G. "Legal Aspects of Care of the Elderly in Egypt to the End of the New Kingdom." In *The Care of the Elderly in the Ancient Near East*, edited by Marten Stol and S.P. Vleeming, 199–221. Studies in the History and Culture of the Ancient Near East 14. Leiden: Brill, 1998.

McDowell, Andrea G. *Village Life in Ancient Egypt: Laundry Lists and Love Songs*. New York: Oxford University Press, 1999.

McElroy, Ann, and Patricia K. Townsend. *Medical Anthropology in Ecological Perspective*. 3rd ed. Boulder: Westview Press, 1996.

McGinnis, J. Michael, Pamela Williams-Russo, and James R. Knickman. "The Case for More Active Policy Attention to Health Promotion." *Health Affairs* 21, no. 2 (2002): 78–93.

Meindl, Richard S., and C. Owen Lovejoy. "Ectocranial Suture Closure: A Revised Method for the Determination of Skeletal Age at Death Based on the Lateral-Anterior Sutures." *American Journal of Physical Anthropology* 68, no. 1 (1985): 57–66.

Miller, Franklin G., Luana Colloca, and Ted J. Kaptchuk. "The Placebo Effect: Illness and Interpersonal Healing." *Perspectives in Biology and Medicine* 52, no. 4 (2009): 518. https://doi.org/10.1353/pbm.0.0115.

Miller, Robert L. "Counting Calories in Egyptian Ration Texts." *Journal of the Economic and Social History of the Orient* 34, no. 3 (1991): 257–269. https://doi.org/10.1163/156852091X00021.

Mitchell, Piers D. "Retrospective Diagnosis and the Use of Historical Texts for Investigating Disease in the Past." *International Journal of Paleopathology* 1, no. 2 (October 2011): 81–88. https://doi.org/10.1016/j.ijpp.2011.04.002.

Mitchell, Piers D, ed. *Sanitation, Latrines and Intestinal Parasites in Past Populations*. London: Routledge, 2016. https://doi.org/10.4324/9781315607603.

Mittler, Diane M., and Dennis P. van Gerven. "Developmental, Diachronic, and Demographic Analysis of Cribra Orbitalia in the Medieval Christian Populations of Kulubnarti." *American Journal of Physical Anthropology* 93, no. 3 (March 1994): 287–297. https://doi.org/10.1002/ajpa.1330930302.

Molleson, Theya. "A Method for the Study of Activity Related Skeletal Morphologies." *Bioarchaeology of the Near East* 1 (2007): 5–33.

Molto, J. E. "The Comparative Skeletal Biology and Paleoepidemiology of the People from Ein Tirghi and Kellis, Dakhleh Oasis, Egypt." In The Oasis Papers: Proceedings of the First International Symposium of the Dakhleh Oasis Project, edited by C.A. Marlow and A.J. Mills, 81–100. Dakhleh Oasis Project: Monograph 6. Oxford: Oxbow Books, 2001.

Montserrat, Dominic, and Lynn Meskell. "Mortuary Archaeology and Religious Landscape at Graeco-Roman Deir El-Medina." *The Journal of Egyptian Archaeology* 83 (1997): 179–197. https://doi.org/10.2307/3822465.

Mosites, Emily, Elizabeth Dawson-Hahn, Judd Walson, Ali Rowhani-Rahbar, and Marian L. Neuhouser. "Piecing Together the Stunting Puzzle: A Framework for Attributable Factors of Child Stunting." *Paediatrics and International Child Health* 37, no. 3 (2017): 158–165. https://doi.org/10.1080/20469047.2016.1230952.

Moss, Gordon Ervin. *Illness, Immunity, and Social Interaction: The Dynamics of Biosocial Resonation*. New York: Wiley, 1973.

Müller, Miriam. "Deir El-Medina in the Dark—the Amarna Period in the History of the Village." In *Deir El-Medina Studies, Helsinki, June 24–26, 2009. Proceedings*, edited by Jaana Toivari-Viitala, Turo Vartiainen, and Saara Uvanto, 154–167. The Finnish Egyptological Society Occasional Publications 2. Helsinki: The Finnish Egyptological Society, 2014.

Musselwhite, Sarah. "Skeletal Health in Early Egypt." In *Current Research in Egyptology 2012*, edited by Carl Graves, Gabrielle Heffernan, Luke McGarrity, Emily Millward, and Marsia Sfakianou Bealby, 128–144. Oxford and Oakville: Oxbow Books, 2013.

Näser, Claudia. "Zur Interpretation Funerärer Praktiken Im Neuen Reich: Der Ostfriedhof von Deir El-Medine." In *Begegnungen Antike Kulturen Im Niltal: Festgabe Für Erika Endesfelder, Karl-Heinz Priese, Walter Friedrich Reineke Und Steffen Wenig*, edited by Caris-Beatrice Arnst, Ingelore Hafemann, and Angelika Lohwasser, 373–398. Leipzig, Germany: Wodtke and Stegbauer, 2001.

Nassar, Mohamed A. "The Wise Woman and the Healing Practice (O. OIM 16974)." *Journal of Ancient Egyptian Interconnections* 24, no. 1 (2019). http://journals.librarypublishing.arizona.edu/jaei/article/id/1396/.

Nerlich, Andreas G., Bettina Schraut, Sabine Dittrich, Thomas Jelinek, and Albert R. Zink. "Plasmodium Falciparum in Ancient Egypt." *Emerging Infectious Diseases* 14, no. 8 (August 2008): 1317–1319. https://doi.org/10.3201/eid1408.080235.

Nerlich, Andreas G., A. Zink, H.G. Hagedorn, U. Szeimies, and C. Weyss. "Anthropological and Palaeopathological Analysis of the Human Remains from Three 'Tombs of the Nobles' of the Necropolis of Thebes-West, Upper Egypt." *Anthropologischer Anzeiger* 58, no. 4 (2000): 321–343.

Nunn, John F. *Ancient Egyptian Medicine*. Norman: University of Oklahoma Press, 1996.

Nutton, Vivian. *Ancient Medicine*. 2nd ed. London: Routledge, 2012.

O'Donnell, Lexi, Jane E. Buikstra, Ethan C. Hill, Amy S. Anderson, and Michael J. O'Donnell Jr. "Skeletal Manifestations of Disease Experience: Length of Illness and Porous Cranial Lesion Formation in a Contemporary Juvenile Mortality Sample." *American Journal of Human Biology* 35, no. 8 (2023): e23896. https://doi.org/10.1002/ajhb.2389.

O'Donnell, Lexi, Ethan C. Hill, Amy S. Anderson Anderson, and Heather J.H. Edgar. "Cribra Orbitalia and Porotic Hyperostosis Are Associated with Respiratory Infections in a Contemporary Mortality Sample from New Mexico." *American Journal of Physical Anthropology* 173, no. 4 (2020): 721–733. https://doi.org/10.1002/ajpa.24131.

Okan, Orkan, Ullrich Bauer, Diane Levin-Zamir, Paulo Pinheiro, and Kristine Sørensen, eds. *International Handbook of Health Literacy: Research, Practice and Policy across the Lifespan*. Bristol: Policy Press, 2019.

Ortner, Donald J. *Identification of Pathological Conditions in Human Skeletal Remains*. 2nd ed. San Diego: Academic Press, 2003.

Papathanasiou, Anastasia, Nicholas J. Meinzer, Kimberly D. Williams, and Clark Spencer Larsen. "History of Anemia and Related Nutritional Deficiencies." In *The Back-*

bone of Europe: Health, Diet, Work and Violence over Two Millennia, edited by Richard H. Steckel, Clark Spencer Larsen, Charlotte A. Roberts, and Joerg Baten, 198–230. Cambridge Studies in Biological and Evolutionary Anthropology 80. Cambridge: Cambridge University Press, 2018.

Pechníková, Markéta, Davide Porta, and Cristina Cattaneo. "Distinguishing between Perimortem and Postmortem Fractures: Are Osteons of Any Help?" *International Journal of Legal Medicine* 125, no. 4 (2011): 591–595.

Peck, William. "Mummies of Ancient Egypt." In *Mummies, Disease and Ancient Cultures*, edited by Thomas Aidan Cockburn, Eve Cockburn, and Theodore A. Reyman, 2nd ed., 15–37. Cambridge: Cambridge University Press, 1998.

Pecotte, Jerilyn K. "Temporal Trends in Biological Stress Indicators from Two Egyptian Mortuary Samples." PhD Dissertation, University of Utah, 1986.

Pestman, Pieter W. *Marriage and Matrimonial Property in Ancient Egypt*. Papyrologica Lugduno-Batava 9. Leiden: Brill, 1961.

Pestman, Pieter W. "Who Were the Owners, in the 'Community of Workmen', of the Chester Beatty Papyri." In *Gleanings from Deir El-Medîna*, edited by Robert J. Demarée and Jac. J. Janseen, 155–172. Egyptologische Uitgaven 1. Leiden: Nederlands Instituut voor het Nabije Oosten, 1982.

Pierrat-Bonnefois, Geneviève. "Cimetière Est Du Village Ou Cimetière à l'est de Deir El-Médineh?" In *Deir El-Médineh et La Vallée Des Rois. Actes Du Colloque Organisé Par Le Musée Du Louvre Les 3 et 4 Mai 2002*, edited by Guillemette Andreu, 49–65. Paris: Musée du Louvre, 2003.

Pilloud, Marin A., and Al W. Schwitalla. "Re-Evaluating Traditional Markers of Stress in an Archaeological Sample from Central California." *Journal of Archaeological Science* 116 (April 2020): 105102. https://doi.org/10.1016/j.jas.2020.105102.

Pinch, Geraldine. "Childbirth and Female Figurines at Deir El-Medina and El-'Amarna." *Orientalia* 52, no. 3 (1983): 405–414.

Piperata, Barbara A., Mark Hubbe, and Kammi K. Schmeer. "Intra-Population Variation in Anemia Status and Its Relationship to Economic Status and Self-Perceived Health in the Mexican Family Life Survey: Implications for Bioarchaeology." *American Journal of Physical Anthropology* 155, no. 2 (2014): 210–220.

Pommerening, Tanja. "Heilkundliche Texte aus dem Alten Ägypten: Vorschläge zur Kommentierung und Übersetzung." In *Translating Writings of Early Scholars in the Ancient Near East, Egypt, Greece and Rome: Methodological Aspects with Examples*, edited by Annette Imhausen and Tanja Pommerening, 175–280. Beiträge zur Altertumskunde 344. De Gruyter, 2016.

Porter, Bertha, and Rosalind L.B. Moss. *Topographical Bibliography of Ancient Egyptian Hieroglyphic Texts, Statues, Reliefs and Painting Volume 1: The Theban Necropolis, Part 1—Private Tombs*. Oxford: Griffith Institute, 1960.

Porter, Roy. *Blood and Guts: A Short History of Medicine*. London: Allen Lane, 2002.

Porter, Roy. *The Greatest Benefit to Mankind: A Medical History of Humanity*. New York: W.W. Norton & Company, 1998.

Prentice, Andrew M., Kate A. Ward, Gail R. Goldberg, Landing M. Jarjou, Sophie E. Moore, Anthony J. Fulford, and Ann Prentice. "Critical Windows for Nutritional Interventions against Stunting." *The American of Clinical Nutrition* 97, no. 5 (2013): 911–918.

Primeau, Charlotte, Laila Friis, Birgitte Sejrsen, and Niels Lynnerup. "A Method for Estimating Age of Medieval Sub-Adults from Infancy to Adulthood Based on Long Bone Length." *American Journal of Physical Anthropology* 159, no. 1 (2016): 135–145.

Qian, Zhiyi, Grace Y. Wang, Marcus Henning, and Yan Chen. "Understanding Health Literacy from a Traditional Chinese Medicine Perspective." *Journal of Integrative Medicine* 21, no. 3 (2023): 215–220. https://doi.org/10.1016/j.joim.2023.03.001.

Quack, Joachim Friedrich. "Beiträge Zu Einigen Religiösen Und Magischen Texte." In *Ramesside Studies in Honour of K.A. Kitchen*, edited by Mark Collier and Steven Snape, 413–416. Bolton: Rutherford Press, 2011.

Quack, Joachim Friedrich. "Nochmals Zum Lautwert von Gardiner Sign-List U 23." *Lingua Aegyptia* 30 (2022): 271–289. https://doi.org/10.37011/lingaeg.30.09.

Rapisidara, Vittoria. "'Indossare' i Tatuaggi: Studio Del Tatuaggio Nell'Antico Egitto Sui Resti Umani, Archeologici e Iconografici." MA Thesis, Università di Pisa, 2020.

Rathbun, Ted A., and Richard H. Steckel. "The Health of Slaves and Free Blacks in the East." In *The Backbone of History: Health and Nutrition in the Western Hemisphere*, edited by Richard H. Steckel and Jerome C. Rose, 208–225. Cambridge: Cambridge, 2002.

Raxter, Michelle H. "Metric Sex Estimation in an Ancient Egyptian Skeletal Sample." *SAS Bulletin: Newsletter of the Society for Archaeological Sciences* 30, no. 4 (2007): 9–12.

Raxter, Michelle H., Christopher B. Ruff, Ayman Azab, Moushira Erfan, Muhammad Soliman, and Aly El-Sawaf. "Stature Estimation in Ancient Egyptians: A New Technique Based on Anatomical Reconstruction of Stature." *American Journal of Physical Anthropology* 136, no. 2 (2008): 147–155. https://doi.org/10.1002/ajpa.20790.

Redfern, Rebecca C. *Injury and Trauma in Bioarchaeology: Interpreting Violence in Past Lives*. Cambridge: Cambridge University Press, 2016.

Reid, D.J., and M.C. Dean. "Variation in Modern Human Enamel Formation Times." *Journal of Human Evolution* 50, no. 3 (March 1, 2006): 329–346. https://doi.org/10.1016/j.jhevol.2005.09.003.

Reitsema, Laurie J., and Britney Kyle McIlvaine. "Reconciling 'Stress' and 'Health' in Physical Anthropology: What Can Bioarchaeologists Learn from the Other Subdisciplines?" *American Journal of Physical Anthropology* 155, no. 2 (2014): 181–185. https://doi.org/10.1002/ajpa.22596.

Ridealgh, Kim. "Polite like an Egyptian? Case Studies of Politeness in the Late Ramesside Letters." *Journal of Politeness Research* 12, no. 2 (July 1, 2016): 245–266. https://doi.org/10.1515/pr-2016-0007.

Ritner, Robert K. *The Mechanics of Ancient Egyptian Magical Practice*. Studies in Ancient Oriental Civilization 54. Chicago: The Oriental Institute of the University of Chicago, 1993.

Ritzman, Terrence B., Brenda J. Baker, and Gary T. Schwartz. "A Fine Line: A Comparison of Methods for Estimating Ages of Linear Enamel Hypoplasia Formation." *American Journal of Physical Anthropology* 135, no. 3 (March 1, 2008): 348–361. https://doi.org/10.1002/ajpa.20750.

Rivera, Frances, and Marta Mirazón Lahr. "New Evidence Suggesting a Dissociated Etiology for Cribra Orbitalia and Porotic Hyperostosis." *American Journal of Physical Anthropology* 164, no. 1 (2017): 76–96. https://doi.org/10.1002/ajpa.23258.

Robins, Gay, and Charles Shute. "Predynastic Egyptian Stature and Physical Proportions." *Human Evolution* 1, no. 4 (August 1986): 313–324. https://doi.org/10.1007/BF02436705.

Roche, Alex F., and Gail H. Davila. "Late Adolescent Growth in Stature." *Pediatrics* 50, no. 6 (December 1, 1972): 874–880. https://doi.org/10.1542/peds.50.6.874.

Rodney, Nicole C., and Connie J. Mulligan. "A Biocultural Study of the Effects of Maternal Stress on Mother and Newborn Health in the Democratic Republic of Congo." *American Journal of Physical Anthropology* 155, no. 2 (2014): 200–209.

Rogers, Juliet, and Tony Waldron. *A Field Guide to Joint Disease in Archaeology*. Chichester: Wiley, 1995.

Rolfe, Steve, Lisa Garnham, Jon Godwin, Isobel Anderson, Pete Seaman, and Cam Donaldson. "Housing as a Social Determinant of Health and Wellbeing: Developing an Empirically-Informed Realist Theoretical Framework." BMC *Public Health* 20, no. 1 (July 20, 2020): 1138. https://doi.org/10.1186/s12889-020-09224-0.

Rösing, Friedrich W. *Qubbet el Hawa und Elephantine: zur Bevolkerungsgeschichte von Agypten*. Stuttgart: Fischer, 1990.

Roth, Ann Macy. *Egyptian Phyles in the Old Kingdom: The Evolution of a System of Social Organization*. Studies in Ancient Oriental Civilization 48. Chicago: The Oriental Institute of the University of Chicago, 1991.

Russo, Barbara. *Kha (TT 8) and His Colleagues: The Gifts in His Funerary Equipment and Related Artefacts from Western Thebes*. GHP Egyptology 18. London: Golden House Publications, 2012.

Rzepka, Sławomir. *Who, Where and Why: The Rock Graffiti of Members of the Deir El-Medina Community*. Warsaw: Pro-Egipt, 2014.

Sabbahy, Lisa. "The People of Deir El-Medineh: A Preliminary Paleopathology Study." *Anthropologie* 48, no. 2 (2010): 117–120.

Sanchez, Jose, and Robert Hoppa. "Is Adulthood Required? Examining the Accuracy of Pelvic Sex Estimation Throughout Pubertal Growth." *Bioarchaeology International* 7, no. 2 (2023): 173–188. https://doi.org/10.5744/bi.2022.0005.

Sarry El-Din, Azza Mohamed. "Bone Fractures in Ancient Egyptians from Giza, Old

Kingdom." *Egyptian Medical Journal of the National Research Center* 2, no. 2 (2003): 1–13.

Sarry, El-Din, and Azza Mohamed. "Bone Fractures in Ancient Egyptians From Giza, Old Kingdom." *Egyptian Medical Journal* 2, no. 2 (2003): 1–13.

Sauer, Norman J. "The Timing of Injuries and Manner of Death: Distinguishing among Antemortem, Perimortem and Postmortem Trauma." Edited by Kathy Reichs. *Forensic Osteology: Advances in the Identification of Human Remains* 2 (1998): 321–331.

Sauneron, Serge. "Le Rhume d'Anynakhte (Pap. Deir El-Medineh 36)." *Kemi* 20 (1970): 7–18.

Sauneron, Serge. *Les prêtres de l'ancienne Égypte*. Le temps qui court 5. Paris: Éditions du Seuil, 1957.

Schaible, Ulrich E, and Stefan H.E. Kaufmann. "Malnutrition and Infection: Complex Mechanisms and Global Impacts." *PLoS Medicine* 4, no. 5 (May 2007). https://doi.org/10.1371/journal.pmed.0040115.

Scheidel, Walter. *Death on the Nile: Disease and the Demography of Roman Egypt*. Leiden: Brill, 2001.

Scheuer, Louise, and Sue M. Black. *The Juvenile Skeleton*. London: Elsevier Academic Press, 2004.

Schousboe, Karoline, P.M. Visscher, Bircan Erbas, Kirsten Ohm Kyvik, J.L. Hopper, Jan Erik Henriksen, B.L. Heitmann, and T.I.A. Sørensen. "Twin Study of Genetic and Environmental Influences on Adult Body Size, Shape, and Composition." *International Journal of Obesity* 28, no. 1 (2004): 39–48.

Schrader, Sarah A. "Activity Patterns in New Kingdom Nubia: An Examination of Entheseal Remodeling and Osteoarthritis at Tombos." *American Journal of Physical Anthropology* 149, no. 1 (September 2012): 60–70. https://doi.org/10.1002/ajpa.22094.

Schrader, Sarah A., and Michele R. Buzon. "Everyday Life after Collapse: a Bioarchaeological Examination of Entheseal Change and Accidental Injury in Postcolonial Nubia." *Bioarchaeology International* 1, no. 1–2 (2017): 19–34. https://doi.org/10.5744/bi.2017.1000.

Schwartz, Gary T., Don J. Reid, M. Christopher Dean, and Adrienne L. Zihlman. "A Faithful Record of Stressful Life Events Recorded in the Dental Developmental Record of a Juvenile Gorilla." *International Journal of Primatology* 27, no. 4 (August 2006): 1201–1219. https://doi.org/10.1007/s10764-006-9051-2.

Schweitzer, Simon D. "Zum Lautwert Einiger Hieroglyphen." *Zeitschrift Für Ägyptische Sprache Und Altertumskunde* 138, no. 2 (2011): 132–149. https://doi.org/10.1524/zaes.2011.0011.

Scott, Amy B., and Robert D. Hoppa. "The Subtleties of Stress: A Comparative Analysis of Skeletal Lesions between the Medieval and Post-Medieval Black Friars Cemetery

Population (13th to 17th Centuries)." *International Journal of Osteoarchaeology* 28, no. 6 (2018): 695–702.

Sebastian Richter, Tonio, Daniel A. Werning, Hans-Werner Fischer-Elfert, and Peter Dils. "Thesaurus Linguae Aegyptiae, Corpus Issue 17, Web App Version 2.1.0," October 13, 2023. https://thesaurus-linguae-aegyptiae.de/.

Selye, Hans. *The Stress of Life*. New York: McGraw-Hill, 1956.

Shalaby, Mostafa Abbas, and Ashraf Abd-Elkhalik Hammouda. "Analgesic, Anti-Inflammatory and Anti-Hyperlipidemic Activities of Commiphora Molmol Extract (Myrrh)." *Journal of Intercultural Ethnopharmacology* 3, no. 2 (2014): 56–62.

Smedley, Brian D., Adrienne Y. Stith, and Alan R. Nelson, eds. *Unequal Treatment: Confronting Racial and Ethnic Disparities in Health Care*. Washington, D.C.: National Academies Press, 2003.

Smith, B. Holly. "Patterns of Molar Wear in Hunter–Gatherers and Agriculturalists." *American Journal of Physical Anthropology* 63, no. 1 (1984): 39–56.

Smith, Stuart Tyson. "Intact Tombs of the Seventeenth and Eighteenth Dynasties from Thebes and the New Kingdom Burial System." *Mitteilungen Des Deutschen Archäologischen Instituts Kairo* 48 (1992): 193–231.

Smith, Stuart Tyson. *Wretched Kush: Ethnic Identities and Boundaries in Egypt's Nubian Empire*. London: Routledge, 2003.

Smith-Guzmán, Nicole E. "Cribra Orbitalia in the Ancient Nile Valley and Its Connection to Malaria." *International Journal of Paleopathology* 10 (September 2015): 1–12. https://doi.org/10.1016/j.ijpp.2015.03.001.

Smith-Guzmán, Nicole E. "The Skeletal Manifestation of Malaria: An Epidemiological Approach Using Documented Skeletal Collections." *American Journal of Physical Anthropology* 158, no. 4 (December 1, 2015): 624–635. https://doi.org/10.1002/ajpa.22819.

Smith-Guzmán, Nicole Elizabeth. "The Paleoepidemiology of Malaria in the Ancient Near East." Ph.D. Dissertation, University of Arkansas, 2015.

Snape, Steven. "Sennedjem: Building and Buying at Deir El-Medina." In *Ancient Egyptian Tombs: The Culture of Life and Death*, 233–244. Chichester: Wiley-Blackwell, 2011.

Sobo, Elisa Janine, and Martha O. Loustaunau. *The Cultural Context of Health, Illness, and Medicine*. 2nd ed. Santa Barbara: Praeger, 2010.

Soliman, Daniel M. "Of Marks and Men: The Functional and Historical Context of the Workmen's Marks of the Royal Theban Necropolis." Ph.D. Dissertation, Leiden University, 2016.

Soliman, Daniel M. "Workmen's Marks in Pre-Amarna Tombs at Deir El-Medina." In *Non-Textual Marking Systems in Ancient Egypt (and Elsewhere)*, edited by Julia Budka, Frank Kammerzell, and Slawomir Rzepka, 109–132. Lingua Aegyptia Studia Monographica 16. Hamburg: Widmaier, 2015.

Sousa, Rogério. *Gilded Flesh: Coffins and Afterlife in Ancient Egypt*. Oxford: Oxbow Books, 2019. https://doi.org/10.2307/j.ctv138wsfh.

Spradley, James P., and Mark Phillips. "Culture and Stress: A Quantitative Analysis." *American Anthropologist* 74, no. 3 (June 1972): 518–529. https://doi.org/10.1525/aa.1972.74.3.02a00190.

Starling, Anne P., and Jay T. Stock. "Dental Indicators of Health and Stress in Early Egyptian and Nubian Agriculturalists: A Difficult Transition and Gradual Recovery." *American Journal of Physical Anthropology* 134, no. 4 (December 2007): 520–528. https://doi.org/10.1002/ajpa.20700.

Steckel, Richard H., C.S. Larsen, P.W. Sciulli, and P.I. Walker. "Global History of Health Data Collection Codebook," 2006. https://economics.osu.edu/sites/default/files/Codebook-01-24-11-em.pdf.

Steckel, Richard H., Clark Spencer Larsen, Charlotte A. Roberts, and Joerg Baten, eds. *The Backbone of Europe: Health, Diet, Work and Violence over Two Millennia*. Cambridge Studies in Biological and Evolutionary Anthropology 80. Cambridge: Cambridge University Press, 2018.

Steckel, Richard H., Clark Spencer Larsen, Paul W. Sciulli, and Phillip L. Walker. "Data Collection Codebook." In *The Backbone of Europe: Health, Diet, Work and Violence over Two Millennia*, edited by Richard H. Steckel, Clark Spencer Larsen, Charlotte A. Roberts, and Joerg Baten, 397–427. Cambridge Studies in Biological and Evolutionary Anthropology 80. Cambridge: Cambridge University Press, 2018.

Steckel, Richard H., and Jerome C. Rose. "Conclusions." In *Backbone of History: Health and Nutrition in the Western Hemisphere*, edited by Richard H. Steckel and Jerome C. Rose, 583–592. Cambridge: Cambridge University Press, 2002.

Steckel, Richard H., and Jerome C. Rose. "Patterns of Health in the Western Hemisphere." In *The Backbone of History: Health and Nutrition in the Western Hemisphere*, edited by Richard H. Steckel and Jerome C. Rose, 563–579. Cambridge: Cambridge University Press, 2002.

Steckel, Richard H., and Jerome C. Rose, eds. *The Backbone of History: Health and Nutrition in the Western Hemisphere*. New York: Cambridge University Press, 2002.

Stevens, Anna, Gretchen Dabbs, Mérat Amandine, and Anna Garnett. "The North Cliffs Cemetery at Amarna." *Egyptian Archaeology*, no. 56 (2020): 4–9.

Stevens, Anna, Gretchen R. Dabbs, Jolanda E.M.F. Bos, Amandine Mérat, Anna Garnett, and Gemma Tully. "Tell El-Amarna, Autumn 2018 to Autumn 2019." *The Journal of Egyptian Archaeology* 106, no. 1–2 (2020): 3–15. https://doi.org/10.1177/0307513320973678.

Stevens, Anna, Corina E. Rogge, Jolanda E.M.F. Bos, and Gretchen R. Dabbs. "From Representation to Reality: Ancient Egyptian Wax Head Cones from Amarna." *Antiquity* 93, no. 372 (December 2019): 1515–1533. https://doi.org/10.15184/aqy.2019.175.

Stinson, Sara. "Sex Differences in Environmental Sensitivity during Growth and Development." *American Journal of Physical Anthropology* 28, no. S6 (1985): 123–147. https://doi.org/10.1002/ajpa.1330280507.

Strouhal, Eugen, and Ladislav Bares. *Secondary Cemetery in the Mastaba of Ptahshepses at Abusir*. Prague: Czech Institute of Egyptology, 1993.

Strouhal, Eugen, and Luboš Vyhnánek. *Egyptian Mummies in Czechoslovak Collections*. Sbórnik Národního Muzea v Praze 35-B 1–4. Praha: Národní Muzeum, 1979.

Stuart-Macadam, Patty. "Porotic Hyperostosis: A New Perspective." *American Journal of Physical Anthropology* 87, no. 1 (1992): 39–47. https://doi.org/10.1002/ajpa.1330870105.

Stuart-Macadam, Patty. "Porotic Hyperostosis: New Evidence to Support the Anemia Theory." *American Journal of Physical Anthropology* 74, no. 4 (1987): 521–526. https://doi.org/10.1002/ajpa.1330740410.

Stuart-Macadam, Patty. "Porotic Hyperostosis: Representative of a Childhood Condition." *American Journal of Physical Anthropology* 66, no. 4 (1985): 391–398. https://doi.org/10.1002/ajpa.1330660407.

Sun, Yue, and Shannon M. Monnat. "Rural-Urban and within-Rural Differences in COVID-19 Vaccination Rates." *The Journal of Rural Health* 38, no. 4 (2022): 916–922. https://doi.org/10.1111/jrh.12625.

Sutphen, James L. "Growth As a Measure of Nutritional Status." *Journal of Pediatric Gastroenterology and Nutrition* 4, no. 2 (April 1985): 169–181. https://doi.org/10.1097/00005176-198504000-00004.

Sweeney, Deborah. *Correspondence and Dialogue: Pragmatic Factors in Late Ramesside Letter Writing*. Ägypten Und Altes Testament 49. Wiesbaden: Harrassowitz Verlag, 2001.

Sweeney, Deborah. "Idiolects in the Late Ramesside Letters." *Lingua Aegyptia* 4 (1994): 275–324.

Sweeney, Deborah. "Women Growing Older at Deir El-Medina." In *Living and Writing in Deir El-Medine: Socio-Historical Embodiment of Deir El-Medine Texts*, edited by Andreas Dorn and Tobias Hofmann, 135–154. Basel: Schwabe, 2006.

Sweeney, Deborah. "Women's Correspondence from Deir El-Medineh." In *Acts of the Sixth International Conference of Egyptology*, 2:523–529. Sesto Congresso Internazionale Di Egittologia. Atti, 1993.

Sweeney, Edward A., Jorge Cabrera, Juan Urrutia, and Leonardo Mata. "Factors Associated with Linear Hypoplasia of Human Deciduous Incisors." *Journal of Dental Research* 48, no. 6 (1969): 1275–1279.

Syed, Samina T., Ben S. Gerber, and Lisa K. Sharp. "Traveling Towards Disease: Transportation Barriers to Health Care Access." *Journal of Community Health* 38, no. 5 (October 2013): 976–993. https://doi.org/10.1007/s10900-013-9681-1.

Taylor, John H. *Death and the Afterlife in Ancient Egypt*. 1st ed. University Of Chicago Press, 2001.

Taylor, John H. *Unwrapping a Mummy: The Life, Death and Embalming of Horemkenesi.* Austin: University of Texas Press, 1996.

Temple, Daniel H. "Bioarchaeological Evidence for Adaptive Plasticity and Constraint: Exploring Life-History Trade-Offs in the Human Past." *Evolutionary Anthropology* 28, no. 1 (January 2019): 34–46. https://doi.org/10.1002/evan.21754.

Temple, Daniel H. "Plasticity and Constraint in Response to Early-Life Stressors among Late/Final Jomon Period Foragers from Japan: Evidence for Life History Trade-Offs from Incremental Microstructures of Enamel." *American Journal of Physical Anthropology* 155, no. 4 (December 2014): 537–545. https://doi.org/10.1002/ajpa.22606.

Temple, Daniel H., and Alan H. Goodman. "Bioarcheology Has a 'Health' Problem: Conceptualizing 'Stress' and 'Health' in Bioarcheological Research." *American Journal of Physical Anthropology* 155, no. 2 (October 2014): 186–191. https://doi.org/10.1002/ajpa.22602.

The Metropolitan Museum of Art. "Cosmetic Box from the Tomb of Sennedjem | New Kingdom, Ramesside." Accessed February 28, 2023. https://www.metmuseum.org/art/collection/search/544701.

"The True Death Toll of COVID-19: Estimating Global Excess Mortality." Accessed May 16, 2023. https://www.who.int/data/stories/the-true-death-toll-of-covid-19-estimating-global-excess-mortality.

Thoits, Peggy A. "Mechanisms Linking Social Ties and Support to Physical and Mental Health." *Journal of Health and Social Behavior* 52, no. 2 (June 2011): 145–161. https://doi.org/10.1177/0022146510395592.

Tilley, Lorna. *Theory and Practice in the Bioarchaeology of Care.* Bioarchaeology and Social Theory. New York: Springer, 2015.

Tilley, Lorna, and Tony Cameron. "Introducing the Index of Care: A Web-Based Application Supporting Archaeological Research into Health-Related Care." *International Journal of Paleopathology* 6 (September 2014): 5–9. https://doi.org/10.1016/j.ijpp.2014.01.003.

Todd, T. Wingate. "Age Changes in the Pubic Bone. I: The Male White Pubis." *American Journal of Physical Anthropology*, no. 3 (1921): 285–334.

Todd, T. Wingate. "Age Changes in the Pubic Bone. III: The Pubis of the White Female." *American Journal of Physical Anthropology*, no. 4 (1921): 1–70.

Toivari-Viitala, Jaana. "Marriage and Divorce." *UCLA Encyclopedia of Egyptology* 1, no. 1 (2013). https://escholarship.org/uc/item/68f6w5gw.

Toivari-Viitala, Jaana. "O. DeM 764: A Note Concerning Property Rights." *Göttinger Miszellen: Beiträge Zur Ägyptologischen Diskussion*, no. 195 (2003): 87–96.

Toivari-Viitala, Jaana. *Women at Deir El-Medina: A Study of the Status and Roles of the Female Inhabitants in the Workmen's Community during the Ramesside Period.* Egyptologische Uitgaven 15. Leiden: Nederlands Instituut Voor Het Nabije Oosten, 2001.

Toivari-Viitala, Jaana, Elina Paulin-Grother, Tanja Alsheimer, and Virpi Perunka. "Preliminary Report of the Work Performed During the Fifth Season in 2012–2013." Workmen's Huts in the Theban Mountains Project. Academy of Finland and University of Helsinki, 2013. https://www.egyptologinenseura.fi/wp-content/uploads/sites/9/2019/09/Report-2012-2013_ACADEMY-OF-FINLAND-AND-UNIVERSITY-OF-HELSINKI_5th-season.pdf.

Tomsová, Julie, and Zuzana Schierová. "Skeletal Material from Deir El-Medina in the Egyptological Collection of the Hrdlička Museum of Man in Prague." *Annals of the Náprstek Museum* 37, no. 1 (2016): 41–69.

Toonen, Willem H.J., Angus Graham, Benjamin T. Pennington, Morag A. Hunter, Kristian D. Strutt, Dominic S. Barker, Aurélia Masson-Berghoff, and Virginia L. Emery. "Holocene Fluvial History of the Nile's West Bank at Ancient Thebes, Luxor, Egypt, and Its Relation with Cultural Dynamics and Basin-Wide Hydroclimatic Variability." *Geoarchaeology* 33, no. 3 (2018): 273–290. https://doi.org/10.1002/gea.21631.

Torras Benezet, Núria. "The Pure Priest of Sekhmet, Between Health and Disease." In *Pharmacy and Medicine in Ancient Egypt: Proceedings of the Conference Held in Barcelona (2018)*, edited by Rosa Dinarès Solà, Mikel Fernàndez Georges, and Maria Rosa Guasch-Jané, 116–124. Oxford: Archaeopress, 2021. https://doi.org/10.2307/j.ctv1r2xx81.

Towle, Ian, and Joel D. Irish. "Recording and Interpreting Enamel Hypoplasia in Samples from Archaeological and Palaeoanthropological Contexts." *Journal of Archaeological Science* 114 (February 2020): 105077. https://doi.org/10.1016/j.jas.2020.105077.

Twaddle, Andrew C. "Influence and Illness: Definitions and Definers of Illness Behavior among Older Males in Providence, Rhode Island." Ph.D Dissertation, Brown University, 1968.

Ubelaker, Douglas H. "The Estimation of Age at Death from Immature Human Bone." In *Age Markers in the Human Skeleton*, edited by Mehmet Yaşar İşcan, 55–70. Springfield: Charles C. Thomas, 1989.

Uchino, Bert N. *Social Support and Physical Health: Understanding the Health Consequences of Relationships*. Yale University Press, 2004. https://doi.org/10.12987/yale/9780300102185.001.0001.

Uchino, Bert N., John T. Cacioppo, and Janice K. Kiecolt-Glaser. "The Relationship between Social Support and Physiological Processes: A Review with Emphasis on Underlying Mechanisms and Implications for Health." *Psychological Bulletin* 119, no. 3 (1996): 488–531.

Umberson, Debra, and Jennifer Karas Montez. "Social Relationships and Health: A Flashpoint for Health Policy." *Journal of Health and Social Behavior* 51, no. Suppl (2010): S54–66. https://doi.org/10.1177/0022146510383501.

Unger, Juliane. "Ancient Egyptian Prescriptions for the Back and Abdomen and Their

Mesopotamian and Mediterranean Counterparts." In *Systems of Classification in Premodern Medical Cultures: Sickness, Health, and Local Epistemologies*, edited by Ulrike Steinert, 122–139. New York: Routledge, 2020.

United Nations. *Age and Sex Patterns of Mortality: Model Life-Tables for Under-Developed Countries*. Population Studies 22. United Nations Department of Social Affairs, Population Branch, 1955.

University of Wisconsin Population Health Institute. "2022 Measures." County Health Rankings & Roadmaps. Accessed July 14, 2022. https://www.countyhealthrankings.org/2022-measures.

Vachala, Břetislav. "Der Brief Einer Gescholtenen Ehefrau an Ihre Schwester (o Prag 1826)." In *Times, Signs and Pyramids: Studies in Honour of Miroslav Verner on the Occasion of His Seventieth Birthday*, edited by Vivienne G. Callender, Bareš Ladislav, Miroslav Bárta, Jiří Janák, and Jaromír Krejčí, 423–427. Faculty of Arts, Charles University, 2011.

Valbelle, Dominique. *Les ouvriers de la Tombe*. Bibliothèque d'Étude 96. Cairo: Institut français d'archéologie orientale du Caire, 1985.

Vercellotti, Giuseppe, Barbara A. Piperata, Amanda M. Agnew, Warren M. Wilson, Darna L. Dufour, Julio C. Reina, Rosa Boano, Hedy M. Justus, Clark Spencer Larsen, and Sam D. Stout. "Exploring the Multidimensionality of Stature Variation in the Past through Comparisons of Archaeological and Living Populations." *American Journal of Physical Anthropology* 155, no. 2 (2014): 229–242.

Vilke, Gary M., Gerard DeMers, Nilang Patel, and Edward M. Castillo. "Safety and Efficacy of Milk and Molasses Enemas in the Emergency Department." *The Journal of Emergency Medicine* 48, no. 6 (June 2015): 667–670. https://doi.org/10.1016/j.jemermed.2015.01.035.

Waldron, Tony. *Palaeopathology*. Cambridge: Cambridge University Press, 2008.

Walker, Phillip L., Rhonda R. Bathurst, Rebecca Richman, Thor Gjerdrum, and Valerie A. Andrushko. "The Causes of Porotic Hyperostosis and Cribra Orbitalia: A Reappraisal of the Iron-Deficiency-Anemia Hypothesis." *American Journal of Physical Anthropology* 139, no. 2 (2009): 109–125. https://doi.org/10.1002/ajpa.21031.

Walker, Phillip L., Gregory Dean, and Perry Shapiro. "Estimating Age from Tooth Wear in Archaeological Populations." In *Advances in Dental Anthropology*, edited by Marc A. Kelley and Clark Spencer Larsen, 169–178. New York: Wiley-Liss, 1991.

Walker, Phillip L., John R. Johnson, and Patricia M. Lambert. "Age and Sex Biases in the Preservation of Human Skeletal Remains." *American Journal of Physical Anthropology* 76, no. 2 (1988): 183–188. https://doi.org/10.1002/ajpa.1330760206.

Wallaker, Kimberley, Ezio Fortuna, Stuart Bradin, Michelle Macy, Michelle Hassan, and Rachel Stanley. "Milk and Molasses Enemas: Clearing Things Up." *Journal of Emergency Nursing* 40, no. 6 (November 2014): 546–551. https://doi.org/10.1016/j.jen.2013.08.012.

Wangui-Verry, Jackline, Michele Farrington, Grace Matthews, and Sharon J. Tucker. "CE: Original Research: Are Milk and Molasses Enemas Safe for Hospitalized Adults? A Retrospective Electronic Health Record Review." *The American Journal of Nursing* 119, no. 9 (September 2019): 24–28. https://doi.org/10.1097/01.NAJ.0000580148.43193.76.

Wapler, Ulrike, Eric Crubézy, and Michael Schultz. "Is Cribra Orbitalia Synonymous with Anemia? Analysis and Interpretation of Cranial Pathology in Sudan." *American Journal of Physical Anthropology* 123, no. 4 (April 1, 2004): 333–339. https://doi.org/10.1002/ajpa.10321.

Warinner, Christina, João F. Matias Rodrigues, Rounak Vyas, Christian Trachsel, Natallia Shved, Jonas Grossmann, Anita Radini, et al. "Pathogens and Host Immunity in the Ancient Human Oral Cavity." *Nature Genetics* 46, no. 4 (April 2014): 336–344. https://doi.org/10.1038/ng.2906.

Watts, Rebecca. "Childhood Development and Adult Longevity in an Archaeological Population from Barton-upon-Humber, Lincolnshire, England." *International Journal of Paleopathology* 3, no. 2 (2013): 95–104.

Weiss, Elizabeth, and Robert Jurmain. "Osteoarthritis Revisited: A Contemporary Review of Aetiology." *International Journal of Osteoarchaeology* 17, no. 5 (2007): 437–450. https://doi.org/10.1002/oa.889.

Wendrich, Willeke. "Entangled, Connected or Protected? The Power of Knots and Knotting in Ancient Egypt." In *Through a Glass Darkly: Magic, Dreams and Prophecy in Ancient Egypt*, edited by Kasia Maria Szpakowska, 243–269. Swansea: Classical Press of Wales, 2006.

Wente, Edward F. "A Goat for an Ailing Woman (Ostracon Wente)." In *Studies in Honor of William Kelly Simpson*, edited by Peter Der Manuelian, 2:855–867. Boston: Boston Museum of Fine Arts, 1996.

Wente, Edward F. "A Letter of Complaint to the Vizier To." *Journal of Near Eastern Studies* 20, no. 4 (1961): 252–257.

Wente, Edward F. *Letters from Ancient Egypt*. Society of Biblical Literature. Writings from the Ancient World 1. Atlanta: Scholars Press, 1990.

Weston, Darlene A. "Investigating the Specificity of Periosteal Reactions in Pathology Museum Specimens." *American Journal of Physical Anthropology* 137, no. 1 (2008): 48–59. https://doi.org/10.1002/ajpa.20839.

Weston, Darlene A. "Nonspecific Infection in Paleopathology: Interpreting Periosteal Reactions." In *A Companion to Paleopathology*, edited by Anne L. Grauer, 492–512. Wiley Blackwell Companions to Anthropology. Hoboken: Wiley-Blackwell, 2011.

White, Peter, ed. *Biopsychosocial Medicine: An Integrated Approach to Understanding Illness*. Oxford: Oxford University Press, 2005.

Whitmore, Katie Marie, Michele R. Buzon, and Stuart Tyson Smith. "Living on the Border: Health and Identity during Egypt's Colonization of Nubia in the New Kingdom

Period." In *Bioarchaeology of Frontiers and Borderlands*, edited by Cristina I. Tica and Debra L. Martin, 135–159. Gainesville: University of Florida Press, 2019.

Wilfong, Terry G. "Menstrual Synchrony and the 'Place of Women' in Ancient Egypt (OIM 13512)." In *Gold of Praise. Studies on Ancient Egypt in Honor of Edward F. Wente*, edited by Emily Teeter and John A. Larson, 419–434. Studies in Ancient Oriental Civilization 58. Chicago: The Oriental Institute of the University of Chicago, 1999.

Wilkinson, Richard G. *Unhealthy Societies: The Afflictions of Inequality*. Routledge, 2002.

Williams, Kimberly D., Nicholas J. Meinzer, and Clark Spencer Larsen. "History of Degenerative Joint Disease in People Across Europe." In *The Backbone of Europe: Health, Diet, Work and Violence over Two Millennia*, edited by Richard H. Steckel, Clark Spencer Larsen, Charlotte A. Roberts, and Joerg Baten, 253–299. Cambridge Studies in Biological and Evolutionary Anthropology 80. Cambridge: Cambridge University Press, 2018.

Winand, Jean. "Identifying Semitic Loanwords in Late Egyptian." In *Greek Influence on Egyptian-Coptic: Contact-Induced Change in an Ancient African Language*, edited by Eitan Grossman, Peter Dils, Tonio Sebastian Richter, and Wolfgang Schenkel, 481–511. Hamburg: Widmaier, 2017.

Winchester, Margaret S., and Brian King. "Decentralization, Healthcare Access, and Inequality in Mpumalanga, South Africa." *Health & Place* 51 (2018): 200–207. https://doi.org/10.1016/j.healthplace.2018.02.009.

Winkler, Eike-Meinrad, and Harald Wilfing. *Tell el-Dab'a VI: anthropologische Untersuchungen an den Skelettresten der Kampagnen, 1966-69, 1975-80, 1985*. Untersuchungen der Zweigstelle Kairo des Österreichischen Archäologischen Institutes 9. Wien: Verlag der Österreichische Akademie der Wissenschaften, 1991.

Winlock, Herbert Eustis. "The Museum's Excavations at Thebes." *The Metropolitan Museum of Art Bulletin* 21, no. 3 (March 1926): 5–32. https://doi.org/10.2307/3254817.

Wisseman, Sarah U. *The Virtual Mummy*. Urbana: University of Illinois Press, 2003.

Wit, Caroline C. de, Theo C.J. Sas, Jan M. Wit, and Wayne S. Cutfield. "Patterns of Catch-Up Growth." *The Journal of Pediatrics* 162, no. 2 (February 2013): 415–420. https://doi.org/10.1016/j.jpeds.2012.10.014.

Wolff, Harold G. *Stress and Disease*. American Lecture Series 166. Springfield: Thomas, 1953.

Wood, James W., George R. Milner, Henry C. Harpending, Kenneth M. Weiss, Mark N. Cohen Cohen, Leslie E. Eisenberg, Dale L. Hutchinson, et al. "The Osteological Paradox: Problems of Inferring Prehistoric Health from Skeletal Samples [and Comments and Reply]." *Current Anthropology*, 1992, 343–370.

World Health Organization. "International Classification of Functioning, Disability and Health (ICF)," 2012. http://www.who.int/classifications/icf/en/.

Wright, Lori E., and Cassady J. Yoder. "Recent Progress in Bioarchaeology: Approaches to the Osteological Paradox." *Journal of Archaeological Research* 11, no. 1 (2003): 43–70. https://doi.org/10.1023/A:1021200925063.

Wyatt, Harold V. "Poliomyelitis." In *The Cambridge World History of Human Disease*, edited by Kenneth F. Kiple, 942–950. New York: Cambridge University Press, 1993.

Yaussy, Samantha L. "The Intersections of Industrialization: Variation in Skeletal Indicators of Frailty by Age, Sex, and Socioeconomic Status in 18th- and 19th-Century England." *American Journal of Physical Anthropology* 170, no. 1 (2019): 116–130. https://doi.org/10.1002/ajpa.23881.

Yaussy, Samantha L., and Sharon N. DeWitte. "Patterns of Frailty in Non-Adults from Medieval London." *International Journal of Paleopathology* 22 (September 2018): 1–7. https://doi.org/10.1016/j.ijpp.2018.03.008.

Yaussy, Samantha L., Sharon N. DeWitte, and Rebecca C. Redfern. "Frailty and Famine: Patterns of Mortality and Physiological Stress among Victims of Famine in Medieval London." *American Journal of Physical Anthropology* 160, no. 2 (2016): 272–283.

Ye, Xinyuan. "Exploring the Relationship between Political Partisanship and COVID-19 Vaccination Rate." *Journal of Public Health*, October 23, 2021. https://doi.org/10.1093/pubmed/fdab364.

Young, Allan. "The Anthropologies of Illness and Sickness." *Annual Review of Anthropology* 11 (1982): 257–285.

Zakrzewski, Sonia R., Robert A. Foley, and Marta M. Lahr. "Change and Continuity over the Predynastic and Early Dynastic Periods of Ancient Egypt." In *Egyptology at the Dawn of the Twenty-First Century: Proceedings of the Eighth International Congress of Egyptologists, Cairo, 2000*, edited by Zahi A. Hawass and Lyla Pinch Brock, 2:587–597. Cairo; New York: American University in Cairo Press, 2003.

Zdilla, Matthew J., Nicholas S. Nestor, Bruce M. Rothschild, and H. Wayne Lambert. "Cribra Orbitalia Is Correlated with the Meningo-Orbital Foramen and Is Vascular and Developmental in Nature." *The Anatomical Record* 305, no. 7 (2022): 1629–1671. https://doi.org/10.1002/ar.24825.

Zhang, Xufan, Matthew E. Dupre, Li Qiu, Wei Zhou, Yuan Zhao, and Danan Gu. "Urban-Rural Differences in the Association between Access to Healthcare and Health Outcomes among Older Adults in China." *BMC Geriatrics* 17, no. 1 (2017): 151. https://doi.org/10.1186/s12877-017-0538-9.

Zimmerman, Michael R. "Mummification Styles as a Guide to the Dating of Egyptian Mummies." In *Dating and Age Determination of Biological Materials*, edited by Michael R. Zimmerman and J. Lawrence Angel, 166–169. London: Croom Helm, 1986.

Index of Topics

Index of Names

Numbering and anglicization follow Davies 1999

Index of Sources

Ostraca

Papyri

Stelae

www.ingramcontent.com/pod-product-compliance
Ingram Content Group UK Ltd.
Pitfield, Milton Keynes, MK11 3LW, UK
UKHW021421091026
15624UKWH00010B/339

9 789004 700864